40 Years of Academic Public Psychiatry

40 Years of Academic Public Psychiatry

Editors

To Elaine. Best wishes

**Selby C. Jacobs, M.D., M.P.H. and
Ezra E. H. Griffith, M.D.**

BICENTENNIAL
1807
WILEY
2007
BICENTENNIAL

John Wiley & Sons, Ltd

Other Wiley Editorial Offices

John Wiley & Sons Inc., 111 River Street, Hoboken, NJ 07030, USA

Jossey-Bass, 989 Market Street, San Francisco, CA 94103-1741, USA

Wiley-VCH Verlag GmbH, Boschstr. 12, D-69469 Weinheim, Germany

John Wiley & Sons Australia Ltd, 33 Park Road, Milton, Queensland 4064, Australia

John Wiley & Sons (Asia) Pte Ltd, 2 Clementi Loop #02-01, Jin Xing Distripark, Singapore 129809

John Wiley & Sons Canada Ltd, 6045 Freemont Blvd, Mississauga, Ontario, L5R 4J3

Wiley also publishes its books in a variety of electronic formats. Some content that appears in print may not be
available in electronic books.

Anniversary Logo Design: Richard J. Pacifico

Library of Congress Cataloging-in-Publication Data

40 years of academic public psychiatry / editors, Selby C. Jacobs and Ezra E.H. Griffith.
      p. ; cm.
   Includes bibliographical references and index.
   ISBN 978-0-470-98767-4 (alk. paper)
1. Connecticut Mental Health Center—History.   2. Community psychiatry—Connecticut—History.
3. Community mental health services—Connecticut—History.   4. Academic medical centers—Connecticut—
History.   I. Jacobs, Selby, 1939–   II. Griffith, Ezra E. H., 1942–   III. Title: Forty years of academic public
psychiatry.
   [DNLM: 1. Connecticut Mental Health Center.   2. Community Mental Health Services—history—
Connecticut.   3. Academic Medical Centers—history—Connecticut.   4. Community Psychiatry—education—
Connecticut.   5. Health Services Research—history—Connecticut.   WM 11 AC8 Z999 2007]
   RA790.65.C8A28 2007
   362.2'209746—dc22

                                                                                                    2007040688

British Library Cataloguing in Publication Data

A catalogue record for this book is available from the British Library

ISBN: 9780470987674

Typeset in 10/12pt Minion by SNP Best-set Typesetter Ltd., Hong Kong
Printed and bound in Great Britain by Antony Rowe, Chippenham, Wiltshire.
This book is printed on acid-free paper responsibly manufactured from sustainable forestry in which at least two trees
are planted for each one used for paper production.

Dedication

To All the Staff and Patients of the Connecticut Mental Health Center

While we have chosen to emphasize the melding of service delivery and academic initiatives in this text, it is still important to acknowledge that the CMHC has been an organization in which both staff and patients have spent significant parts of their lives. There are many patients who have obtained most of their psychiatric care at this one locale. Some physicians, nurses, psychologists and social workers have spent almost all their professional lives at the Center. Other support staff can make the same claim. Consequently, many individuals can recount life narratives that place this mental health facility at the center of their work lives. Those stories are not part of this text. Nevertheless, as editors, we recognize that the CMHC in its 40-year history has not just been a crucible where intellectuals contemplated their ideas. Some people, among those the Center serves, have lived out their personal stories in this place and have had their lives intertwined inextricably with the history of the Center. This fortieth anniversary therefore celebrates, too, all those who have made use of the Center as a place that offered succor and hope, while also serving as a buffer against the slings and arrows encountered in the external environment. On a particular and final note, the editors would like to acknowledge their profound debt of gratitude to Dr Boris M. Astrachan, an inspiring mentor, a Professor of Medicine at the Yale University School of Medicine, and the Director of the Connecticut Mental Health Center from 1970 to 1987.

Selby C. Jacobs and Ezra E. H. Griffith

Table of contents

Contributors

George K. Aghajanian, MD
Foundations' Fund Professor of Psychiatry and Professor of Pharmacology, Yale
University School of Medicine

Nancy Anderson, MSN, APRN
Lecturer, Yale School of Nursing
Director of Education and Training, Connecticut Mental Health Center

Luis Añez, PsyD
Associate Professor of Psychiatry, Yale University School of Medicine
Director, Hispanic Services, Connecticut Mental Health Center

Madelon V. Baranoski, PhD
Associate Professor of Psychiatry, Yale University School of Medicine
Director, New Haven Diversion Program, Connecticut Mental Health Center

Richard Belitsky, MD
Associate Professor of Psychiatry and Deputy Dean for Education, Yale University
School of Medicine

Dinesh Bhugra, FRCPsych. PhD
Professor of Mental Health and Cultural Diversity, Institute of Psychiatry,
London

Howard C. Blue, MD
Assistant Clinical Professor of Psychiatry, Yale University School of Medicine
Director of Clinical Services, Department of Mental Health and Counseling, Yale
University Health Services

Malcolm B. Bowers, Jr., MD
Professor Emeritus of Psychiatry and Senior Research Scientist, Yale University
School of Medicine

Benjamin S. Bunney, MD
Charles B.G. Murphy Professor of Psychiatry and Chairman, Department of
Psychiatry; Professor of Neurobiology and Pharmacology, Yale University School of
Medicine

Kathleen Carroll, PhD
Professor of Psychiatry, Yale University School of Medicine
Director of Psychosocial Research, Division of Substance Abuse, Veterans
Administration Medical Center, West Haven, CT

Robert A. Cole, MHSA
Lecturer, Yale University School of Medicine
Chief Operating Officer, Connecticut Mental Health Center

Wayne F. Dailey, PhD
Assistant Clinical Professor of Psychiatry, Yale University School of Medicine
Senior Policy Advisor, Connecticut Department of Mental Health and Addiction
Services

Larry Davidson, PhD
Associate Professor of Psychiatry, Yale University School of Medicine
Director, Program for Recovery and Community Health, Connecticut Mental
Health Center

Rani Desai, PhD
Associate Professor of Psychiatry, Yale University School of Medicine
Director, Program on Psychiatric Public Health, Connecticut Mental
Health Center

Paul J. Di Leo, MS
Lecturer, Yale University School of Medicine
Chief Operating Officer, Connecticut Department of Mental Health and Addiction
Services

Ronald S. Duman, PhD
Elizabeth Mears and House Jameson Professor of Psychiatry and Professor of
Pharmacology, Yale University School of Medicine
Director, Ribicoff Research Facilities, Connecticut Mental Health Center

Ezra E. H. Griffith, MD
Professor of Psychiatry and of African American Studies; Deputy Chairman,
Department of Psychiatry, Yale University School of Medicine

Dietra Hawkins, PsyD
Clinical Instructor of Psychiatry, Yale University School of Medicine
Clinical Director, Dixwell Newhallville Community Mental Health and Family
Support Services

George R. Heninger, MD
Professor Emeritus of Psychiatry and Senior Research Scientist, Yale University
School of Medicine

Michael Hoge, PhD
Professor of Psychiatry, Yale University School of Medicine
Director, Yale Behavioral Health

Selby C. Jacobs, MD, MPH
Professor of Psychiatry and of Public Health, Yale University School of
Medicine
Director, Connecticut Mental Health Center

Thomas A. Kirk, Jr., PhD
Commissioner, Connecticut Department of Mental Health and Addiction
Services

Herbert Kleber, MD
Professor of Psychiatry, College of Physicians and Surgeons, Columbia
University of the City of New York
Director, Division on Substance Abuse, New York State Psychiatric Institute

Thomas Kosten, MD
Professor of Psychiatry and Neuroscience, Baylor University College of Medicine,
Houston, TX

John H. Krystal, MD
Robert L. McNeil Jr. Professor of Clinical Pharmacology, Professor of Psychiatry and
Deputy Chairman for Research, Department of Psychiatry, Yale University School of
Medicine

Martha L. Mitchell, RN, MSN
Associate Clinical Professor, Yale School of Nursing
Clinical Nurse Specialist and former Director of Nursing, Connecticut Mental
Health Center

Stephanie O'Malley, PhD
Professor of Psychiatry, Yale University School of Medicine
Director, Division of Substance Abuse Research, Substance Abuse Treatment Unit,
Connecticut Mental Health Center

Robert Page, MSW, LCSW
Executive Director, Dixwell Newhallville Community Mental Health and Family
Support Services
Clinical Instructor of Social Work, Southern Connecticut State University School of
Social Work

Manuel Paris, PsyD
Assistant Professor of Psychiatry, Yale University School of Medicine
Director of Program Development, Connecticut Mental Health Center

Bruce Rounsaville, MD
Professor of Psychiatry, Yale University School of Medicine
Director, VISN 1 Mental Illness Research Education and Clinical Center, VA
Connecticut Healthcare, West Haven, Connecticut

Richard Schottenfeld, MD
Professor of Psychiatry, Yale University School of Medicine

Rajita Sinha, PhD
Professor of Psychiatry, Yale University School of Medicine
Director, Research Program on Stress, Addiction and Psychopathology, Connecticut
Mental Health Center

William H. Sledge, MD
George D. and Esther S. Gross Professor of Psychiatry, Yale University School of
Medicine
Assistant Chief of Psychiatry, Yale New Haven Hospital

David L. Snow, PhD
Professor of Psychiatry, Yale University School of Medicine
Director, The Consultation Center, Connecticut Mental Health Center

Jeanne Steiner, DO
Associate Professor of Psychiatry, Yale University School of Medicine
Medical Director, Connecticut Mental Health Center

John Strauss, MD
Professor Emeritus of Psychiatry, Yale University School of Medicine

Thomas Styron, PhD
Associate Professor of Psychiatry, Yale University School of Medicine
Executive Director, Community Services Network of Greater New Haven

Ajoy Thachil, MBBS, DPM, MRCPsych
Specialty Registrar, Section of Cultural Psychiatry, Institute of Psychiatry, London

Kenneth S. Thompson, MD
Medical Director, Center for Mental Health Services, Substance Abuse and Mental
Health Services Administration, Washington, DC
Associate Professor of Psychiatry and Public Health, University of Pittsburgh

Gary Tischler, MD
Professor Emeritus of Psychiatry, University of California, Los Angeles

Sophie Tworkowski, LCSW, MPH
Assistant Clinical Professor of Psychiatry, Yale University School of Medicine
Former Director, Social Work, Connecticut Mental Health Center

Bruce Wexler, MD
Professor of Psychiatry, Yale University School of Medicine
Associate Medical Director for Rehabilitation Therapies, Connecticut Mental Health
Center

Howard V. Zonana, MD
Professor of Psychiatry, Yale University School of Medicine and Adjunct Clinical
Professor of Law, Yale Law School
Director, Law and Psychiatry Division, Connecticut Mental Health Center

Foreword

Kenneth S. Thompson

In 1987, after finishing my residency in psychiatry at Albert Einstein College of Medicine in the Bronx, I became a Post-Doctoral Fellow in Mental Health Services Research at Yale University. I asked if I could continue my clinical work. Given my interest in community psychiatry, I was assigned to the outpatient department of the Connecticut Mental Health Center (CMHC). For the next four and a half years, at a point just over half way through the forty-year history this volume captures, I had the privilege of being a participant in the work of this remarkable institution.

First as a Fellow, and then as a member of the junior faculty, I was exposed to the cutting edges of mental health services research, psychiatric epidemiology, substance abuse treatment, forensics, psychopharmacology, cultural psychiatry and public mental health policy. I learned how to work in an outpatient team and I helped create and initiate a project, funded by the National Institute for Alcohol Abuse and Alcoholism and the State of Connecticut, to serve homeless men. In 1992, when I left to return to my hometown, Pittsburgh, to focus on promoting public psychiatry there, I was very well prepared.

Looking back now, I can see how my time at the CMHC changed my life. My professional and personal horizons expanded in multiple directions. I had some extraordinary teachers. The clinical staff I worked with—clerical staff, mental health workers, nurses, social workers, psychologists—supervised and mentored me. The psychiatrists and social scientists who instructed me and with whom I worked taught me lessons that I have never forgotten and which I call on every day. Of course the patients were more than patient with me.

As I write this, I can easily picture the people and live through the moments again. I would love to list them and pay them the respect I owe them for giving me so much, especially to recognize those who are no longer with us. But the list would be too long and therefore not personal enough.

No doubt there are others who will read these words and be carried on their own wave of nostalgia. But riding my own wave further is not the intent of this foreword.

Rather, my objective is to reflect on this institution that supported my growth and that of countless others. I want to comment on its nature and on its accomplishments, and perhaps a bit on what the future may hold. The production of this book provides an important focus for this. This book is an example of what the CMHC aspires to be and largely is—a learning center for research, scholarship and public service in the context of a community. It is a unique place in that it actually manages to keep itself balanced on all aspects of this mission. Academic medical centers that attend fully and earnestly to public service are relatively rare. Nor are there many public services that fully embrace scholarship.

The partnership developed between the State of Connecticut and Yale University has been a highly adaptive one, as the evolution of the CMHC attests. But it has always maintained its focus on ensuring that the results of scholarship, research and innovation found their way into the practice of psychiatry for the benefit of the patients and communities served by the Center.

This book contains a record of the Center's multiple achievements and some of its struggles. There is no question that people at the CMHC have given shape nationally to the development of public psychiatry. The accomplishment that I want to highlight, which is not heralded strongly enough elsewhere in this volume, is the fact that so many of the authors have dedicated their careers to the Center and its missions—and therefore to each other and their community. Many of the people whose words appear here were in New Haven when I was there. Such persistence and commitment is also very rare and reflects a unique blending of leadership and "followership." This is an institution that insists on participating in and contributing to the development of its community. It is, I believe, rooted in a love of work, scholarship, each other and suffering humanity that somehow suffuses this very human institution and keeps it fresh and alive.

This is not to say that there haven't been conflicts and feuds in the family. There is no way for these to be avoided, given the stresses and strains of attempting to achieve the Center's multiple goals. In this sense, it is worth noting that not all voices are heard from within these covers. Wouldn't it be fascinating to have a chapter written by consumers? But the recovery movement is just getting underway and the CMHC is leading the way (see Chapter 1). No doubt the next volume will have one, if not many such chapters! In fact, I would not be surprised if this volume becomes the basis for an ongoing wikipedia on the evolution of the Center. We may not need to wait 40 years for the next installment.

Which brings us to the future, a future that is just not that far away. Our communities and how we live in them continue to change rapidly. The opportunities and demands of modern life proliferate as our economy changes and we grow older, more diverse and, unfortunately, less equal in assets. Without further improvements in our science and our services and changes in our society, there is every reason to expect that the burdens of psychiatric disorders will grow, especially for people with the least resources. To serve the nation and to serve humanity, we must continue to struggle to learn more, improve services, develop personnel, refine public policy and figure out how to support these efforts.

Let us hope that the groundbreaking work of the Center continues. Let us also hope that it helps to lead the nation in transforming public service psychiatry. I don't know where the next wave of innovation and passion will come from beyond furthering its essential current work. Perhaps there will be a drive to deepen connections with primary care and physical health or perhaps to improve links with child, geriatrics and family services. Maybe there will be a greater focus on mental health promotion and protection in the unique social environment of post-industrial cities, now dependent on "eds and meds" (educational and medical institutions) for economic survival. Or maybe there will be further forays into supporting global health initiatives. Or perhaps there will be a breakthrough in quality improvement and the role of information technology.

Whatever it is, it will be something, if not several things! The point is that we are lucky to have sustained an institution like the CMHC and the people in it (and by extension, those who have passed through it) because the evidence in this book suggests that somehow they will find a way to be relevant, innovative, timely and of public service.

For this, for the vision and work of Fritz Redlich and those who have and will come after, we can all be grateful. For those of us not at the CMHC, we must think hard about how we can create and sustain more institutions like it.

Introduction: The Connecticut Mental Health Center as a public psychiatry initiative

Selby C. Jacobs and Ezra E. H. Griffith

This text celebrates the fortieth anniversary of the Connecticut Mental Health Center (CMHC). The CMHC, from its very inception, represented a collaborative effort of the State of Connecticut and Yale University. This unique connection between state and academic interests attended to the psychiatric interests of the public while focusing on ways to advance knowledge and to train students of the mental health professions. It is our contention that this unusual hybrid has had a remarkable history. Further, the CMHC has had a significant impact on psychiatric service models because of the very nature of the organization's identity. The CMHC represents forty years of sustained commitment to the provision of outstanding clinical services to patients in the public sector. These services have also been informed and buttressed by academic initiatives and a focus on the education of future psychiatrists as well as other mental health professionals.

In this volume, we focus on the psychiatric subspecialty of public psychiatry that was practised in a mental health center integrally connected to an academic department of psychiatry and its parent medical school. While this perspective may limit a comprehensive picture of community mental health, we believe it is important to develop the history of academic public psychiatry for both service and academic reasons. We return at the end of this introduction to a discussion of the significance of our effort.

Definition of public psychiatry

Public psychiatry is that part of psychiatry practised in the public sector and funded by a state's general funds as well as by reimbursement from entitlements such as Medicaid. Services provided by public sector clinicians serve as a safety net for disadvantaged, vulnerable, mentally ill and addicted individuals in the community. For disabled, chronically ill individuals, Medicare may fund services after disability is established

40 Years of Academic Public Psychiatry. Edited by Selby C. Jacobs and Ezra E. H. Griffith
© 2007 John Wiley & Sons, Ltd.

by the Social Security Administration. Public psychiatry is practised in many loci: mental health and addiction agencies; community behavioral health centers and programs; residential and nursing care facilities; rehabilitative and support service agencies; and organizations offering forensic and public health programs. Considering its funding sources, its targeted attention to the poor and seriously, chronically ill, and its breadth of services, the CMHC is clearly a public psychiatry service.

We contend that public psychiatry is a subspecialty of general psychiatry and should be identified as such for educational purposes. In the past 25 years, psychiatry has seen the development of several subspecialties. These include addictions, forensic psychiatry, consultation psychiatry, emergency psychiatry and geriatric psychiatry. All of these have special educational requirements. It is clear to us that public psychiatrists also require specialized education in order to practise competently. Public psychiatrists must understand psychiatric disability and how to complete functional assessments. They must also be knowledgeable about psychosocial and vocational rehabilitation in order to integrate these concepts into comprehensive plans of care. They should appreciate the principle of recovery and should be at ease in their interactions with consumers so as to respond effectively to the needs and aspirations of their patients. Public psychiatrists are expected to collaborate with other community-based professionals providing residential and money management services that support patients outside of the hospital. They must be competent, if not qualified, in the evaluation of addictions and should have a working understanding of legal problems commonly encountered by patients seeking services in the public sector. Psychiatrists working in this arena must be effective members of interdisciplinary teams, often as leaders of a team, and confident about medical roles in both clinic and community settings as well as aware of the roles of other professional groups. Indeed, they must understand how non-traditional mechanisms are employed beyond the clinic for reaching out and serving patients. Psychiatrists in public settings optimally achieve an understanding of systems dynamics and a population perspective on the use of clinical resources. Though these areas of knowledge and competence are obvious to the average psychiatrist in public sector practice and constitute a substantial domain of expertise, we are unaware of any movement at present to define public psychiatry as a subspecialty. Perhaps this volume will give some impetus to such a movement.

Academic public psychiatry concerns itself with the educational preparation of young psychiatrists and other mental health professionals to confront the challenges of public sector practice. It is this young cadre who also will carry out research into pressing questions raised by public sector practice. We wish to emphasize that such scholarship is necessary if public psychiatry is to advance and if its practitioners are to become progressively more skilled. An important task for this text is to show how academic public psychiatrists and other mental health professionals housed at the CMHC have engaged in such scholarly efforts over the past 40 years. They have done so always with an eye on improving practice, thereby benefiting the patients served.

Brief history of public psychiatry

The origins of public psychiatry can be traced to Dorothea Dix and the 19th Century. She was instrumental in a movement to bring to a wider public the benefits of moral psychiatry, which had been responsible for the opening of large, famous private hospitals such as the Institute of Living in Connecticut and Brattleboro Retreat in Vermont. In 1854, President Pierce vetoed legislation passed by Congress that would have created a federal role in providing for seriously ill psychiatric patients, leaving responsibility for the mentally ill in the hands of the states and local communities.

Over the next 50 years, many states opened large hospitals or asylums. The State of Connecticut constructed the Connecticut Valley Hospital and four other state-owned facilities. These became the cornerstones of public sector psychiatric care. Owing to the combination of ineffective treatments, the chronicity of serious disorders and eventual overcrowding, it was difficult to maintain a high level of care in these state facilities. In one reaction to the poor quality of care in large state facilities during the early 20th Century, the Yale University graduate Clifford Beers championed development of the mental hygiene movement. Mr. Beers suffered from bipolar disorder and had been hospitalized at Connecticut Valley Hospital. On recovery from his illness, he promoted early intervention and community clinics.

Before World War II, the majority of psychiatric practice occurred in large state hospitals and mental hygiene clinics. The post-World War II era saw the rise of another major reaction to state hospitals, culminating in the community mental health movement of the 1960s and 1970s. That movement was driven by federal policy and initiative as a result of converging forces that included wartime lessons in early intervention, the emergence of new treatments such as chlorpromazine, and considerable optimism. The passage of the Community Mental Health Centers Act in 1963 signaled that a fundamental transformation of psychiatric practice was underway. It heralded the emergence of a new system of care focused on community-based services and predicated on public health concepts. The transformation included the development of 675 community mental health centers. The Hill-West Haven Division, a part of the Connecticut Mental Health Center, was one of them. Meanwhile, state departments of mental health continued to provide services, largely through state hospitals and, to some extent, in newly developed, outpatient clinics supported by the National Institute of Mental Health. In this period, federal policy initiative and investment in the construction and staffing of community mental health centers eclipsed state roles. In the first phase of the community mental health center movement until the mid-1970s, there was little coordination between the new community mental health centers and the old state hospitals and clinics. The public practice of psychiatry during this time was divided between federal and state initiatives.

It is important to note that reimbursement by the newly enacted Medicaid and Medicare legislation in the 1960s led to a significant expansion in the role played by general hospitals in the institutional care of psychiatric patients. Also, the number of nursing homes for long-term care of chronically ill and elderly mentally ill grew enormously. In this way, federal entitlements fostered the development of alternatives to institutional care in large state hospitals. General hospital units and nursing homes became major building blocks in the modern system of care for patients treated in the public sector. As a result of the role played by federal entitlements, it is sometimes difficult to discern where the public sector ends and the private sector begins.

The contemporary concept of public psychiatry emerged during the 1980s. More precisely, it reemerged, as the Community Mental Health Centers Act and movement wound down. Probably the passage of mental health block grants to states under President Reagan in 1982 marked the change. Public psychiatry in state departments of mental health and state hospitals did not disappear between 1963 and 1982; it receded into the background. Deinstitutionalization was the most prominent movement within state public psychiatry from the 1960s to the 1990s. With the replacement of categorical federal funding with block grants to states in 1982, reinforced by the Community Support Program of the National Institute of Mental Health, state departments of mental health began once again to play a leading role in public psychiatry. In addition, while academic programs organized around community psychiatry were developed and dominated the 1970s, so-called public sector academic programs slowly began to emerge, notably at Columbia University, the University of Massachusetts, the University of Colorado and the University of Oregon. At Yale University, a more gradual transition occurred from academic programs in community psychiatry to programs now called public psychiatry.

During the 1990s, as states pursued federal reimbursement for mental health services, Medicaid policies and regulations began to define the public sector more prominently. This was a time of federal–state collaboration as states submitted plans that were reviewed by the Center for Medicare and Medicaid Services. The types of services and parameters of service were defined by Medicaid regulations, even as states exercised considerable choice over the extent and shape of Medicaid programs. This heralded the reemergence of an indirect federal role as a payer in defining the public sector. The role of payer would prove indicative of future development of services under the assumptions of managed care and privatization.

Progressively, state departments of mental health increasingly transitioned from the role of providing services in state-owned facilities to purchasing services in the community. A large number of private, non-profit agencies thrived because of this change. Their budgets were predominantly made up of state, public money supplemented by revenue from Medicaid and other payers. Tracing the evolution of state budgets for mental health starting in the 1980s, a shift occurred from predominant support for inpatient services to ambulatory services and from state-provided services to services purchased and provided in the community by private, non-profit agencies. Similar to the effects of Medicaid and Medicare in the 1960s, the boundaries and distinctions between public and private sector services blurred even more. It became progressively difficult to discern when, during patients' careers in treatment, they were in the private or public domain.

A federal New Freedom Commission reported in 2003 that the mental health system was in "shambles" and called for a transformation of the system, particularly in the public sector. The New Freedom Commission recommended bringing about systems change by pursuing the following principles: (1) mental health is essential to overall health; (2) mental health is consumer and family driven; (3) disparities in mental health services are eliminated; (4) early mental health screening, assessment and referral to services are common practice; (5) excellent mental health care is delivered and research is accelerated; and (6) technology is used to access mental health care and information. The exact implications of transformation for the public psychiatric system of services in which community mental health centers operate are still unclear.

The Connecticut Mental Health Center and public psychiatry

The idea of creating the CMHC originated in the 1950s in discussions between the Chairman of the Yale Department of Psychiatry, Fritz Redlich, and Connecticut's Governor Abraham Ribicoff. Initially, the intent was to develop an academic, state institute for clinical demonstration projects and research. The New York State Psychiatric Institute was a reference model in the original discussions. By the time the CMHC opened in 1966, the original concept was already changing under the influence of federal policy. At the CMHC's opening, the relationship between the State of Connecticut and Yale University was codified in a memorandum of agreement, which still serves as a reference point for definition of the missions of the Center as well as the respective responsibilities of the two parties.

The passage of the Community Mental Health Centers Act in 1963 created incentives for Connecticut and Yale University to seek federal support for a "catchmented" center, one that would have responsibility for a specific geographic area. Eventually, the federally funded center known as the Hill-West Haven Division was opened as a clinical division within the larger administrative entity known as the CMHC. Over time the Hill-West Haven Division and federal policies under the 1963 Act dominated the evolution of clinical services at the CMHC. The clinical services of the CMHC also influenced the agenda for education and research.

With block grants starting in 1982 and the reemergence of the Connecticut Department of Mental Health, the CMHC gradually realigned its clinical programs and academic missions with the goals of the state agency. In the early part of this new phase, the principles and policies of the Community Support Program of the National Institute of Mental Health, which disseminated system concepts and clinical programs for chronically ill persons, were a guiding force. Though program diversification began in the 1970s, it was not until the 1990s that the CMHC's services were clearly diversified. This occurred with the emergence of forensic and substance abuse services.

The relationship of the CMHC to the Connecticut Department of Mental Health and Addiction Services and the Yale Department of Psychiatry continues to define the CMHC. It is the State–Yale collaboration that shapes a definition of the multiple missions of the CMHC. The four major missions are clinical services, education, research and community development. This last mission is a function of the Center's location in an urban setting with typical social problems that impinge on the recipients of care. The multiple missions give the CMHC its particular character as an academic community mental health facility.

A staffing contract between the State of Connecticut and Yale University provides for the leadership, medical staff and psychologists (with some nurses and social workers) at the CMHC to be hired by Yale University. All of these professionals are also faculty in Yale's Department of Psychiatry or the School of Nursing. By virtue of this, the CMHC serves as the principal location of faculty in the Department of Psychiatry who concern themselves with academic public psychiatry.

Within the historical framework outlined above, the CMHC presently is a state-owned community mental health center located in a medium-sized urban setting. As noted, the professional and medical staff of the CMHC hold faculty appointments in the Yale Department of Psychiatry or the School of Nursing while most nurses and other operational personnel are state employees. The CMHC serves over 5000 individuals per year through a variety of clinical programs. The majority of the patients in treatment have disabilities, co-occurring substance abuse problems and legal problems. The clinical programs include acute inpatient services (20 beds); sub-acute, transitional services to housing (10 beds); 12 research beds; a walk-in, evaluation service; an outreach service to homeless persons and to individuals in crisis; a classical, assertive community treatment team; and ambulatory treatment and case management, organized into diagnostic teams. In addition, through satellites, the CMHC has a clinic for substance abuse treatment and a Hispanic clinic dispensing care to monolingual Latinos. The satellites include three community-based clinics in local communities. In one satellite, the CMHC provides services to children and families and operates a special program for late teenagers and young adults from the city who are aging out of child care. Further, the CMHC is a lead mental health agency for 16 community-based agencies that provide vocational and psychosocial rehabilitation, residential services, case management, and family education and support services. The CMHC's budget for clinical services from state general fund dollars was approximately $26M in fiscal year 2006. The total budget for the CMHC in the same year exceeded $50M. This latter amount included not only state general fund dollars but also grants obtained by individual faculty.

This text offers a history and an intensive case study of the CMHC, one community mental health center that has highly developed academic programs. While the example of the CMHC is particular, we believe there are both national and international implications and applications of this parochial experience. For example, the book's discussion of the special knowledge, experiences and education in public psychiatry for trainees at the CMHC has implications, joining with other academic centers and the field at large, for national discussions of the value of added qualifications in public psychiatry. Another example is the implication of the discussion in the chapter on chronic mental illness for other community mental health centers, which might be concerned about preserving a focus on a core, target population of patients, while the current agenda in public psychiatry diversifies and multiplies. In general, much of the knowledge and many of the programs described in this book, such as in the chapters on substance use disorders or law and psychiatry, might be applied in public practice.

Academic programs in public psychiatry

In the past 25 years, several fellowships in public psychiatry have emerged for post-residency training of psychiatrists. While not numerous, they reflect recognition of the particular problems that confront professionals in the public sector. Examples of such programs are found at Columbia University, the University of Maryland, the University of Massachusetts and the University of Oregon, to mention a few. The CMHC also offers advanced psychiatric training for research and practice in public psychiatry.

Academic public psychiatry has evolved over the past 40 years. The chapters in this volume provide a summary of where public psychiatry academic programs stand at present in the CMHC and in the field generally. We will outline our existing programs below as we introduce the chapters in this volume. The present configuration of programs does not represent the service system of the CMHC at its inception. At that time, subjects originating from the 1960s community mental health center movement dominated the agenda. These topics included evaluation of community-based services and catchmenting; organization and management theory; studies of crisis theory; prevention and community services; the role of faith-based services; services research and epidemiology; and the search for new and more effective treatment interventions. Slowly during the early 1970s, research on addictions emerged. It was followed in the late 1970s by an academic program on forensic psychiatry. In the early 1980s, research on chronic illness was consolidated. Each of these recent, academic programs, missing at the outset, now constitutes a major stream of research and teaching at the Center as outlined in chapters that follow.

Certain themes in public psychiatry cut across the organization of our academic programs. These include concern with treatment in the community as opposed to that meted out in the hospital, the debate concerning outpatient commitment, comparisons between old and new antipsychotic medications, the integration of clinical treatments and rehabilitation, challenges evoked by the recovery and the consumer movements, the introduction of patient-centered care, the integration of mental health and addictions treatments to address the problems of co-occurring disorders, the utility of service systems, state-owned versus private non-profit ownership, and the problem of shrinking mental health care budgets. These subjects, more or less particular to public psychiatry, are supplemented by general movements in American health care that include patient safety, discrepancies in health care outcomes for ethnic minorities, quality management and ownership of health benefits. These themes will be considered in more than one chapter. The concluding section will create a synthesis of these threads and will ultimately suggest a direction for the evolution of public psychiatry.

The book has been structured so as to represent, through its chapters, major programs at the CMHC. These programs encapsulate at once both clinical and academic initiatives. All of the chapters' authors have had extensive connections to the CMHC.

Chapter 1, Severe and Persistent Mental Illness, will trace the development of an academic program that started with John Strauss and Courtney Harding in the 1980s. It will cover both theoretical and practical approaches to care and will consider the long-term impact of mental illness on individuals. It will explore research on the non-acute phases of illness, psychosocial treatments, rehabilitation, recovery, and the integration of clinical and community care.

Chapter 2, Addictions, will describe the development of an academic Division of Substance Abuse that started with the pioneering work of Herbert Kleber and culminated in the construction of a Substance Abuse Center within the CMHC. This program is now the largest academic component of the CMHC. The chapter will tell the story of how an academic program may lead the way for development in a community mental health center by redefining the target population and practice in an essential area. It will summarize the role of the academic program in developing treatment approaches for addictions and co-occurring disorders.

Chapter 3, Forensic Services, relates the development of a law and psychiatry program that has flourished to the present point of annually offering subspecialty training targeted at four graduate psychiatry fellows. This chapter will cover the development of competency evaluations and jail diversion programs and contributions to the debate on involuntary outpatient treatment. In addition, it will describe its critical role in risk management and the ethics of community practice.

The fourth chapter, Neurobiological Research, describes the development of the Ribicoff Research Facility and the contributions of neurobiological research to new and improved treatments. The chapter will highlight the translation of basic work into clinical research and clinical research into practice. It will summarize the impact of research on treatment of the seriously mentally ill and will review the current debate on old versus new antipsychotic drugs.

Chapter 5, Epidemiology, Services Research, Prevention and Public Health, will follow the history of services research starting in the 1970s leading to and including studies of early detection, prevention, community development, the epidemiology of psychiatric disorders in the community and services utilization. The chapter will highlight the influence of a population perspective on services and the impact of a public health approach on patient care.

In Chapter 6, Ethnicity, Health Disparities and Cultural Competence, the authors will cover the concept of multicultural care in a community setting. The chapter traces the origins of special services such as the Hispanic and Hill clinics that developed as programmatic responses to the problem of barriers to care. It also highlights the relationship of professional services to the faith-based community. It discusses disparities in health care outcomes for minorities and offers strategies, including cultural competence, to eliminate them.

Chapter 7, A Public–Academic Partnership, will discuss 40 years of partnership between the State of Connecticut and the CMHC and will suggest how policy for our academic mental health center should be formulated. It will summarize the State's view of the academy and will define approaches to defining the mission of the CMHC. The authors will provide a brief history of major policy periods such as the community support programs of the 1980s, Medicaid and privatization in the 1990s, and the current transformation agenda stemming from the federal government's New Freedom Commission.

Chapter 8, Public Psychiatry Training and Education, provides a history that starts in the 1970s and traces the introduction of social and community psychiatry into general psychiatric training. It will discuss the relationship of public psychiatry to general psychiatric education. It will also provide an overview of training public sector professionals for the unique public sector context.

In Chapter 9, the Future of Academic Public Psychiatry, the authors will offer a summary and a vision of the future of the CMHC and of public psychiatry. They will discuss the viability of the community mental health center model of academic–state partnership, while clarifying commitments to the partnership that are necessary for the collaboration to have some chance of success.

Significance

It is our contention that academic contributions to the development of public psychiatry have been manifold and important. Two obvious examples of this are the contributions of academic programs in substance abuse and forensic services to the evolution of systems and services over the past two decades. Twenty years ago, the target population of community mental health centers was practically and exclusively made up of individuals with serious mental illness. Few, if any, individuals with substance abuse problems or legal problems entered treatment. Now, most patients at the CMHC have co-occurring disorders and are involved in some way in the criminal justice system. It was academic programs in these two arenas that prepared the CMHC for present public sector practice.

Other academic programs have also made signal contributions. Neurobiological research has contributed new, effective pharmacologic treatments, when 40 years ago, psychotherapy was the norm. Research on chronic illness has enhanced our understanding of the possibility of recovery and strategies for achieving it. Epidemiology has placed disorders in a population perspective and emphasized the concept of disease burden, which highlights the problem of psychosocial disability in society. Services research has evaluated the significance of system development, among other matters, and found it wanting, contributing to the movement to transform the "de facto," "fragmented" system of care as we presently know it. These are examples that come to mind as we enter the process of documenting the academic programs at the CMHC. In the chapters that follow we intend to reemphasize the idea that academic programs make substantial contributions to public psychiatry.

Further, academic programs and the initiative of academic psychiatrists in seeking grant support are instrumental in leveraging resources to supplement existing state-funded programs. A good example of this is the development of housing resources over the past 11 years at the CMHC. Through the initiative of faculty and staff at the Center, residential slots for patients have been doubled from approximately 250 slots funded by state dollars to 500 slots. These additional housing resources have been funded through successful grant applications to the federal Department of Housing and Urban Development. The federal resources amount to about $25M over the 11-year period.

Given the limitations of current knowledge, not least of the contributions that academic programs can make to public psychiatry is the catalytic role academic programs play in the translation of new research and discoveries into practice. Translation is a challenge for everyone. Academic centers embrace it. At the CMHC, for instance, the professional staff now engage in a perennial process of reviewing current knowledge and recent discoveries, not only within the Center itself but nationwide, to consider which practices merit implementation. We now conceptualize this process on three levels: the patient, specific practices and programs. For example, at the individual patient and clinician level, we are progressively implementing a center-wide program of evidence-based medicine. We also introduce new practices when we believe research has documented their efficacy; a current example is a locally proven, neuro-cognitive enhancement therapy for individuals in vocational rehabilitation. At the program level, we now have introduced eight best-practice packages ranging from an ACT team and Integrated Dual Diagnosis Treatment, to an Early Intervention Program for Psychotic Disorders. Periodically, we conduct fidelity studies, when the technology exists, to assure adherence to models.

It is our hope that the vision and ideas about directions for public psychiatry, which emerge from the descriptions and analysis in the sections that follow, will be useful not only to the CMHC but also to public psychiatry in general.

1

Severe and persistent mental illness

Bruce Wexler, Larry Davidson, Thomas Styron and John Strauss

Individuals treated in public sector community mental health centers often have chronic or recurrent illnesses and difficulties in housing, employment and social activities that compound one another. Understanding that this complex of clinical symptoms and functional compromise constitute the illnesses we treat, researchers at the Connecticut Mental Health Center (CMHC) described the variability in long-term course and experience of patients as they lived with their illnesses, engaged patients in their own treatment and that of others, and documented scientifically the value of an integrated network of clinical and community services. As part of an academic department of psychiatry, the CMHC has provided opportunities for translational research that brings basic neuroscience to bear on community care, and for training researchers and clinicians able to address the complexity of the illnesses and humanity of the patients.

Most people treated in public sector community mental health centers are suffering from chronic or recurrent mental illness, and most are faced with difficulties in housing, employment and social activities. Their illnesses and their problems with housing, employment and social activities compound one another, and all compromise general well-being and quality of life. It is this complex of clinical symptoms and functional deficits that constitute the illnesses we treat. Chronic and recurrent psychiatric illnesses take their greatest toll during the 95% of our patients' lives when they are out of the hospital and "clinically stable." In studying and working with patients during the long periods between symptom exacerbations and hospitalizations, researchers at the Connecticut Mental Health Center (CMHC) have made important contributions to public psychiatry.

Appreciation of the interrelation of illness and community function in the lives of our patients has led to two general principles that guide public sector treatment and research programs at the CMHC:

1. Manifestations of chronic and recurrent mental illnesses are much broader than the clinical symptoms (such as hearing voices) highlighted in diagnostic manuals and include compromise and complication of many aspects of community functioning (such as holding a job).

---

40 Years of Academic Public Psychiatry. Edited by Selby C. Jacobs and Ezra E. H. Griffith
© 2007 John Wiley & Sons, Ltd.

2. Treatment of chronic and recurrent illnesses must include components that address housing, employment and social function, both because compromise in these areas is part of the illness and because addressing these aspects of the illnesses is necessary to limit clinical symptoms and prevent clinical decompensation and hospitalization.

The first principle is reflected in the pioneering research of John Strauss and Courtney Harding, who described the long-term course and experience of patients as they and their clinicians sought to deal with their multifaceted illnesses (Harding et al., 1987; Strauss et al., 1985). These studies showed that the course of illness was anything but linear or uniform. Periods of little change could be followed by bursts of improved function. Symptom flare-ups and hospitalizations could be frequent in one stretch of time and rare in another. More people had better outcomes than many providers concluded from their cross-sectional views of patients in treatment at a particular moment. The extent of functional recovery varied widely from person to person despite the fact that they had the same diagnosis and received the same medications.

These observations raised important questions and pointed to areas of needed research. Why did people move forward in fits and starts? What was happening during periods of little overt change and during periods of increased community activity, success and independence? What was occurring during periods of symptom exacerbation and functional losses? Why did some people have smoother or more successful courses than others? In pursuing these questions, Strauss (1992, 1994) found and reasserted the importance of the person in their illness. People managed their illnesses differently, and some individuals did so better than others. Some were strong partners in their treatments. Strauss asked what clinicians and treatment centers do to enable and disable a patient's sense of his own independence? Strauss's work approached these issues through the relationship between objectivity and subjectivity in understanding, experiencing and treating mental illness.

The shift in focus to the person as the center of the experience and treatment of chronic and recurrent mental illnesses provided a foundation for what has become the recovery movement: treatment that aims to improve quality of life in the community, follows the patient's lead as to the goals of treatment, and focuses more on an individual's strengths and aspirations than on his weaknesses and losses. Larry Davidson, one of Strauss's early collaborators, has written about the recovery movement from a policy and practice point of view, beginning with its roots in the work of Strauss et al. and the consumer movement to its most recently taking center stage with the New Freedom Commission on Mental Health report that called for a transformation of the health care system with recovery as the overarching aim. Davidson put the research he and colleagues have done at the CMHC in a national and international context.

The second principle cited above has influenced the CMHC's involvement in the work of the Community Service Network (CSN). The CSN is a community-based, integrated care system that brings together providers of different professional disciplines, employed by different agencies, funded by different sources and focused on different facets of our clients' problems related to housing and social and vocational rehabilitation. Evidence gathered at the CMHC demonstrates the worth of these component community-based services as well as the value of integration of those services, particularly as they enhance the importance of "social capital/valued social roles" in the recovery process.

As an academic community mental health center and an integral part of a large academic department of psychiatry, the CMHC also provides opportunities for translational research that brings findings of more basic neuroscience to bear on community care. Some of these opportunities are discussed in the chapters on clinical neuroscience, substance use and other types of research at the CMHC. In the final portion of this chapter, we will describe work done at the CMHC that draws on the neuroscience of brain plasticity to develop new treatments for the cognitive deficits associated with severe mental illnesses. Wexler and Bell developed and provided these treatments to patients who were also participating in supported employment programs. They found their neuroscience-based treatments resulted in greater employment success and marked improvement in patient quality of life. Based on these results, treatments they developed are being applied at the CMHC and other community mental health centers in Connecticut.

The nature of the problem

When considering psychiatric disorders, that old, simple, but basic question about any area of concern, "what is going on here anyway?" underlies practice, treatment systems, even research. When Kraepelin identified the disorder "dementia praecox," the earliest label for what is now called schizophrenia, by defining what he considered to be a disease process, not merely a syndrome, he established the foundation for modern psychiatry. This foundation was based on the view that the course of a disorder, not merely a group of symptoms, identified a disease process. Kraepelin believed that this group of problems identified an illness, presumably organic in nature, because these people had an inevitable downhill course. This view dominated much of twentieth century psychiatry implying, as well, that custodial treatment would be required for the presumably helpless individual caught in the tentacles of the malady.

More recently, evidence has shown that this disorder, or group of disorders, in fact has an extremely heterogeneous course and outcome. Thus the founding rationale of much of modern psychiatry theory and treatment systems was in fact inaccurate. Initiated by the World Health Organization in 1969, over thirty years of rigorous clinical research conducted in more than a dozen countries and involving thousands of individuals with schizophrenia has now demonstrated that this disorder manifests considerable heterogeneity. Strauss's Center for the Study of Prolonged Psychiatric Disorder at the CMHC was one of the first such programs in the world to document the fact that recovery was not only possible in serious mental illness, but that it was in fact just as common, if not more so, than the progressive, deteriorating course first described by Kraepelin at the turn of the 20th century. Most recently, the CMHC faculty have collected and published this extensive body of research in the two-volume anthology (Davidson et al., 2005, 2006b).

Kraepelin, who was a fine observer in spite of his limited access to the sampling and statistical methodologies of modern science, also noted that some patients with chronic illness who continued to work did not get worse. He thus opened the way for considering social and psychological factors as important in even the supposedly most severe psychiatric conditions. New data suggest that the psychiatric patient, even one afflicted by schizophrenia, does not appear to be just a passive victim of the disorder. In fact, as should have been suggested by Kraepelin's early observation regarding the role of work, there appears to be important effects of social, psychological and biological factors on the course of these disorders. Indeed, Bell and Wexler at the CMHC established that work is itself therapeutic and able to alter as well as reflect the course of illness. Combined biosocial treatments can enhance the ability to work.

The patient as active agent

The data go even further. During a series of research interviews conducted during the 1990s, concerning course of disorder and its determinants such as treatment and social contexts, one patient with schizophrenia said, "Why don't you ever ask me what I do to help myself?" The answer (simple enough in retrospect, but difficult to accept) was "because what the patient does to help himself does not fit into our model, often implicit, of severe mental illness, its nature and its course." That is, it does not fit into the model of "you have this disease for which you can do essentially nothing except 'comply' with our treatments as we develop and improve them."

The possibility that people can often help themselves revolutionizes the way of viewing not only the disorder itself, but also treatment systems and research. We can no longer ignore it when a patient says, "I looked around me at the other patients on the ward and knew that I had to do better." Or, "I had to get better because they were going to take my daughter away." Or, "The most important thing in my improvement was someone who cared about me." Or, "The most important thing in my improvement was someone who didn't just see me as a patient, but who took me seriously as a person." Considering the number of such statements from patients of various ages and with various syndromes and degrees of chronicity seen in follow-up interviews from various countries around the world, it would be a very dubious assumption to consider these statements as peripheral or irrelevant in our understanding, practice and research.

The next step indicates that it is crucial to consider the patient's subjectivity: his desire to improve and feelings about doing so, his feelings about such things as people caring for him or taking him seriously, his understanding of possible actions he can take on his behalf, and his desire and ability to do so. These feelings and actions are strongly influenced of course by his past experiences and his social context, including the treatment environment, his family and other social contacts, and even that old Kraepelin variable, the possibility for work. Patients are often told by a doctor, "You have a disease like diabetes. You will have it all your life. You will have to take medications all your life, and there are certain things you will never be able to do." Understandably, for many patients that is a message of despair, a message to give up hope. And even when the treatment system does not convey such a message overtly, the covert message is often the same.

Attention to the theater and other arts can help us to learn more about and sensitize ourselves to people's subjective experiences of their situations and our role in assisting or destroying hope and possibilities for action. It is after all a main goal of the arts to understand and reflect how people experience their world and see their place in it. The actor, for example, in playing a role is constantly asking himself what he is trying to do in the role that he is playing.

Our way of viewing mental illness is determined by our society and our training. It often includes explicit and implicit but inadequate beliefs that form the foundation for how we develop treatment systems and carry out research. Often, for the socially disadvantaged who already have extra difficulties in leading their lives, rather than helping, these beliefs add an overwhelming burden interfering with improvement. Recent developments in treatment systems and research are increasingly recognizing the possibility of improvement for even the most severe and long-standing disorder. The role of the patient, including the role of the patient's subjective experience (of life, treatment and possibilities), is being recognized also as a crucial aspect of the disorder and improvement process. Recognizing and understanding our many roles influencing those subjective experiences mark the progress in our field.

Recovery as the goal

In 1999 U.S. Surgeon General David Satcher issued an unprecedented report on mental health (DHHS, 1999). This report took the first substantial step since the Carter Commission of the 1970s in reconceptualizing the nature of mental health care and, as a result, recasting the fate of individuals with serious mental illness and the future of their loved ones. The Carter Commission had recognized how little progress had been made in fulfilling the promises of deinstitutionalization twenty years after there had begun to be a steady flow of people out of centuries-old, overcrowded state hospitals. The community support movement arose out of the stark recognition that people were being discharged literally to the streets. The movement envisioned offering an array of outpatient services to allow people, who in the past would have lived out the majority of their adult lives in distant institutions, to remain in their local communities (Parrish, 1989; Turner and Tenhoor, 1978). According to the surgeon general, and confirmed more extensively by the 2003 Presidential New Freedom Commission on Mental Health that followed, the U.S. has not only failed to keep the promises of deinstitutionalization and the Carter Commission by not funding needed community services, it also has set the bar too low. As described in the New Freedom Commission Report, entitled *Achieving the Promise: Transforming Mental Health Care in America* (DHHS, 2003), even the services that were being provided in community settings "simply manage[d] symptoms and accept[ed] long-term disability." With the surgeon general's report, this was no longer considered adequate, and the aim of mental health care shifted from managing symptoms to promoting recovery. Allowing the patients' views of their illnesses, their wishes for their lives and their ongoing participation in the treatment process helped alter the goals as well as the process of treatment. In this way, it contributed to the "recovery model of care" being increasingly adopted by community mental health agencies across the country.

What led the federal government, and the various experts it had called upon in drafting the surgeon general and New Freedom Commission reports, to believe that recovery from mental illness was not only possible, but that it should be stipulated as the overarching aim of all mental health care? Following as it did on the heels of 150 years of pessimism, institutionalization and neglect, what led the New Freedom Commission, for example, to envision a day "when all adults with serious mental illnesses . . . will live, work, learn, and participate fully in their communities" (DHHS, 2005).

The convergence of two historical and scientific developments, both of which passed through the CMHC, partly accounted for these exciting, landmark advances in mental health policy and practice. First, mentioned above, was the groundbreaking research conducted by John Strauss, Courtenay Harding and others beginning in the early 1970s examining the course and outcome of serious mental illness. Second was the emergence of patients as providers of care for others.

Patients as providers

People living with and recovering from these conditions provided the second, and equally important, impetus to the shift to recovery currently taking over the field. As people with serious mental illnesses began living outside of institutional settings, many of them became active in advocating for changing the conditions from which they had been liberated and also became active in establishing self-help, mutual support and peer-run programs across the country. They became living proof of the heterogeneity in course and outcome that Strauss, Harding and others had discovered and demonstrated, by example, that it was possible to live with, manage and overcome serious mental illness. As role models for others, they also advocated for a mental health system that both expected and promoted this kind of recovery, and began to pursue mental health care careers in order to bring about such a transformation. A series of initiatives at the CMHC was informed by, and has since contributed to, these developments.

The first so-called "consumer initiative" arose as part of the creation of the Community Support Network at the CMHC in the early 1990s. Following shortly on the success of a pilot program in Colorado, a first class of people with histories of serious mental illness graduated from a "community living specialist" program sponsored by the CSN (Strauss and Davidson, 1996). Since that time, thousands of people around the country with a history of serious mental illness have been trained and employed to provide a range of services and help to others in what has since come to be referred to as "peer support." Peer support differs both from self-help and from mutual support in that it refers to a non-reciprocal relationship in which one person who has managed to live with and/or recover from a serious mental illness offers role modeling, mentoring and other services to another person who is currently having more difficulty. Since Davidson developed the first training program for peer staff in 1992, faculty of the CMHC have been central in the articulation, implementation and evaluation of a variety of peer-delivered services. They have been able to demonstrate the variety of ways in which people with serious mental illnesses can play an active and valuable role in the recovery of their peers (e.g., Chinman et al., 2000, 2001; Davidson et al., 1997a, 1997b, 1997c, 1999, 2000, 2001, 2004b; Stayner et al., 1996; Weingarten et al., 2000), and most recently reviewed this increasingly important body of work for a special issue of *Schizophrenia Bulletin* on the evidence base for recovery-oriented interventions (Davidson et al., 2006a).

Concurrent with this emphasis on the role of people in promoting the recovery of their peers, CMHC faculty have been instrumental in identifying, examining and then promoting the role of the person with a serious mental illness in his own recovery. Beginning within the context of the longitudinal studies led by Strauss, Davidson and colleagues, a body of qualitative research has developed describing the role of the person in containing and minimizing the deleterious effects of the illness while reconstructing an effective sense of social agency and a meaningful and productive life based on his remaining assets, interests, and areas of health and competence (e.g., Chinman et al., 1999b; Davidson, 1997, 2003; Davidson and Stayner, 1997; Davidson and Strauss, 1992, 1995; Davidson et al., 1995; 2004a; Sells et al., 2003). Development of this body of research required establishing a rigorous approach to studying subjectivity (e.g., Davidson, 1987, 1988, 1992, 1993, 1994, 1997, 2003; Fossey et al., 2002), as well as making room within policy debates for the voices of people in recovery (e.g., Chinman et al., 1999b; Davidson et al., 1996), resulting most recently in two special issues of journals devoted to these topics.

This last issue, of eliciting and incorporating the voices of people in recovery in shaping mental health policy and practice, provides a useful illustration of the practical implications of this line of research. As the field has devoted the majority of its efforts to figuring out how to get rid of mental illness, we have learned very little about how people can manage to live with an illness and reclaim a life despite having the illness. In this respect, who better to educate us about what is entailed in living with, managing and reclaiming a life despite the illness than the people living with the illness themselves? This has been the focus of much of the work of these faculty during the previous decade.

As a first example, when asked in the mid-1990s to facilitate the discharge of a cohort of people with extended stays in the state hospital, CMHC faculty recognized that this policy decision had not benefited from the input of the people affected most directly by it: the patients themselves. When they subsequently asked this cohort of individuals about their experiences of long-term hospitalization and discharge, the faculty were surprised to find that life in the hospital was more alike than different from life outside of the hospital. While life in the community had the advantages of offering people freedom, privacy, safety, and proximity to family and their home communities, life in the hospital was associated with better access to health care (both psychiatric and primary care) and less social isolation. In the community, participants spent many hours alone in their apartments, with only a television or radio for company; whereas in the hospital, as one participant in this study explained, you were at least "confined together" with others (Davidson et al., 1995).

Other than these differences, participants' lives were described in strikingly similar terms across hospital and community settings. These were the terms of impoverishment, emptiness, loneliness and despair. More important than where they lived, participants were most concerned with the losses they had endured, both of important and caring people in their lives and of meaningful ways to spend their time (Davidson et al., 1995). And rather than providing a simple answer to the straightforward question "where would you rather receive treatment, in the hospital or in the community?" participants in this study suggested that the investigators and clinicians were posing the wrong questions.

This recognition led to further innovations in methodology, so that by the time a second opportunity was presented for input, people with mental illness were included as full partners in the research enterprise, helping to shape the questions themselves as well as the solutions. This opportunity was presented by a subpopulation of adults with serious mental illnesses who cycled in and out of acute inpatient care. For these adults who were living in the post-institutional era, the failure to establish and main-tain tenure outside of institutional settings was typically attributed to the severity of their illness, their abuse of alcohol or other substances, and/or their refusal to take medications as prescribed and attend scheduled outpatient appointments. These assumptions had yet to be assessed; furthermore, these individuals had not themselves been asked about possible solutions.

In this case, as well, participants defied conventional expectations when asked how they might be better helped to remain out of the hospital. Far from viewing hospitali-zations as crises or failures—and therefore to be avoided—participants described their stays in the hospital as offering them respite and a "vacation" from their impoverished, lonely and empty lives on the streets. It thus made no sense to them that they should try to stay out of the hospital, as it was the only place left for them to go when all other doors had been closed. In addition, and in contrast to clinicians' usual concerns that each subsequent hospitalization leads to further deterioration and a worsening outcome, one representative participant described how his experiences in the hospital had actually improved over time:

"The first time I was scared, the second time I had been here before and I knew what to expect, the third time it was like coming home again. Everyone was like greeting me at the door. . . . The third time was the best."—Man describing his successive hospitalizations (Davidson et al., 1997c, p. 774).

This picture of the hospital and its role only make sense in the context of the "home-less, broke, unemployed . . . same harsh" everyday lives participants described, which made the system's goal of preventing their re-hospitalization extremely difficult, if not impossible, to achieve (Davidson et al., 1997b). In addition to being destitute, study participants described a basic sense of powerlessness, not just over their illnesses but over their lives as a whole, along with an overwhelming sense of hopelessness and demoralization. Given the pervasive sense of helplessness which had participants trapped, they could think of nothing that they—or anyone else, for that matter—could do that would help them to stay out of the hospital.

This is not to suggest, however, that these participants could not think of many other things which would have improved their lives in the community. Fortunately, we had learned from the prior study that we did not even know the right questions to ask, and had therefore included our participants this time more as collaborators than as subjects in this research. In addition to answering our questions about their experi-ences of hospitalization, participants were invited to tell us about their lives in general, the things they considered important, and the things that would make their lives better. In this way, they painted a much fuller picture of their day-to-day lives, their experiences of poverty, discrimination and isolation, and their struggles both with mental illness and with unresponsive mental health services and providers. Whereas in the earlier study we still considered ourselves to be the experts in designing inter-ventions to address the issues the participants identified (e.g., supported socialization to address their loneliness), in this study we asked the participants to be our partners in designing new ways of addressing their unmet needs. Participants identified as most pressing, in this regard, their isolation and demoralization and the lack of responsiveness they found in the mental health services they were offered or mandated to receive.

About these unmet needs, participants had many ideas and suggestions. Meeting these needs creatively through mechanisms that they then helped to develop has since been shown to decrease readmissions and substance use, and to increase social functioning and participants' active role in and use of mental health care (Davidson et al., 2000; O'Connell et al., 2005).

Is it surprising that from people with such severe disabilities should come such effective strategies for improving their everyday lives in the community and, as a result, for increasing their community tenure? Only if such people are equated with, or subsumed by, their disabilities; not, on the other hand, if they are viewed as knowledgeable about their disabilities and about developing ways to bypass, compensate for, or overcome them in pursuit of a meaningful, gratifying and productive life.

These two studies provide examples of the ways in which adults with serious mental illnesses, including those significantly disabled by these illnesses, retain the capacity to speak for themselves, both in identifying their needs and in suggesting strategies for addressing those same needs. In this respect, we suggest that people with serious mental illnesses themselves represent a highly valuable and yet relatively untapped resource for accumulating psychiatric knowledge and informing the development of clinical and rehabilitative interventions. A central component of the transformation process should thus be the inclusion of people with serious mental illnesses in all phases and aspects of the research, treatment, rehabilitative and policy enterprises. In this way, we will support the pursuit of a common agenda and enable the mental health system in the words of the *Federal Action Agenda*, to "better meet the needs of the individuals and families it is designed to serve" (DHHS, 2005, p. 5).

Putting it all together in the service system

Appreciation of the importance of social contact, good housing and opportunities for productive activities led to a broad range of services to address these needs. Initially these services were each separate programs with independent staff and funding. However, research at the CMHC and the Greater Bridgeport Community Mental Health Center soon demonstrated that patients benefited more from services that were integrated. In 1990, based on this important research, DMHAS established the Community Services Network (CSN) which is central to DMHAS' and the Department of Psychiatry's partnership to provide an integrated system of recovery-oriented services for people with psychiatric disabilities in the Greater New Haven community. A consortium of 16 community-based not-for-profit organizations funded by DMHAS and for which the CMHC serves as the lead agency, the CSN provides a wide variety of rehabilitation and support programs in the following service areas: clinical, residential, vocational, social rehabilitation, crisis, respite, family support and case management. Consistent with DMHAS' Standards and Practice for Recovery-Oriented Care, the overarching goal of all CSN activities is to promote a system of care that identifies and builds upon each individual's assets, strengths, and areas of health and competence. In this way, the patient achieves mastery over his condition while regaining a meaningful, constructive sense of membership in the broader community.

Fundamental to achieving this goal are efforts on the part of CSN leadership to find new and creative ways to promote social capital or valued social roles for the individuals served by the CSN. Although the academic literature does not clearly define social capital and ways to measure it, it has been well established that people of any background who lack positive social roles are at significant risk for a host of negative life experiences (including lower perceptions of self-esteem and self-worth), such as rejection, poverty, lack of opportunity, and physical or emotional victimization (Huppert and Whittington, 2003; Katschnig and Krautgartner, 2002; Schaie and Schooler, 1998; Stein and Wemmerus, 2001; Wolfensberger, 2000). People with serious psychiatric disabilities, who frequently experience intense social isolation and report having few, if any, friends or significant relationships, consistently identify meaningful community activities and socially valued roles as critical elements of the recovery process. They express a strong preference to live in typical housing, to have friendships and intimate relationships with a wide range of people, to work in regular employment settings, and to participate in school, worship, recreation, shopping and other pursuits alongside other (non-disabled) community members (Breier et al., 1991; Davidson and Stayner, 1997; Reidy, 1992). And it has been demonstrated that through such activities, individuals often gain access to the valued roles that can provide the foundation for their recovery (Ridgway, 2001; Walsh, 1996).

In addition to numerous CSN programs that promote independent housing, competitive employment, education and recreation, faculty and staff associated with the CMHC and the CSN have engaged in a number of innovative research demonstration programs to promote valued social roles through other means as well. Three recent examples of such initiatives follow.

The partnership project: a supported socialization study

The Partnership Project was a New Haven-based, SAMHSA-funded psychiatric rehabilitation study that found that volunteers could support people with psychiatric disabilities to increase their participation in community activities, thereby enhancing their social supports and quality of life (Davidson et al., 2001). The project was the first randomized, controlled trial of a supported socialization intervention that matched participants either with a volunteer having a personal history of psychiatric disability (a "consumer partner") or with a volunteer with no such history (a "community partner"). All pairs were given a $28/month stipend and asked simply to participate in social and recreational activities of their choosing over a nine-month period. In addition, the study employed a control condition in which individuals were assigned to a "stipend only" group where they received the financial supplement but not the community or consumer partner. The initial phase of data analysis relied on qualitative data analytic procedures that examined themes obtained from participant interviews. Overall findings suggest that all participants desired, and responded to, opportunities for friendship, i.e., opportunities to occupy the role of "friend." Participants regularly described valuing their experiences of being able to go out and do "normal" things and of regaining parts of themselves that they had lost since the onset of their illnesses. Isolation and loneliness decreased, while social networks, confidence, self-esteem and quality of life all increased.

The recovery is for everyone grants program (RIFE)

RIFE offers mini-grants to individuals in recovery from mental health and substance abuse problems for innovative projects to help them take steps forward in achieving their life aspirations (Tracy et al., 2004). The grant application is open-ended and maximizes the individual's originality and initiative for independent projects that do not fit either a standard format or a treatment intervention. Typical awards allow grantees to develop volunteer civic organizations (e.g., making quilts and toys for newborns in a local hospital), start personal businesses (e.g., starting and marketing a DJ company), or to re-enroll in educational pursuits (e.g., finishing a nursing assistant program). Each of these awards allows individuals to develop a meaningful role that they perceive as being critical to their well-being and recovery (e.g., the roles of volunteer, business owner, or student). Quantitative outcome evaluation of the project yielded the following results: 91% of participants reported improvements in daily life, 82% in thoughts of self, 80% in belief in capabilities, 60% in social roles, 80% in socializing and 50% in values. These areas were assessed through the administration of the Making Decisions Scale (MDS), a validated tool that measures the construct of empowerment, and the Evaluation of Program Questionnaire (EPQ), a questionnaire that evaluates the impact of the program on the participant in the multitude of areas noted above.

The leadership project

This project links the theories of citizenship and "social capital" in the design of a pilot intervention supporting homeless or formerly homeless individuals with behavioral health disorders (Rowe et al., 2003). Within this intervention, participants were trained for internships on boards and action groups that provide services to people who are homeless. It was designed in response to the fact that many service organizations are required to include people with psychiatric disabilities on their boards and action groups. However, this requirement rarely resulted in successful, ongoing representation. Thus, the board or action group loses the valuable contributions of individuals with first-hand experiences, and the individual loses the opportunity to "give back" by occupying the socially valued role of board member or community activist.

The preparatory classes in the pilot Leadership Project met for seven weeks, twice a week for three hours each and covered such topics as interpersonal skills, public speaking, assertiveness training, negotiation and conflict resolution, board and committee training, the legislative process, networking and advocacy, and homelessness. Evaluation methods of the project included brief surveys (given both to participants and to board mentors or support persons), collection of demographic and other information, and participant observation.

Preliminary findings suggested that the Leadership Project was overall a successful intervention. Students who graduated from the class and moved on to board internships were almost uniformly positive about their experiences. In addition, many individuals who did not complete the training have maintained contact with the project coordinator and have stated that their experience was a positive one. The response of board members was similarly positive and has prompted interest from other service providers and boards in New Haven and other areas of Connecticut. Given the promising preliminary findings of this pilot project, it has recently been modified and is being applied in the context of a study on jail diversion among mental health clients. The project/study compares individuals who receive mental health treatment alone to individuals who receive mental health treatment along with peer support, group "citizenship" classes, and opportunities to participate in an internship involving a socially valued role, e.g., being an intern on a board for a social service agency.

Cognitive remediation and vocational rehabilitation: a translational neuroscience research program

The important work initiated by Strauss and colleagues, and developed further by Davidson and colleagues, has helped provide a foundation for a treatment philosophy and procedures that assume the following: people with psychiatric illnesses can lead lives enriched by the relationships and activities important to those without illness. It does not deny that our patients have serious illnesses, nor question the potential value of also addressing those illnesses from medical or neurobiological perspectives. The fact that the CMHC is part of an academic department of psychiatry with strong biomedical research provides opportunities to integrate biomedical and psychosocial research.

At a joint DMHAS-CMHC-Yale conference for the academic and general community in the early 1990s, Wexler reported the results of research on problems with concentration, memory and problem-solving in patients with serious psychiatric illnesses. He called it the "hidden problem" since diagnosis and treatment focused on clinical symptoms, like loose associations, hallucinations and delusions, and many clinicians were unaware of the nature and severity of their patients' cognitive deficits. In a pioneering 1997 publication, he demonstrated that when cognitive tasks with which patients have marked difficulty were first made easy enough for patients to do successfully, and then made incrementally more difficult as patient performance improved through simple drill and practice, patients could attain normal and supernormal levels of performance (Wexler et al., 1997). He conceived of this cognitive remediation as engaging underactive neurocognitive systems and producing "activity-dependent" neural recruitment and functional enhancement.

At the same time, another Yale faculty member, Morris Bell, was conducting randomized controlled clinical trials at the West Haven VA Medical Center that demonstrated the power of paid employment to reduce patient symptoms and improve quality of life (Bell et al., 1993; Bell and Lysaker, 1997). Bell and colleagues noted, however, that patients with greater cognitive deficits were less able to work (Bell and Lysaker, 1995; Lysaker et al., 1995). Wexler and Bell then joined in a series of large studies to develop cognitive remediation treatments and evaluate their ability to produce generalized and durable improvements in cognition, improved work function and better quality of life.

Most aspects of cognitive, motor and sensory function have been shown to be abnormal in patients with schizophrenia, schizoaffective disorder or other major mental illnesses. Functional magnetic resonance (fMRI), and other available brain imaging methods have demonstrated regional brain activation abnormalities associated with the observed cognitive deficits. Multiple studies have shown under-activation of the frontal cortex in patients (Ganguli et al., 1997; Weinberger et al., 1988; Yurgelun-Todd et al., 1996), sometimes as part of a broader activation failure of a cortical-cerebellar-thalamic-cortical system (Crespo-Fracorro et al., 1999). Under-activation has also been reported in primary and secondary sensory areas during tasks requiring sustained attention and simple sensory processing. Other studies report abnormal increases in parietal or temporal activation (Callicott et al., 1998; Curtis et al., 1998; Yurgelun-Todd et al., 1996), and even frontal areas, suggesting inefficiency of neural processing. It is, of course, no surprise that there are neural activation abnormalities associated with the cognitive deficits. But the brain imaging studies help identify targets for therapeutic intervention and provide important measures of treatment effects, and are an additional component of the Wexler-Bell research program.

Cognitive dysfunctions have been associated with poor psychosocial function in several studies (Green, 1996; Green et al., 2000) and several investigators (Carter and Flesher, 1995; Green, 1996; Liberman, 1996) have described neurocognitive deficits as "rate limiting factors" in work capacity. Bell and colleagues found that cognitive impairment affects the rate of improvement on work performance measures (Bell and Lysaker, 1995; Lysaker et al., 1995) and that neuropsychological testing can predict 78% of the variance in individual improvement in work quality (Bell et al., 1997). Moreover, they identified a subgroup for whom these impairments are particularly severe. These subjects had more difficulty on the job, worked fewer hours and fewer weeks, and made fewer clinical gains than other patients in our work program. Cognitive deficits also distinguished subjects who completed the program from those who did not (Bell et al., 2003), raising the possibility that such deficits may limit the ability of patients to take full advantage of a variety of psychosocial treatments. For multiple reasons, then, treatment of the cognitive deficits is important for full and effective implementation of a community or public psychiatry approach.

Pharmacotherapy has, unfortunately, proved to have very limited effect on the cognitive deficits of psychiatric illness. Faced with the clinical importance of cognitive deficits, and the absence of available treatments, Wexler took note of new animal research demonstrating that even in adult monkeys, unusually intensive and extended activation of a particular neural system led to "activity-dependent" recruitment of neural resources by the system. Wexler reasoned that if it were possible to engage and exercise under-functioning neurocognitive systems in patients, it may be possible to produce an activity-dependent enhancement of function. He also noted that the animal studies suggested that patients might also be limited by "disuse atrophy" of cognitive functions (Wexler et al., 1997), because activities that involve areas of deficits are often avoided and unrewarded. Therapeutic exercise or practice of these functions and activation of the associated neural centers could, at the least, reverse such atrophy and, at best, decrease the initial deficit.

The first test of this physiologically based treatment approach was done at the CMHC in 1996 (Wexler et al., 1997). Twenty-two clinically stable, medicated outpatients with schizophrenia participated in four or five training sessions per week for 10 weeks, doing visual reading and spatial memory tasks. Healthy and successfully employed individuals were tested on the training tasks in order to determine whether patients were able to achieve normal performance levels after training. After 10 weeks of exercises, 16 of the 22 patients performed as well or better than the best healthy subject on the verbal reading and spatial memory tasks. For example, by the end of training, over half of the patients were able to read words with stimulus exposures less than or equal to 100 milliseconds; response periods of 800 milliseconds during which they had to say the words out loud before the next stimulus appeared; continuous task durations of 10 minutes; and performance accuracies ranging from 93% to 99%.

This initial study demonstrated that on two tasks with which patients with schizophrenia have repeatedly been found to have significant difficulty (sustained and rapid language processing and spatial memory), repeated practice with incremental adjustments of difficulty led to normal or even supernormal performance. Apparently the necessary neural substrates were not missing or destroyed. Subsequent studies were designed to determine whether performance gains generalized to tasks that were not themselves practiced, persisted after the treatment ended, were associated with normalization of brain activation abnormalities, and led to functional gains in the community. Wexler teamed up with Bell in two large studies to address these questions. The first was located at the West Haven VA Hospital and included patients from the CMHC. The second was located at the CMHC.

Patients in both studies received vocational services: work therapy (WT) in the first and supported employment (SE) in the second. Half the patients were randomly assigned also to receive computerized exercises for cognitive remediation therapy (CRT) and two weekly cognition focused therapy groups. In the first study, the active treatment was for six months with follow-up at one year. In the second study, active treatment was for 12 months with follow-up at two years. Both studies recruited outpatients, with schizophrenia or schizoaffective disorder as determined by structured clinical interviews, who were in a post-acute phase of illness. The WT study included 145 patients and the SE study 77. Both samples of individuals had severe and persistent illness, were about 40 years old on average, and had average IQ scores of about 85.

The effects of the CRT on cognition were evaluated by comparing neuropsychological test performance before and after the active intervention periods. To reduce experiment-wise error in analyses of the first study, 21 neuropsychological variables were subjected to factor analysis to produce four groupings of variables: executive function, working memory, thought disorder, and visual and verbal recall. Patients receiving CRT + WT showed greater improvements than those in the WT only group on executive function ($p < 0.006$) and working memory clusters ($p < 0.01$). The thought disorder and visual and verbal recall factors had non-significant trends favoring CRT + WT. Significant individual variables included Wisconsin Card Sorting Test Conceptual Level ($p < 0.002$), WCST Categories Correct ($p < 0.04$), WCST Non-perseverative Errors ($p < 0.004$), Bell Lysaker Emotion Recognition Test (BLERT, $p < 0.001$) and Digit Span Backward (WAIS-III, $p < 0.05$). For many patients the functional gains were substantial, with improvements greater than 0.8 SD in 35% of patients on the WCST Conceptual Level, 39% on Digits Backward and 39% on the BLERT. Analyses of the second study focused on the effects observed in the first study. Again the group that received CRT showed significantly greater improvement on the WSCT measures ($p < 0.005$–0.05) and Digit Span ($p < 0.03$). Self-report measures yielding scores on coping styles and personality traits, and interview assessment of quality of life were added to the second study. The patients who received CRT showed significantly greater post-treatment gains in quality of life ratings, conscientiousness and use of coping styles. The durability of cognitive gains was demonstrated six months after the end of treatment in the first study, with CRT patients still showing significantly greater increases in WCST and Digit Span performance and showing new evidence of greater gains in working memory. Similar analyses from the second study have not yet been done.

Employment data were collected six months after the end of the six-month WT program ($N = 145$) and 12 months after the cessation of the 12-month SE program in the patients who have thus far completed the two-year follow-up in the SE study ($N = 43$). Hours worked and the number of percentages of patients employed were compared in the groups with and without CRT, using repeated measures ANOVA and looking for differences between groups over time. For hours worked, the time by condition interaction was significant in both studies. The patients receiving CRT maintained or increased the number of hours they worked during the follow-up period while hours worked decreased in the other conditions ($p < 0.05$ for WT study, and $p < 0.05$ for SE study. Results are similar when the percentages of patients employed are. Employment rates are much higher in the WT study because of placement in non-competitive jobs in the medical center rather than community employment. There is still a suggestion that CRT + WT patients were more likely to remain employed after the end of treatment than WT-only patients. With the greater demands of competitive community employment and longer post-treatment follow-up in the SE study, this difference is much greater.

Summary and future direction

Strauss's ability to look at the big picture, to value subjective as well as observer-based objective assessments of clinical state and outcomes, and to spend the time and effort to talk and listen to people with major psychiatric illnesses led to a major reconceptualization of the role of the person with the illness in setting the goals of treatment. Davidson took things another step by demonstrating the value of patients as providers of services to others. Together, the work of Strauss and Davidson, and their students and colleagues, were major factors in the development of a "recovery" model of care that increasingly guides organization and provision of services nationwide. By operating within an academic environment, a premium was placed on describing and evaluating this work, and then disseminating results to others through scholarly and research publications. By operating as part of an integrated state mental health agency, it was possible to integrate the new services that grew out of the recovery model into an integrated community services network as described by Styron. By working within a biomedical research environment, current basic science work on neuroplasticity could be brought to bear on issues of work and community function so important in the recovery model. Toward this end, the translational research program of Bell and Wexler extends from basic neuroscience to community function and cost-benefit analyses and includes outcome measures ranging from functional brain imaging to two-year follow-up of work hours and quality of life.

The great future challenge of this field is not only to continue the empirical study of practice applied to helping individuals with severe and persistent mental illness but also to evaluate a better integration of the disparate parts of this field. With regard to empirical studies, work is already under way at the CMHC to study essential practices of the recovery model such as illness management and recovery (IMR) and person-centered care. With regard to integration, development of the relationship of the patients' qualitative and lay points of view, embodied in the recovery model, to the academic clinician's professional and scientific perspectives will produce smoother long-term care. Evaluation of integrated clinical services at the CMHC and rehabilitative services provided through the CSN in the community will establish a foundation for practice, which is at present taken largely for granted. As new knowledge is developed, such as neurocognitive enhancement therapies, prompt evaluation in the community services of the CSN will enhance the task of incorporating discoveries into practice.

The CMHC is ideally suited to accomplish such a future agenda. It is poised to conduct future research that incorporates biomedical advances, including new pharmacotherapies, as well as new knowledge of person-centered care and IMR, into the framework of the recovery model. Based on longer time frames and sophisticated measures of clinically meaningful outcomes, collaborative research efforts will be able to evaluate and best adapt advances in biotechnology and empirically tested knowledge to benefit actual human lives.

References

Bell MD, Lysaker PH: Clinical benefits of paid activity in schizophrenia: one year follow-up. Schizophr Bull 23:317–28, 1997

Bell MD, Lysaker PH: The relationship of psychiatric symptoms to work performance for persons with severe mental disorders. Psychiatr Serv 46:508–11, 1995

Bell MD, Lysaker P, Bryson G: A behavioral intervention to improve work performance in schizophrenia: work Behavior Inventory feedback. J Vocational Rehabil 18:43–50, 2003

Bell MD, Milstein RM, Lysaker PH: Pay and participation in work activity: clinical benefits for clients with schizophrenia. Psychiatr Rehabil J 17:173–7, 1993

Breier PL, Schreiber JL, Dyer J, et al.: National Institute of Mental Health longitudinal study of chronic schizophrenia. Arch Gen Psychiatry 48:239–46, 1991

Callicott JH, Ramsey NF, Tallent K, et al.: Functional magnetic resonance imaging brain mapping in psychiatry: methodological issues illustrated in a study of working memory in schizophrenia. Neuropsychopharmacology 18:186–96, 1998

Carter M, Flesher S: The neurosociology of schizophrenia: vulnerability and functional disability. Psychiatry 58:209–24, 1995

Chinman M, Allende M, Bailey M, et al.: Therapeutic agents in assertive community treatment. Psychiatr Q 70:137–62, 1999a

Chinman M, Allende M, Weingarten R, et al.: On the road to collaborative treatment planning: consumer and provider perspectives. J Behav Health Serv Res 26:211–18, 1999b

Chinman M, Rosenheck R, Lam JA, et al.: Comparing consumer and non-consumer-provided case management services for homeless persons with serious mental illness. J Nerv Ment Dis 188:446–53, 2000

Chinman MJ, Weingarten R, Stayner D, et al.: Chronicity reconsidered: improving person-environment fit through a consumer-run service. Community Ment Health J 37:215–30, 2001

Crespo-Fracorro B, Paradiso S, Andreasen NC, et al.: Recalling word lists reveals "cognitive dysmetria" in schizophrenia: a positron emission tomography study. Am J Psychiatry 156:386–92, 1999

Curtis VA, Bullmore ET, Brammer MJ, et al.: Attenuated frontal activation during a verbal fluency task in patients with schizophrenia. Am J Psychiatry 155:1056–63, 1998

Davidson L: What is the appropriate source for psychological explanation? The Humanistic Psychol 15:150–66, 1987

Davidson L: Husserl's refutation of psychologism and the possibility of a phenomenological psychology. J Phenomen Psychology 19:1–17, 1988

Davidson L: Developing an empirical-phenomenological approach to schizophrenia research. J Phenomen Psychology 23:3–15, 1992

Davidson L: Story telling and schizophrenia: using narrative structure in phenomenological research. The Humanistic Psychol 21:200–20, 1993

Davidson L: Phenomenological research in schizophrenia: from philosophical anthropology to empirical science. J Phenomen Psychol 25:104–30, 1994

Davidson L: Vulnérabilité et destin dans la schizophrénie: prêter l'oreille à la voix de la personne (Vulnerability and destiny in schizophrenia: harkening to the voice of the person). L'Evolution Psychiatrique 62:263–84, 1997

Davidson L: Living Outside Mental Illness: Qualitative Studies of Recovery in Schizophrenia. New York: New York University Press, 2003

Davidson L, Chinman M, Kloos B, et al.: Mental illness as a psychiatric disability: shifting the paradigm toward mutual support. The Community Psychologist 30:19–21, 1997a

Davidson L, Chinman M, Kloos B, et al.: Peer support among individuals with severe mental illness: a review of the evidence. Clinical Psychology: Science and Practice 6:165–87, 1999

Davidson L, Chinman M, Sells D, et al.: Peer support among adults with serious mental illness: report from the field. Schizophr Bull 32:443–50, 2006a

Davidson L, Haglund KE, Stayner DA, et al.: "It was just realizing . . . that life isn't one big horror": a qualitative study of supported socialization. Psychiatr Rehabil J 24:275–92, 2001

Davidson L, Harding CM, Spaniol L: Recovery from Severe Mental Illnesses: Research Evidence and Implications for Practice, Volume 1. Boston, MA: Center for Psychiatric Rehabilitation of Boston University, 2005

Davidson L, Harding CM, Spaniol L: Recovery from Severe Mental Illnesses: Research Evidence and Implications for Practice, Volume 2. Boston, MA: Center for Psychiatric Rehabilitation of Boston University, 2006b

Davidson L, Hoge MA, Godleski L, et al.: Hospital or community living? Examining consumer perspectives on deinstitutionalization. Psychiatr Rehabil J 19:49–58, 1996

Davidson L, Hoge MA, Merrill M, et al.: The experiences of long-stay inpatients returning to the community. Psychiatry 58:122–32, 1995

Davidson L, Shahar G, Stayner DA, et al.: Supported socialization for people with psychiatric disabilities: lessons from a randomized controlled trial. J Community Psychol 32:453–77, 2004a

Davidson L, Stayner D: Loss, loneliness, and the desire for love: perspectives on the social lives of people with schizophrenia. Psychiatr Rehabil J 20:3–12, 1997b

Davidson L, Stayner DA, Lambert S, et al.: Phenomenological and participatory research on schizophrenia: recovering the person in theory and practice. J Social Issues 53:767–84, 1997c

Davidson L, Stayner DA, Chinman MJ, et al.: Preventing relapse and readmission in psychosis: using patients' subjective experience in designing clinical interventions, in Outcome Studies in Psychological Treatments of Psychotic Conditions. Edited by Martindale B. London: Gaskell Publishers, pp 134–56, 2000

Davidson L, Stayner DA, Nickou C, et al.: "Simply to be let in": inclusion as a basis for recovery from mental illness. Psychiatr Rehabil J 24:375–388, 2001. Reprinted in Ausienetter 20:10–15, 2004b

Davidson L, Strauss JS: Sense of self in recovery from severe mental illness. Br J Med Psychol 65:131–45, 1992

Davidson L, Strauss JS: Beyond the biopsychosocial model: integrating disorder, health and recovery. Psychiatry 58:44–55, 1995

Davidson L, Weingarten R., Steiner J, et al.: Integrating prosumers into clinical settings, in Consumers as Providers in Psychiatric Rehabilitation. Edited by Mowbray CT, Moxley DP, Jasper CA, et al. Columbia, MD: International Association for Psychosocial Rehabilitation Services, pp 437–55, 1997a

Department of Health and Human Services (DHHS). Surgeon General's Report on Mental Health. Rockville, MD: Substance Abuse and Mental Health Services Administration, 1999

Department of Health and Human Services (DHHS). Achieving the Promise: Transforming Mental Health Care in America. President's New Freedom Commission on Mental Health. Final Report (Pub. No. SMA-03–3832). Rockville, MD: DHHS, 2003

Department of Health and Human Services (DHHS). Transforming Mental Health Care in America. Federal Action Agenda. First steps. Rockville, MD: Substance Abuse and Mental Health Services Administration, 2005

Fossey E, Harvey C, McDermott F, et al.: Understanding and evaluating qualitative research. Aust NZ J Psychiatry 36:717–32, 2002

Ganguli R, Carter C, Mintun M, et al.: PET brain mapping study of auditory verbal supraspan memory versus visual fixation in schizophrenia. Biol Psychiatry 41:33–42, 1997

Green M: What are the functional consequences of neurocognitive deficits in schizophrenia? Am J Psychiatry 153:321–30, 1996

Green MF, Kern RS, Braff DL, et al.: Neurocognitive deficits and functional outcome in schizophrenia: are we measuring the 'right stuff'? Schizophr Bull 26:119–36, 2000

Harding CM, Zubin J, Strauss JS: Chronicity in schizophrenia: fact, partial fact, or artifact? Hosp Comm Psychiatry 38:477–86, 1987

Huppert FA, Whittington JE: Evidence for the independence of positive and negative well-being: implications for quality of life assessment. Br J Health Psychol 8(1):107–22, 2003

Katschnig H, Krautgartner M: Quality of life: a new dimension in mental health care, in Psychiatry in Society. Edited by Sartorius N, Gaebel W, Lopez-Ibor JJ, et al. New York: John Wiley & Sons, Ltd, pp 171–91, 2002

Liberman R: "Rate-Limiting" factors in work capacity in schizophrenia: psychopathology and neurocognitive deficits. A presentation of the Vocational Rehabilitation Research Colloquium, Boston, MA, 1996

Lysaker P, Bell M, Beam-Goulet J: Wisconsin Card Sorting Test and work performance in schizophrenia. Psychiatry Res 56:45–51, 1995

O'Connell M, Rowe M, Davidson L: Increasing treatment adherence through social engagement for adults with co-occurring psychiatric and substance use disorders. Presented at the National Institute of Health Conference on Interventions to Increase Adherence to Medications, Bethesda, MD, June 2005

Parrish J: The long journey home: accomplishing the mission of the community support movement. Psychosocial Rehabilitation Journal 12:107–24, 1989

Reidy D: Shattering illusions of differences. Resources 4:3–6, 1992

Ridgway P: Restorying psychiatric disability: learning from first person recovery narratives. Psychiatr Rehabil J 24:335–43, 2001

Rowe M, Benedict P, Falzer P: Representation of the governed: leadership building for people with behavioral health disorders who are homeless or were formerly homeless. Psychiatr Rehabil J 26:240–8, 2003

Schaie KW, Schooler C: Impact of work on older adults. New York: Springer Publishing, 1998

Sells D, Stayner DA, Davidson L: Recovering the self in schizophrenia: an integrative review of qualitative studies. Psychiatr Q 75:87–97, 2003

Stayner DA, Davidson L, Tebes JK: Supported partnerships: a pathway to community life for persons with serious psychiatric disabilities. The Community Psychologist, 29:14–7, 1996

Stein CH, Wemmerus VA: Searching for a normal life: personal accounts of adults with schizophrenia, their parents and well-siblings. Am J Community Psychol 29:725–46, 2001

Strauss JS, Davidson L: Mental disorder, work and choice, in Mental Disorder, Work Disability, and the Law. Edited by Bonnie R, Monahan J. Chicago: University of Chicago Press, pp 105–30, 1996

Strauss JS, Hafez H, Lieberman RP, et al.: The course of psychiatric disorder: III. Longitudinal principles. Am J Psychiatry 142:289–96, 1985

Strauss JS: The person—key to understanding mental illness: towards a new dynamic psychiatry. Br J Psychiatry 161:19–26, 1992

Strauss JS: The person with schizophrenia as a person: II. Approaches to the subjective and the complex. Br J Psychiatry 164:103–7, 1994

Tracy K, Weingarten R, Mattison E, et al.: Moving beyond illness to recovery: the Recovery Is for Everyone grants program, 2004

Turner JC, Tenhoor WJ: The NIMH community support program: pilot approach to a needed social reform. Schizophr Bull 4:319–49, 1978

Walsh D: A journey toward recovery: from the inside out. Psychiatr Rehabil J 20(2):85–90, 1996

Weinberger DR, Berman KF, Illowsky BP: Physiological dysfunction of dorsolateral prefrontal cortex in schizophrenia. Arch Gen Psychiatry 45:609–15, 1988

Weingarten R, Chinman M, Tworkowski S, et al.: The Welcome Basket project: consumers reaching out to consumers. Psychiatr Rehabil J 24:65–8, 2000

Wexler BE, Hawkins KA, Rounsaville B, et al.: Normal neurocognitive performance after extended practice in patients with schizophrenia. Schizophr Res 26:173–80, 1997

Wolfensberger W: A brief overview of Social Role Valorization. Mental Retardation 38:105–23, 2000

Yurgelun-Todd DA, Waternaux CM, Cohen BM, et al.: Functional magnetic resonance imaging of schizophrenic patients and comparison subjects during word production. Am J Psychiatry 153:2000–5, 1996

2

Connecticut Mental Health Center: clinical, research and training programs in the addictions

Richard Schottenfeld, Kathleen Carroll, Thomas Kosten, Stephanie O'Malley, Bruce Rounsaville, Rajita Sinha and Herbert Kleber

This chapter describes the innovative clinical services, training programs and clinical research developed by the Substance Abuse Treatment Unit (SATU) of the Connecticut Mental Health Center. Since its establishment in 1968, at the onset of an emerging epidemic of drug abuse in the U.S., SATU has pioneered in the development of multi-component and multi-modality substance abuse treatment programs, research aimed at improving addictions treatment, and training of psychiatrists, psychologists, social workers, drug counselors and other health care providers. SATU's clinical, research and training programs have been conducted through a creative partnership involving Yale University, the State of Connecticut, and the APT Foundation, a private, not-for-profit organization. In collaboration with the APT Foundation, the broad range of treatment services currently provided includes: centralized intake and evaluation; methadone, buprenorphine and naltrexone treatment for opioid dependence; specialized ambulatory treatment services for alcohol, cocaine, marijuana and other primary substance use disorders, co-occurring substance use and psychiatric disorders, and opioid detoxification; residential therapeutic communities for adults and adolescents; a primary care medical unit serving the medical needs of patients with substance use disorders; and a specialized vocational services program.

Addiction treatment services

The founding of the Connecticut Mental Health Center (CMHC) in 1966 coincided with an emerging epidemic of drug abuse in the U.S. Heroin addiction among enlisted

* The introductory sections of this chapter, including the descriptions of the early development of SATU clinical programs and the research on narcotic antagonists and strategies to improve opiate detoxification, are excerpted from Kleber HD, The Nathan B. Eddy Award Lecture: "A Passion to Improve Treatment." Problems of Drug Dependence, 1995: Proceedings of the 57th Annual Scientific Meeting, The College on Problems of Drug Dependence, Inc. NIDA Research Monograph 162, pages 24–33.

40 Years of Academic Public Psychiatry. Edited by Selby C. Jacobs and Ezra E. H. Griffith
© 2007 John Wiley & Sons, Ltd.

men in Vietnam and in urban settings and the explosive use of marijuana, psychedelic drugs and stimulants (amphetamine and cocaine) during the 1960s, especially among young people, led to a fast-rising need to develop treatment services for the casualties of these epidemics. Although very few psychiatrists at the time had received any formal training in addictions, the CMHC was fortunate to have recruited back to Yale Herbert Kleber, following his two-year assignment to the Public Health Service Hospital at Lexington, Kentucky. Prior to enlisting in the Public Health Service, Kleber developed an interest in drug abuse during his psychiatry residency training at Yale when he came in contact with psychedelic drugs and was one of the first to document the extent and problems arising from such use (Kleber, 1965, 1967). The Lexington hospital was one of only two facilities in the U.S. devoted to research and treatment of drug addiction. During his time at Lexington, Kleber learned about addiction from the patients, from his mentors, Bill Martin and John Ball, and from colleagues, including George Vaillant and Everett Ellinwood.

Back at Yale, Kleber helped to open both the inpatient and outpatient divisions of the CMHC. Because of his experience at Lexington, he was sought out by addicts, family members and physicians for treatment, advice and consultation. The limits of knowledge at the time about addictive disorders and the realization that what the patients needed was improved and diversified treatment led to his decision to pursue a career in clinical addiction research. With the help of his friend and mentor, Gerald Klerman, then heading the CMHC, Kleber wrote his first grant application to the National Institute of Mental Health (NIMH) and received a five-year grant in 1968 establishing the Drug Dependence Unit (DDU) of the CMHC.

The DDU, which became the Substance Abuse Treatment Unit (SATU) in 1975, when an alcohol program was added is one of the oldest and probably the only continuously operating multi-modality treatment, research and training center for substance abuse in the U.S. Expansion of treatment services was facilitated by the entrepreneurial ingenuity of the founders and administrators of the program and the formation by them of the APT Foundation (initially named the Addiction Prevention and Treatment Foundation) in 1970. The APT Foundation is a private, not-for-profit organization, with a dedicated community board tying it closely to the needs of New Haven, that was founded and, for its first 30 years, directed and operated by the SATU leadership team. This early example of a public–private partnership between the DDU and the APT Foundation provided the flexibility to obtain funds more readily for treatment expansion and program development while also ensuring coordination of service and research activities.

Research aimed primarily at improving treatments for addictive disorders has been central to the mission of the DDU since its inception. The diversity of addictive disorders and patient populations treated and the rich array of clinical services and programs have provided a ready platform for conducting research and training clinicians and clinical researchers.

The initial components of the DDU were a Central Intake Unit, a Methadone Maintenance Program, and a community outreach storefront called NARCO. Shortly after the inauguration of the DDU, and with the same initial grant, an adult residential therapeutic community modeled after Daytop Village in New York, and an outpatient drug-free program for adolescents were also established; these programs eventually formed the initial core of the APT Foundation. From the outset, the Central Intake

Unit served to triage patients to the appropriate level and type of treatment, a process facilitated by the availability of several different treatment modalities within the same system of care. The early leadership team of the DDU/SATU included, in addition to Kleber, Roslyn Liss, who served as Administrator of SATU and Executive Director of the APT Foundation; Charles Riordan, who served as Medical Director of the DDU/SATU and the APT Foundation; and a formidable team of other clinicians and administrators, including Kevin Kinsella, Leroy Gould and Mark Hurzeler, among many others. Throughout her tenure at SATU and APT, Liss played a central role in developing and expanding treatment services for individuals with addictive disorders and in managing the complex relationships among SATU, APT, Yale and the State of Connecticut. Liss originated and carried through to success a number of the innovative ancillary programs, including the Central Vocational Unit and the Center of Progressive Education (COPE), an accredited therapeutic school for adolescents.

The Methadone Maintenance Program, one of the oldest in the country, pioneered day treatment induction onto methadone (Kleber, 1970) and also planned detoxification protocols for patients who had made sustained changes in lifestyle (Riordan et al., 1976). The inpatient induction method of Dole and Nyswander, in vogue at the time, seemed too costly and inefficient, while the outpatient approach Wieland was using in Philadelphia did not appear to make a major dent in one's critical lifestyle. With the day induction approach, individuals who needed an intensive approach came in daily for four to six weeks after starting methadone. Issues addressed were diverse: getting to the program on time, vocational readiness, use of leisure time, breaking the code of the street, and learning to cope more effectively and refrain from acting-out behaviors that could get them fired from jobs. In the early 1970s, many methadone programs believed that individuals could not be successfully detoxified from methadone maintenance. However, follow-up studies of the specialized detoxification program for methadone maintained patients, who had achieved sustained heroin abstinence and psychosocial stability while on methadone, demonstrated that it was possible for many patients to detoxify and remain abstinent (Riordan et al., 1976). Two of these patients, Raymond and Geraldine Bryant, went on to assume leadership roles in the expanded methadone programs: he directed the Legion Avenue Clinic, which was initially operated as part of the CMHC; and she directed the Orchard Clinic, which has been continuously operated as part of the APT Foundation. A formidable husband and wife team, the Bryants were tireless advocates for improved treatment services for addicted individuals and widely respected in the drug treatment programs and wider community for their wisdom and clinical acumen. Other successfully detoxified patients, as well as many more patients who achieved sustained remission from addiction while remaining on methadone maintenance, went on to resume or assume positions of responsibility in many other fields.

At the heart of their success, the methadone program differed from many other such programs in the country in insisting on a high level of psychosocial rehabilitative efforts (Kleber, 1977) and involving patients with clinic governance. In 1986 the limited vocational services initially provided in the methadone program were transformed into a full-scale vocational services program, providing job counseling, job readiness training, job seeking skills, job development and continuing post-employment vocational support services to patients with addictive disorders treated in any treatment program (Schottenfeld et al., 1992). The vocational services unit, developed under the auspices of the APT Foundation, was the first such unit in the country affiliated with a drug program to be accredited by a national accrediting body. Similarly, after frustrating battles with hospital and free-standing medical clinics to obtain adequate medical care for recovering patients, the APT Foundation opened its own Central Medical Unit to provide medical care to patients treated in SATU or APT clinical programs. The Central Medical Unit, a licensed primary care clinic, subsequently pioneered protocols for coordinating drug abuse treatment and medical care for patients with HIV (O'Connor et al., 1992a, 1994) as well as protocols for expanding addiction treatment services into primary care clinics and physician offices, as described below.

When the initial methadone programs were no longer sufficient to handle the volume of patients remaining in treatment and out of treatment, a third program was added by the APT Foundation in the early 1980s. When third-party reimbursements finally permitted expansion of the methadone programs beyond the set number of treatment "slots" funded by state grants, a rapid admissions procedure facilitated admission to methadone treatment within 72 hours of seeking treatment (compared to a waiting period of several months or longer previously) and a dramatic expansion over a short period, during the late 1990s, of the number of patients treated over a short period, from less than 600 to more than 1200 patients at any time. Such a rapid expansion of services was possible because the programs were operated by the APT Foundation, a not-for-profit that could retain and use for program expansion the revenue generated by reimbursement for services. Subsequently, however, capacity expansion stalled, partly as a result of the continuing difficulties of finding locations for new treatment programs.

The initial adult residential therapeutic community, Daytop, seeded by staff, graduates and some current patients from Daytop Village in New York, opened without the benefit of a facility to house the program. While the initial facility was being outfitted, community board members and others provided housing for patients in their own homes. When it became clear that the initial outpatient approach for adolescents was not sufficiently intensive, a day program for adolescents, Veritas, was added in 1969. When day treatment proved insufficient, an adolescent therapeutic community, Alpha House, was added in 1970. An accredited therapeutic school for adolescents, Center of Progressive Education (COPE) was opened in 1976 and used therapeutic insights to improve academic performance as well. The victim of a severe NIMBY (Not In My Backyard) syndrome, the residential programs survived a suspicious fire in one early location and evictions from subsequent locations, until the residential programs found a more secure longer-term location on the campus of the state-owned and operated Fairfield Hills Hospital in Newtown, Connecticut. When Fairfield Hills Hospital closed, the last programs to be relocated were Daytop, Alpha House and COPE, all of which moved to a converted nursing home in Bridgeport, Connecticut. Daytop was for many years under the dedicated leadership of Vincent Nuzzo, one of the first Daytop graduates.

The residential programs have evolved over time from their roots in a relatively "hard concept" approach, in which addicts, living and working together in a hierarchical, structured and closed community, are repeatedly confronted by their peers about their maladaptive behaviors and learn to tolerate emotional distress and recognize their actual, as opposed to fantasized and extreme, strengths and vulnerabilities without resorting to "acting out" or maladaptive behavior. Without losing the power-ful impact of this approach, the programs have incorporated an increasingly profes-sional staff; treatments have been individualized to address the unique strengths and vulnerabilities of each patient; and the programs are now capable of treating success-fully a more fragile and vulnerable patient population, including younger adolescents and many patients with co-occurring psychiatric and substance use disorders.

Additional clinical services have been added over time by the SATU or the APT Foundation to meet identified, unmet treatment needs of patients in the community. The lack of adequate alcohol treatment in the community led to the formation of the Alcoholism Treatment Unit in 1975. A long-term research program aimed at develop-ing narcotic antagonist treatment as an alternative to methadone maintenance or long-term residential treatment finally came to fruition in 1984 with the approval of the long-acting antagonist, naltrexone, for the treatment of opioid dependence. Sub-sequently, the naltrexone program, operated as a clinical research program by the APT Foundation, was transferred to the CMHC, which was able to provide subsidized medications to patients without prescription medication coverage or the financial means to pay for naltrexone. In exchange, the Legion Avenue methadone program was transferred from the CMHC to APT, which was able to use reimbursements to expand the number of patients treated beyond the fixed number of grant-supported "treatment slots." As with so many of the innovative solutions to problems related to funding, resources and service gaps, Liss played an instrumental role in identifying and executing the solution. In the early 1980s, the emergence of cocaine abuse led to development of a cocaine treatment program, and cocaine and crack's devastating effects on pregnant women led, in the late 1980s, to the development of a special program for pregnant addicts (Schottenfeld et al., 1994). More recently, treatment services and clinical research have expanded to focus on nicotine dependence, gambling disorders, and co-occurring psychiatric and substance use disorders. At present, the SATU and APT clinical programs treat more than 1800 patients at any time.

Satu leadership, faculty development and training

Focusing on addictive disorders was a lonely endeavor for psychiatrists and psycholo-gists throughout the 1960s and 1970s. Training in addictions was rarely if ever pro-vided in medical or psychology graduate schools or internship or residency training. Addictions were treated as an unwanted component of an already stigmatized mental health profession, and few psychiatrists or psychologists chose to pursue academic, research or clinical work focusing on addictions. With the continued successful devel-opment of clinical services closely connected to the Yale University School of Medicine and the expansion of clinical research opportunities addressing addictive disorders, however, by the early 1980s several full-time junior faculty members were recruited to SATU, including Bruce Rounsaville, Thomas Kosten, Richard Schottenfeld, Stephanie O'Malley and Kathleen Carroll. Rounsaville was brought in to work on studies of co-occurring affective and other psychiatric disorders among treatment-seeking heroin-dependent individuals and eventually became director of research. Kosten started in 1984 as the director of the Naltrexone Program. He then went on to lead the Medications Development Research Center before leaving the CMHC to become Chief of Psychiatry at the West Haven Veterans Administration Medical Center (VAMC). He also founded a coordinated clinical research program on addictions. Schottenfeld was brought in as director of the Alcohol Treatment Unit in 1984, and O'Malley joined him as associate director shortly thereafter. Together, they supervised first the merger of the Alcohol Treatment Unit, Central Intake Unit and Evaluation/Brief Treatment Unit, and then the eventual incorporation of the naltrexone program into a single, coordinated ambulatory program, SATU. Schottenfeld took the lead in developing the Vocational Services Program and the Central Medical Unit and then became the medical director of the SATU and the APT Foundation clinical programs following the departure of Charles Riordan, who became become chief of psychiatry at the Hospital of St. Raphael. With the subsequent departure in August 1989 of Kleber, who was appointed by President George Bush as the first deputy director for demand reduction of the Office of National Drug Control Policy, Schottenfeld was appointed Director of the SATU and Chief Executive Officer of the APT Foundation, and O'Malley took over as Clinical Director of the SATU. Carroll completed her pre-doctoral clinical research with Kleber and Rounsaville and along with Rounsaville subsequently led the development of drug abuse psychotherapy research at SATU and in the Department of Psychiatry. With the appointment of O'Malley as director of the Division of Substance Abuse Research in the Department of Psychiatry, Rajita Sinha became Clinical Director of SATU. Subsequently, when Schottenfeld was appointed Master of Davenport College in 2001, Sinha became director of the SATU and associate director for addiction services of the CMHC.

The availability of a critical mass of faculty psychiatrists and psychologists and of the extensive clinical programs and clinical research activities at the SATU provided an ideal opportunity to develop formal training programs in addictions and drug abuse clinical research. The SATU was the first program in the country to develop a post-doctoral drug abuse clinical research training program for physicians. This program has been continuously funded by NIDA since 1988. Subsequently, the SATU also launched a Mentored Clinician Scientist Training Program for beginning investigators, which has also been continuously funded by NIDA since its inception. The SATU was among the first academic programs in the country to develop an addictions training program for faculty in pediatrics and internal medicine. These medical school faculty members have continued to provide addictions training to residents in their departments and to medical students during their clerkships. More recently, the SATU has served as a primary training site for Yale's ACGME-accredited Addiction Psychiatry Residency Training Program.

Research accomplishments

Research at the SATU has been directed at improving the efficacy and effectiveness of addictions treatment, making use of clinical observations and capitalizing on close collaborations with basic, preclinical researchers to identify promising pharmacological or behavioral strategies for subsequent clinical investigation. Some of the major areas and themes of the research will be described in the following sections.

Narcotic antagonist treatment for opiate dependence

Investigation of narcotic antagonists for the treatment of opioid dependence was a natural outgrowth of clinical experience. Many addicts did not want methadone maintenance and were not willing to enter a long-term residential community, yet they failed miserably in an outpatient drug-free approach. This led to investigations of narcotic antagonists that could block the effects of heroin and might thus protect against relapse and overdose risk. The first study evaluated very large doses of the short-acting antagonist, naloxone, which at an oral dose of 1000 mg per day provided an 18-hour blockade and was used in the context of a day-treatment program to cover the unblocked hours (Pierson et al., 1974). The lack of a full 24-hour blockade led to the investigation of cyclazacine, which had a longer duration of action and was better than placebo. Unfortunately, it was not well tolerated by patients (Kleber, 1974). Subsequent work with the long-acting opiate antagonist, naltrexone (Hurzeler et al., 1976), including a study showing that tolerance did not develop to naltrexone's opioid blockading effect even after regular use for up to two years (Kleber et al., 1985a), contributed to the eventual approval of this medication in 1984 for the treatment of opioid dependence.

Despite its pharmacological efficacy for blocking opioid effects, poor adherence to naltrexone and problems with high attrition have reduced its effectiveness in clinical practice and prevented widespread dissemination. Early studies conducted in the SATU attempted to develop improved methods of clinical delivery that would improve the acceptability of naltrexone (Kosten and Kleber, 1984). Family therapy was found to double the retention rate over a six-month period (Anton et al., 1981). More recently, contingency management, using monetary vouchers that could be exchanged for goods or services, was found to improve retention and reduce illicit opioid use. Involvement of a significant other in treatment was also associated with improved retention and drug use outcomes (Carroll et al., 2001, 2002).

Strategies to improve opiate detoxification

Research on strategies to improve opiate detoxification procedures complemented the long-standing interests of the SATU in opiate antagonist treatment, since patients can only be inducted onto naltrexone after detoxification. The initial research on detoxification was aimed at facilitating detoxification from methadone maintenance for patients who were interested and ready to transition off methadone maintenance. While a variety of opioid detoxification approaches had been tried, including specialized detoxification groups and short-term or long-term open or blind detoxification, many patients experienced considerable difficulties coming off methadone or avoiding subsequent relapse (Kleber, 1977). The use of clonidine to treat withdrawal symptoms was the first major breakthrough in 1978 (Gold et al., 1978). The idea for using clonidine to treat opioid withdrawal came from a third-year psychiatry resident, Mark Gold, who at the time was working in the methadone programs helping with the detoxification projects and also working with Eugene Redmond examining basic mechanisms associated with indicators of anxiety in rhesus monkeys. In pioneering studies, George Aghajanian had found that clonidine decreased the spontaneous firing of single cell neurons in the locus coeruleus, a brain region regulating physiological signs of anxiety and also affected by opiates. Gold therefore hypothesized that opioid withdrawal symptoms resulted from rebound overactivity of the locus coeruleus and suggested evaluating clonidine to treat opioid withdrawal. Studies carried out over the next seven years refined the method, showed its efficacy for treating withdrawal from heroin or methadone, demonstrated its strengths and weaknesses, and established it as a widely accepted alternative to methadone tapering (Charney et al., 1982b; Gold et al., 1980; Kleber et al., 1985b). For their early work with clonidine, Aghajanian, Gold, Redmond and Kleber were awarded the 1981 American Psychiatric Association Foundation Fund Prize for psychiatric research.

While clonidine is effective for treating many of the symptoms of withdrawal, it does not shorten the time period of withdrawal or the time patients need to remain abstinent before beginning treatment with naltrexone. Subsequent work pioneered techniques to shorten the time period of withdrawal and naltrexone induction by pre-treating with clonidine to block the symptoms of withdrawal and using small doses of naltrexone to precipitate withdrawal. Kleber and other colleagues worked to develop a safe, well-tolerated and effective protocol (Charney et al., 1982a, 1986; Kleber et al., 1987; Vining et al., 1988). Subsequent studies evaluating detoxification using clonidine and clonidine/naltrexone in the Central Medical Unit have facilitated more wide-spread dissemination of these protocols into primary care medical settings (O'Connor et al., 1992b).

Depression and other psychiatric disorders in addicted individuals

An important theme of research in SATU involves the impact and treatment of psychopathology among patients with addictive disorders. The initial studies of methadone safety conducted in SATU showed a high prevalence of anxiety and depressive disorders in these patients. In the late 1970s, SATU was awarded a major grant to evaluate psychiatric disorders in opiate addicts. The landmark study discovered unexpectedly high rates of a number of disorders, most notably Major Depression (Rounsaville and Kleber, 1985b; Rounsaville et al., 1982a, 1982b). Subsequent studies have confirmed these initial reports of high rates of psychiatric disorders in other clinical samples of drug abusers, including cocaine abusers (Rounsaville et al., 1991a).

Given the general responsiveness of depression to psychotherapy and pharmacotherapy in patients who do not abuse drugs, SATU investigators began clinical trials to evaluate the efficacy of psychotherapy and pharmacotherapy for depression in opioid addicts (Kleber et al., 1983; Rounsaville et al., 1983). Promising findings regarding the responsiveness of depression to treatment (Rounsaville and Kleber, 1985a; Rounsaville et al., 1985) and the prognostic significance of depression in opioid addicts and alcoholics (Gawin et al., 1989; Rounsaville et al., 1986, 1987) led to the evaluation of depression as a matching or prognostic variable in subsequent clinical trials of treatments for opioid addicts and cocaine abusers (Gawin et al., 1989).

Another line of investigation that has followed from the initial findings regarding high rates of psychopathology in treated opioid addicts has been a series of family/genetic studies in collaboration with Kathleen Merikangas at Yale's Genetic Epidemiology Unit. These studies have evaluated the role of psychopathology as a potential familialy transmitted contributor to the development of drug abuse by evaluating rates and patterns of psychiatric disorders in the parents and siblings of drug abusers (Rounsaville et al., 1991b). We have followed up this work with adult relatives in investigations of the high risk children of drug abusers. These children are identified prior to the initiation of drug abuse in an attempt to identify familialy transmitted risk factors that are associated with later drug abuse (Luthar et al., 1998).

In more recent studies, we have addressed issues related to the diagnosis of Axis II disorders in substance abusers (Rounsaville et al., 1998) and of the relationship between Axis I and Axis II disorders (Verheul et al., 2000). An exciting aspect of our more recent work has been the development of a close collaboration with a molecular geneticist, Joel Gelernter. He has used data derived from our diagnostic comorbidity samples to assess the association of specific genetic risk factors with comorbid psychopathology in drug abusers including cocaine-induced paranoia (Gelernter et al., 1994) and the personality trait of novelty seeking (Gelernter et al., 1997).

Naltrexone and psychotherapy for alcohol dependence

A programmatic sequence of investigations has followed from a SATU study evaluating naltrexone and cognitive behavioral/coping skills training therapy as treatment for ambulatory alcoholics. Approved by the FDA for treatment of opioid dependence, the use of naltrexone for other drugs of abuse is novel and suggests a role for opioidergic mediation of drug effects that is far wider than expected prior to work at Yale and the University of Pennsylvania. Initial findings demonstrated a robust effect of naltrexone over placebo in reducing relapse to heavy drinking, an effect which endured at follow-up six months after the end of study treatment (O'Malley et al., 1992). In the initial treatment period, coping skills training had efficacy that was equivalent to the comparison treatment, Supportive Therapy (ST), and there was a trend for patients receiving coping skills treatment to take a first drink sooner than those receiving ST. However, at six-month follow up, patients receiving coping skills training displayed delayed treatment effects in prevention of relapse (O'Malley et al., 1996). In our initial study, coping skills treatment and the supportive treatment were delivered by doctorate level therapists. A follow-up study demonstrated that an abbreviated medical management approach delivered by nurses was as effective as more intensive cognitive behavioral treatment combined with naltrexone for the first 10 weeks of treatment. This finding suggests that naltrexone may be effectively delivered in primary care settings (O'Connor et al., 1997a, 1997b). We have also completed the first study to examine whether maintenance with naltrexone is needed when patients respond positively to an initial 10 weeks of medications. We found that maintenance on naltrexone for an additional six months improved outcomes when patients received medical management during their initial treatment, but was not necessary when patients received cognitive behavioral therapy during their initial treatment. This research has spelled out how behavioral therapy and naltrexone can complement and/or substitute for each other to treat alcoholism.

We found that naltrexone was particularly effective in preventing relapse for patients who took an initial drink. This finding has also served as the impetus for a laboratory study to evaluate the psychological and behavioral mechanism of naltrexone's effect on drinking. Specifically, we have shown that naltrexone reduces self-administration of alcohol following receipt of an initial priming drink. Thus, we have moved from the clinic to the behavioral pharmacology laboratory to provide clues about how naltrexone works in humans. Overall, in this series of studies we have followed up on our initial findings regarding the efficacy of a treatment, naltrexone, with studies evaluating the mechanism of action, the optimal duration of treatment and the psychotherapeutic context in which the treatment can be utilized.

Our work on combining behavioral treatments with naltrexone for alcoholism prepared our group to play a key role in Project COMBINE, a multisite project that evaluated two medications, naltrexone and acamprosate, alone and in combination with low-intensity and high-intensity behavioral treatment for alcoholic patients. Although it was initially hypothesized that these two medications would have additive, complementary effects as naltrexone prevents relapse when patients take a priming drink while acamprosate appears to reduce initial drinking in those who have been detoxified, the findings supported the efficacy of naltrexone, but not of acamprosate. There were no added benefits of combining acamprosate with naltrexone compared to using naltrexone alone (Anton et al., 2006).

Opioid antagonists and nicotine dependence

From a clinical observation of greater naltrexone-induced side effects in smokers, O'Malley became interested in the opioid system as it relates to tobacco dependence and the possible role of naltrexone in treatment of this disorder. She and Suchitra Krishnan-Sarin conducted a nicotine challenge laboratory study demonstrating greater dose-related increases in opiate-like withdrawal signs and symptoms, such as tearing, nasal congestion, restlessness, muscle tension and sweating, in smokers compared with non-smokers (Krishnan-Sarin et al., 1999). The finding that the opioid system is altered by tobacco use is likely to be of significance in understanding dependence on other drugs of abuse, such as heroin and cocaine, and the development of treatments for nicotine dependence. Substance abusers have exceedingly high rates of nicotine use compared to the general population (over 90% of heroin users are dependent on nicotine). In a pilot trial of naltrexone combined with the nicotine patch as aids to cigarette smoking cessation, O'Malley found that naltrexone improved success rates and prevented weight gain (Krishnan-Sarin et al., 2003). This combined medication treatment may be especially important for women because female smokers have been demonstrated to have lower treatment success rates and to be concerned about weight gain. O'Malley and Krishnan-Sarin are now conducting integrated treatment and laboratory studies as part of a newly organized Transdisciplinary Tobacco Use Research Center focused on treating tobacco dependence in groups at high risk for relapse, especially women, heavy alcohol users and individuals with depression.

In two clinical trials of naltrexone for alcohol dependence (Jaffe et al., 1996; O'Malley et al., 1998), our group has shown that naltrexone is particularly effective for patients with a positive family history of alcohol dependence. This suggests the possibility that genes that code for variability in opioidergic activity may play a role in the heritability of alcoholism and in detecting patients particularly likely to respond to naltrexone treatment. Bruce Rounsaville and geneticist Joel Gelernter are currently collaborating on studies to identify genetic markers for treatment responsiveness in alcoholics.

Research on medications for smoking cessation has also focused on smokers with serious mental illness (SMI), with a special focus on schizophrenia, and most recently bipolar disorder. The Program for Research in Smokers with Mental Illness (PRISM) group, under the direction of Tony George has conducted several trials of medications for smoking cessation in smokers with SMI, including three controlled trials of nicotine patch, bupropion (Zyban), and their combinations in cigarette smokers with schizophrenia and schizoaffective disorder. The first study (George et al., in press) was an open-label trial of nicotine patch (21 mg/day) and two levels of behavioral group therapy. While we found no differences in group therapy outcomes, treatment with atypical antipsychotics led to a tripling of smoking abstinence rates compared to typical (neuroleptic) agents. Second, we completed the first placebo-controlled trial of sustained-release bupropion (Zyban) for smoking cessation in schizophrenia (George et al., 2002) where we showed that sustained-release bupropion significantly enhanced end of trial quit rates as compared to placebo (50 versus 12.5% abstinence rates, p < 0.05). Our third recently completed study compared treatment with nicotine patch and bupropion SR versus placebo, and we observed that the combination of bupropion SR and nicotine patch significantly enhanced abstinence rates for short- and long-term (six-month) outcomes as compared to placebo plus nicotine patch. In each of these trials, we have found that treatment with atypical antipsychotic drugs enhances overall cessation outcomes and treatment retention, which approaches 80%. In addition to smoking cessation trials and tobacco control assessments in mental health populations, our Cognitive Psychopharmacology Laboratory has conducted groundbreaking work on the role of nicotinic receptor mechanisms, cigarette smoking, and cognitive and clinical dysfunction in patients with schizophrenia and mood disorders (George et al., in press; Sacco et al., 2004, 2005; Weinberger et al., in press).

Pharmacologic treatments for cocaine dependence

By 1982, cocaine abuse was becoming a major public health problem in New Haven as well as the rest of the country, and it was quickly apparent that there was no adequate treatment for it. SATU became the leader in systematic pharmacologic methods that might increase the success of such treatment. The first seven years of this took place under the inspiration of Frank Gawin, who had also completed his psychiatric residency at Yale, and then, when Gawin left for the University of California, by Thomas Kosten. Our early attempts at treating cocaine were based on models of treating heroin addiction. Instead of methadone, we tried methylphenidate, which bore a relation to cocaine that was similar to that between methadone and heroin. Methylphenidate was orally effective, longer acting and produced less euphoria. Unfortunately, it was not methadone—and, though it proved to be effective in treating cocaine abusers who had Attention Deficit Disorder (Khantzian et al., 1984), in individuals without such a diagnosis, it appeared to serve primarily as a cue to more cocaine use (Gawin et al., 1985). We tried lithium as a naltrexone model, since there was animal literature showing that it could block the effects of amphetamine. Unfortunately, it, too, did not pan out, although it was of use in treating bipolar cocaine abusers (Kleber and Gawin,

1986). Desipramine, our third drug, seemed to be useful for cocaine addicts, even those without an affective disorder. The trial was initiated because of our theory about the effects of chronic cocaine on regulation of the dopamine receptor and the similarity of the effects produced to that of the chronic depressive state (Gawin and Kleber, 1988). The open clinical trial was followed by a successful double-blind placebo-controlled trial, with desipramine reducing both craving and use (Gawin et al., 1989). Desipramine remains one of the best-studied drugs for the treatment of cocaine addiction, but, unfortunately, there are both positive and negative studies. In retrospect, it appears that desipramine may indeed be useful for the group of cocaine addicts we studied in the mid-1980s, namely the middle- and working-class individuals taking cocaine by the intranasal route, but its effectiveness may be overwhelmed, both by the social pathology of crack addicts as well as by the smoked and injected routes of administration. Marian Fischman has shown in the human laboratory that desipramine decreases the positive subjective effects of cocaine and cocaine craving without, however, decreasing the frequency of use (Fischman et al., 1990). If one has an individual with social supports such as a job and a family, the decreased hedonic value of the cocaine may be sufficient to help the person give up the habit. With the faster routes of administration and the presence of less social support, this desipramine effect may not be adequate. Gawin's clinical experiences with cocaine addicts led to a theory of a cocaine withdrawal syndrome (Gawin and Kleber, 1986) which has support from clinicians treating outpatient cocaine addicts, but has not been confirmed in inpatient settings, the difference perhaps relating to the availability of cocaine and cocaine-related cues in the outpatient world. The work with cocaine was aided throughout by the research skills and knowledge of stimulants of Robert Byck, who had been studying cocaine long before it had become a major problem in the U.S.

Another series of programmatic studies has arisen from our long history of collaboration between psychopharmacology and psychotherapy researchers. Our work on disulfiram as treatment of cocaine dependence illustrates the synergistic power of this approach. Part of the rationale for targeting alcohol use in cocaine abusers arose from the high rates of comorbid alcohol and cocaine use found in our epidemiological surveys of psychiatric comorbidity in treated cocaine abusers (Rounsaville et al., 1991a) performed in collaboration with epidemiologists, Myrna Weissman and Kathleen Merikangas. Another part of the rationale for targeting alcohol use came from findings by other collaborating Yale investigators, Thomas Kosten and Elinor McCance-Katz, experts in psychopharmacology; and Peter Jatlow, an expert in pharmacodynamics and pharmacokinetics. They showed that combined alcohol and cocaine use at usual doses leads, in vivo, to the production of a potent new compound, cocaethylene which is more slowly metabolized than cocaine and which may reduce the severity of the post-cocaine "crash." Our pilot trial (Carroll, 1998) comparing disulfiram and naltrexone for comorbid cocaine and alcohol abusers demonstrated the promise of disulfiram for these patients. This finding, in turn, provided the impetus for a series of laboratory studies conducted by psychopharmacology investigators, Faiq Hameedi and McCance-Katz, which showed that disulfiram increases dysphoric symptoms associated with administration of cocaine. This finding, in turn, provided the rationale for evaluating effects of disulfiram in cocaine abusers who do not also use alcohol. We have now conducted five additional clinical trials supporting the efficacy of disulfiram for the treatment of cocaine dependence in primary cocaine users (Carroll et al., 1998,

2004a) and methadone or buprenorphine-maintained opioid-dependent patients with co-occurring cocaine dependence (George et al., 2000a, 2000b; Petrakis et al., 2000; Schottenfeld et al., 2005b).

Following an independent line of research, a collaborating geneticist, Joseph Cubbells, has discovered that low levels of the enzyme dopamine beta hydroxylase (DBH) are linked to cocaine-induced paranoia. DBH converts dopamine to norepinephrine. Based on the findings in the clinical trials, laboratory studies and genetic studies, we hypothesized that disulfiram's effects on cocaine might be mediated by its inhibition of DBH and the consequent alteration of the rewarding or aversive effects of cocaine or by the amelioration of the mood instability associated with chronic cocaine use. Based on this hypothesis, we predicted that individuals with the polymorphism coding for low DBH would be more responsive to the effects of disulfiram on cocaine. Two recent studies have provided support for this hypothesis (Hughes et al., 2004; Schottenfeld et al., 2005a, 2005b).

Behavioral treatments for cocaine and other addictive disorders

Recognition of the importance of behavioral, psychological and environmental factors in initiating and sustaining drug use or abstinence, as well as recognition of the limitations of pharmacologic approaches on their own for treating addictive disorders intensified our search for psychosocial and behavioral approaches. Early advances included the work of Bruce Rounsaville with Weissman in developing interpersonal therapy for cocaine abusers. More recent work, led by Kathleen Carroll, has focused on cognitive and behavioral treatment (CBT).

Based on social learning theories of substance use disorders, cognitive behavioral coping skills therapy (CBT) focuses on the implementation of effective coping skills for recognizing, avoiding and coping with situations associated with drug use. CBT is one of comparatively few empirically supported therapies that has been demonstrated to be effective across a range of substance use disorders (Carroll, 1996; DeRubeis and Crits-Christoph, 1998; Irvin et al., 1999; NIDA, 1999, 2000), and the CBT manual developed at SATU was published by NIDA as the first in its series of manuals describing empirically supported treatments (Carroll, 1998). In well-controlled, randomized clinical trials conducted at SATU, CBT has been found to be effective among alcohol-dependent populations (Morgenstern and Longabaugh, 2000; O'Malley et al., 1996; Project Match Research Group, 1997), marijuana-dependent populations (Carroll et al., in press; MTP Research Group, 2004) and cocaine-dependent populations (Carroll et al., 1994a,b, 1998, 2000, 2004a). The mounting empirical support for CBT in the field of substance abuse is consistent with studies demonstrating the effectiveness of cognitive-behavioral-oriented treatments across a range of other psychiatric disorders that frequently co-occur with substance use disorders. Several studies suggest that CBT also appears to be particularly effective among higher-severity drug abusers (Carroll et al., 1991, 1994b; Maude-Griffin et al., 1998). Moreover, CBT is highly compatible with pharmacotherapy and has been used as a psychotherapy "platform" in a number of pharmacotherapy trials (Carroll et al., 2004a, 2004b).

A particularly distinctive feature of CBT is that its benefits appear not only to be durable, but in many cases become stronger after treatment ends. That is, reductions in drug use associated with short-term (e.g., 12-week) CBT may continue to increase over a year after treatment termination. Delayed emergence of effects after CBT has been demonstrated in several trials by our group (Carroll et al., 1994b, 2000, in press; O'Malley et al., 1996). These "sleeper effects" have subsequently been replicated by other research groups (McKay et al., 1999; Rawson et al., 2002). As continuing improvement has generally not been documented among other behavioral therapies for substance use disorders, it is possible that sleeper effects may be associated with distinctive features of CBT. Distinguishing features of CBT that are likely candidates for its enduring effects include skills training and homework assignments that provide opportunities to implement, practice and generalize new coping skills as behavioral alternatives to drug use (Carroll et al., 2005).

No pharmacotherapies are sufficiently comprehensive in their effects to be a sole treatment for most substance users (Leshner, 1999; McLellan et al., 1993; O'Brien, 1997). Moreover, there is consensus that behavioral interventions can broaden, strengthen and extend the effects of even powerful pharmacotherapies (Uhlenhuth et al., 1969), and that effective pharmacotherapies can dramatically enhance treatment retention and outcome for behavioral therapies. Nevertheless, there remains a paucity of systematic investigation on identifying the most effective psychotherapy–pharmacotherapy combinations for treating substance users. Moreover, although factorial designs (where the intensity or type of behavioral therapy is manipulated to identify the most effective, or cost-effective, psychotherapy/pharmacotherapy combination) are efficient strategies for evaluating combination therapies (COMBINE Study Research Group, 2003; O'Malley and Carroll, 1996), there remain but a handful of such studies in the substance abuse treatment literature, many of which were conducted by the SATU group (Carroll et al., 1991, 1994a, 1994b, 2001, 2004a, 2004b; O'Malley et al., 1992, 1996, 2003; Schottenfeld et al., 1997, 2005b).

Work by the SATU group has expanded to cover a wide range of behavioral therapies, including contingency management (Petry et al., 2004, in press; Schottenfeld et al., 2005b), motivational interviewing (Carroll et al., 2006; Martino et al., 2000) and Twelve Step Facilitation (Project Match Research Group, 1998), and most recently has extended to evaluation of methods to train clinicians to use empirically supported therapies effectively (Sholomskas and Carroll, 2006; Sholomskas et al., 2005).

Buprenorphine in the treatment of drug abuse

Buprenorphine is a partial agonist at the mu opiate receptor. As the dosage of buprenorphine is increased, its effects initially increase, but then reach a plateau or diminish. Because of its unique pharmacological properties, including a decreased risk of overdose, long duration of action and possibly decreased abuse liability compared to methadone, we began a programmatic series of studies on buprenorphine in 1986. The aim of the first study was to evaluate buprenorphine as a bridge between an opioid-dependent state on methadone or heroin and the antagonist naltrexone. The initial project involved 41 patients on buprenorphine dosages varying from 2 to 8 mg/day. We examined one-month stabilization on buprenorphine followed by transition to the opioid antagonist naltrexone, and found that transition to naltrexone could be accomplished by precipitating withdrawal using high dosages of the antagonist naloxone. This detoxification protocol from buprenorphine can be completed within one day, although the initial inpatient work to develop this procedure involved a one-week hospitalization. This work led directly to the development of a follow-up project for an outpatient randomized clinical trial comparing clonidine/naltrexone detoxification of opioid addicts to a buprenorphine/naltrexone detoxification protocol in approximately 150 patients. Subsequent studies have shown that the detoxification protocol using buprenorphine can be implemented in primary care clinics and may be advantageous when compared to standard clonidine or clonidine/naltrexone protocols (O'Connor et al., 1997c).

Other work with this group of patients suggested that buprenorphine might be effective in reducing cocaine as well as opioid abuse and led to a series of studies evaluating buprenorphine as an alternative to methadone for maintenance treatment of opioid dependence. The first study was a randomized clinical trial comparing buprenorphine at 2 or 6 mg to methadone 35 mg or 65 mg maintenance. This six-month randomized clinical trial of 120 patients found that higher dose buprenorphine (6 mg) was more effective than low dose (2 mg), but methadone at either 35 mg or 65 mg daily was superior in reducing opioid abuse (Kosten, 1993). The early clinical trials of buprenorphine for maintenance treatment used daily sublingual liquid maintenance doses ranging from 2 mg to 8 mg. To evaluate optimal buprenorphine dosing for maintenance treatment, we conducted a buprenorphine dose-ranging study in patients with concurrent opioid and cocaine dependence and found orderly dose-dependent effects on illicit opioid use (significantly lowest at 12 mg and 16 mg daily) and less robust dose effects on cocaine use (Schottenfeld et al., 1993). These findings suggested the need for higher buprenorphine maintenance doses than were being investigated at the time. We then compared higher- and lower-dose daily buprenorphine (12 mg and 4 mg) and methadone (65 mg and 20 mg) in a randomized, double-blind clinical trial in subjects (N = 116) with co-occurring opioid and cocaine dependence (Schottenfeld et al., 1997). Higher doses of methadone and buprenorphine were superior to lower doses for reducing illicit opioid use, but the study results did not support the hypothesis that buprenorphine was superior to methadone for reducing cocaine; instead, a trend was found favoring methadone.

These findings led to studies evaluating adjunctive pharmacological and behavioral treatments for cocaine dependence. In one six-month trial, examining buprenorphine or methadone in combination with desipramine or placebo, we found that desipramine augmentation was associated with reductions in cocaine use in buprenorphine-maintained but not methadone-maintained patients (Kosten et al., 1992). Another study compared higher-dose buprenorphine and methadone and evaluated the efficacy of adjunctive contingency management when combined with maintenance treatment. Contingency management subjects received monetary vouchers for opioid- and cocaine-negative urine tests, collected thrice weekly; voucher value escalated during the first 12 weeks for consecutive drug-free tests and was reduced to a nominal value in weeks 13–24. Subjects treated with methadone remained in treatment significantly longer and achieved significantly longer periods of sustained abstinence and a greater proportion of drug-free tests compared to those assigned to buprenorphine. Subjects receiving contingency management achieved significantly longer periods of abstinence and a greater proportion of drug-free tests during the period of escalating voucher value, but these effects dissipated after the voucher value was reduced (Schottenfeld et al., 2005a, 2005b).

Gender differences

Until recently, research on addictions has largely focused on men and ignored gender differences, possibly because of the higher prevalence of addictive disorders among men. Nevertheless, the progression to addiction following initiation of substance use is often accelerated, and the severity of addictive disorders may be even higher among women. In recent findings, the SATU faculty examined factors that may contribute to the sex difference in the risk for cocaine dependence. Sinha and Rounsaville (2002) hypothesized that early trauma and chronic distress states increase the risk of drug abuse in women. In a series of studies, the SATU investigators have shown that sex differences in childhood maltreatment affect both the development of drug abuse and treatment outcomes. Results indicate that cocaine-dependent women report greater severity of childhood maltreatment compared to men, and these childhood maltreatment histories are associated with an earlier age of onset of gateway drug use as compared to men with such histories (Hyman et al., 2005). In addition, recent results show that childhood maltreatment history significantly predicts cocaine relapse outcomes in women more so than men (Paliwal et al., 2005). Animal studies (Lynch and Taylor, 2004, 2005a, 2005b; Lynch et al., 2002) have shown that female rats self-administer cocaine at higher rates than male rats with greater evidence of disruption of their diurnal cycle compared to male rats. Follow-up studies are underway to examine the molecular basis for these results, and the role of estrogen in modulating these sex differences is also being examined.

As increased drug craving is one of the key factors that could mediate relapse and course of illness in addicted individuals, SATU investigators are examining whether there are sex differences in stress-induced cocaine craving and reactivity, and the association between these measures and cocaine relapse. In previous research, we developed a novel, individualized, guided imagery technique and were the first to show that stress exposure reliably induces drug craving and arousal in substance-abusing individuals (Sinha et al., 1999, 2000, 2003). Sinha, O'Malley and Carolyn Mazure have collaborated on laboratory studies showing heightened stress reactivity in samples of alcoholic and cocaine-abusing women compared with controls (Sinha et al., 1998, 1999). Recently, we have reported that stress-induced increases in drug craving and HPA axis responses predict cocaine and alcohol relapse outcomes (Breese et al., 2005; Sinha et al., 2006). Although we find no sex differences in stress-induced cocaine craving, women show a more specific anxiety response to stress cues while men show a generalized stress/anxiety response to both stress and drug cues (Fox et al., 2005). Sex differences in the association of these measures and cocaine relapse are currently being examined. In brain imaging studies, SATU and other Yale investigators have shown that cortico-striatal-limbic pathways are activated when imaging neural activity associated with emotional stress (Sinha et al., 2004). In one of the first studies examining neural activity in stress-induced drug craving, Sinha and colleagues have demonstrated that cocaine addicts show reduced frontal and limbic activation during stress compared to controls, but increased caudate/striatal activity, which in turn is associated with stress-induced cocaine craving states (Sinha et al., 2006). Cocaine-dependent women show greater frontal limbic activity during stress compared to men, a finding that may contribute to better treatment outcomes reported in women (Li et al., 2005). Preliminary results also show that drug cue-induced and stress-induced brain activity can reliably predict cocaine treatment and relapse outcomes (Kosten et al., 2006; Sinha et al., 2005).

We are also exploring the relevance of gender differences to the development of sex-specific treatment approaches in drug addiction. Following up on the findings of the benefit of disulfram treatment for cocaine addiction (Carroll et al., 2004a, 2004b), sex differences in these findings were found with regard to the efficacy of disulfram primarily seen in men and not in women (Nich et al., 2004). Sinha, Kosten, Rounsaville and Malison are now conducting follow-up human laboratory studies to examine the basis for these sex differences in treatment response. Another example of these collaborations is found in the laboratory and treatment studies that Sinha and Kosten are conducting to assess the efficacy of lofexidine, an alpha2-adrenegic agonist that inhibits central norepinephrine, for preventing stress-related drug craving and relapse. In preliminary work, we have shown that lofexidine increases abstinence rates in naltrexone-treated opiate addicts possibly via reducing stress-induced drug craving (Sinha et al., 2003). As our earlier findings indicate that women may show greater vulnerability to stress cues and relapse, sex-specific strategies would become the basis for developing medications, such as lofexidine, specifically for the treatment of cocaine addiction in women.

Two separate behavioral therapy initiatives have focused on improving treatment and health outcomes for mothers who use cocaine and/or heroin, and their children. The first series of projects focused on cocaine-using women during pregnancy and their children's early development. In collaboration with Linda Mayes of the Child Study Center and investigators in the Department of Obstetrics and Gynecology, Schottenfeld carried out surveys and clinical trials of behavioral interventions for pregnant, cocaine-using women presenting for pre-natal care or delivery at Yale-affiliated hospitals (Schottenfeld et al., 1994). In a three-year voluntary drug-screening survey of more than 3000 pregnant women, 16% were found to be using cocaine during pregnancy (Jantzen et al., 1998). Schottenfeld, Carroll and Kosten (Chang et al., 1992) have collaborated on two clinical trials of enhanced behavioral treatments, the first of which contrasted primary care and specialty clinical care for substance abuse, and the second of which evaluated the addition of contingency management and community reinforcement treatment to standard pre- and post-natal care. Schottenfeld and Mayes also collaborated on an innovative set of longitudinal studies of children of cocaine-using women and control group women from this setting, extending previous work that focused exclusively on the neonatal period. They demonstrated cognitive and behavioral deficits persisting three and six months, delays in language development, and less maternal attentiveness and sensitivity in studies of mother–child interactions (Ball and Schottenfeld, 1997; Ball et al., 1997; Kain et al., 1995; Malakoff et al., 1994; Mayes et al., 1993). To assess parent–child interactions in greater depth, Mayes and Luthar developed an interview using specific parenting vignettes designed to elicit affective tone and understanding of parenting roles in high- and low-risk women.

Suniya Luthar and Rounsaville have collaborated on studies assessing and intervening with substance-abusing women and their children. They demonstrated that children of drug-abusing parents are at high risk for both internalizing and externalizing behavioral dysfunction (Luthar et al., 1998). In the families of drug abusers, exposure to a substance-abusing mother was associated with higher rates of mental disorders than to a substance-abusing father (Kosten et al., 1991; Luthar et al., 1996). As both a developmental and a clinical psychologist, Luthar felt compelled to do more than simply document dysfunctional elements of substance abusers' families. In collaboration with Carroll and Rounsaville, she developed a manual-guided parenting intervention specifically for drug-abusing mothers called Relational Psychotherapy Mothers' Group (RPMG) (Luthar and Suchman, 1999, in press). Results of a controlled pilot trial under the auspices of the behavioral therapies Clinical Research Center at Yale indicated that RPMG mothers showed both significant reductions in maltreating behaviors and more positive parenting as reported by both mothers and their children. The promise of these findings led to funding for a full-scale clinical trial that continues.

Addictions treatment protocols in primary care medical clinics

One of the great public health challenges in the area of addictions involves developing feasible and cost-effective mechanisms for making evidence-based treatments available to the large numbers of addicted individuals in need of treatment. With regard to heroin dependence, for example, it is estimated that only about 200,000 of the estimated one million heroin addicts in the U.S. are currently treated, and many never receive treatment. The problem is even more severe when considering the even larger number of individuals with prescription opioid abuse or dependence who do not receive treatment. Similar issues pertain to alcohol dependence and other addictive disorders. The public health challenges are even more complex in developing countries that do not have any established infrastructure for treating addictive disorders.

One promising approach for increasing the accessibility and reach of addictions treatment is to utilize office-based physicians and primary care medical settings to provide addictions treatment. This approach would obviate the need for greatly expanding stand-alone, specialty addictions-only treatment programs (and avoid the many problems inherent in finding suitable locations for such programs or supporting the infrastructure needed for them). Since addictions often cause medical problems, many addicts are already receiving treatment in office-based medical practices or primary care settings. Providing addictions treatment in these settings would thus facilitate access to addictions treatment; it could also facilitate better coordination of medical and addictions care. Additionally, this approach would also help to reduce the stigma associated with addictions and addictions treatment.

Our initial studies of primary medical care services for addicted individuals developed and evaluated clinical protocols for improving HIV and other infectious disease management of patients with substance use disorders (O'Connor et al., 1992a, 1994). The studies also evaluated ambulatory opiate detoxification (O'Connor et al., 1992b, 1995, 1997a, 1998).

We have been conducting a program of research on opioid agonist maintenance treatment with methadone or buprenorphine in physicians' offices and primary care medical settings in the U.S. and internationally. Our first study was the first randomized controlled clinical trial of medical maintenance for stabilized methadone-maintained patients (Fiellin et al., 2001). Transferring stabilized methadone-maintained patients to physician office-based treatment (referred to as medical maintenance) may improve patient satisfaction and increase the availability of maintenance treatment by freeing up "slots" in narcotic treatment programs (NTP). The study targeted patients who had been free of illicit drug use for at least one year, were without significant untreated psychiatric comorbidity, and had stable psychosocial functioning. We trained primary care internists to provide the treatment out of their regular practice setting. Patients were randomized to office-based care, where they received methadone maintenance from primary care physicians who received brief training in the care of opioid-dependent patients, or usual care at the NTP. Drug use and most other outcome measures were comparable for patients receiving medical maintenance or continuing treatment in the NTP, but patients receiving medical maintenance rated the quality of care they received higher than those treated in the NTP. The study results support the feasibility and efficacy of medical maintenance and suggest that patients may prefer medical maintenance. The results also suggest that this approach will not substantially improve availability of treatment, since relatively few patients met the eligibility criteria, and support the importance of careful clinical monitoring to identify and respond promptly to relapse.

We are also evaluating office-based and primary care settings for initiation as well as maintenance of treatment. We completed several pilot studies demonstrating the feasibility and potential efficacy of buprenorphine maintenance in a primary care clinic (Fiellin et al., 2002; Pantalon et al., 2004). The pilot studies suggested that drug counseling is feasible to implement in this setting and leads to greater reductions in illicit drug use compared to brief medical management only (Fiellin and O'Connor, 2002; Fiellin et al., 2002; Pantalon et al., 2004). We have recently completed a randomized clinical trial of counseling intensity in this setting. Patients were assigned to nurse-provided brief, standard medical management or more extended, enhanced medical management and buprenorphine medication dispensing either weekly or three times per week. Brief weekly counseling and once-weekly dispensing had efficacy on all outcome measures that was comparable to more extended counseling with either weekly or three times per week buprenorphine dispensing (Fiellin et al., 2006). There was wide variability in adherence to buprenorphine, and increased adherence was associated with improved treatment outcomes, suggesting the importance of monitoring and encouraging adherence to reduce potential misuse and improve outcomes. Findings from the study suggest that primary care and office-based buprenorphine was attracting a population different from the one enrolled in nearby methadone maintenance programs during the same period (Sullivan et al., 2005). Notably, the proportion of patients reporting use only of non-medical prescription opiates increased significantly in successive years of the study, and these patients, who tended to be younger and have no prior history of methadone maintenance treatment, remained in treatment longer and had greater reductions in illicit opiate use compared to heroin-dependent patients (Moore et al., 2007).

The lack of accessibility and availability of treatments for heroin and other opioid dependence is a problem not only in the U.S. but also internationally. In Malaysia, Iran and across many developing nations in the Western Pacific, Southeast Asia, Asia, and Eastern and Central Europe, heroin and injection-drug use are even more prevalent in the adult population than in the U.S., and injection-drug use in these countries is the main driver of the AIDS epidemic. Consequently, over the past five years, Schottenfeld and Marek Chawarski have initiated a program of research aimed at developing, evaluating and disseminating evidence-based treatments internationally. Working in collaboration with psychiatrists in Malaysia and in Iran who received training in addictions research at the CMHC, Schottenfeld and Chawarski are conducting a placebo-controlled study of naltrexone and buprenorphine in Malaysia and a head-to-head comparison of naltrexone and buprenorphine in Iran. The study in Malaysia introduced agonist maintenance treatment to Malaysia, and currently, it is estimated that more than 20,000 heroin addicts are being treated with buprenorphine in Malaysia (Chawarski et al., 2006; Mazlan et al., 2006; Schottenfeld et al., 2006). The behavioral drug and HIV risk-reduction counseling manual developed for these studies is serving as the basis for training drug counselors in Malaysia and Iran and is also now being used as the manual for training drug counselors in Thailand and China as part of efforts to evaluate and disseminate buprenorphine maintenance treatment in those countries.

Implications for public psychiatry

The remarkable accomplishments of the SATU, in conjunction with its longtime partner, the APT Foundation, have important implications for public psychiatry with regard to clinical services, education and clinical research. First, the close collaboration between the CMHC'S SATU and the APT Foundation established a benchmark for the importance of public–private partnerships. The APT Foundation has provided considerable flexibility with regard to new program development, rapid response to emerging problems with new drugs of abuse (e.g., at the start of the cocaine epidemic) or problems affecting new patient population (e.g., development of programs for drug-dependent women who are pregnant or have child-rearing responsibilities), and pilot funding for research studies. Close collaboration has facilitated coordination rather than duplication of services. Coordination of intake to addictions treatment improves access to treatment and identification of service gaps and emerging service needs. Additionally, much of the research of the SATU investigators has been conducted in APT clinical programs.

Second, many of the advances made in developing and improving treatments for addictive disorders have benefited enormously from the dual roles of faculty psychiatrists and psychologists, who treat patients, direct clinical services and develop research addressing the clinical problems experienced by patients, clinical dilemmas faced by clinicians and treatment service needs. Clinician researchers working in the clinical programs are able to identify emerging drug epidemics, problems of co-occurring disorders, service gaps and gaps in our understanding about effective treatments. The advances in treatment have also resulted from the close collaboration between clinical and basic sciences researchers. This collaboration is greatly facilitated by the close proximity of basic scientists located in the Ribicoff Center and clinical researchers in the SATU and the Clinical Neurosciences Research Unit (CNRU). Throughout its history, the SATU has been committed to translating research into new treatments and clinical practice.

Third, in order to meet the public health needs of communities regionally, nationally and internationally, it is critical to train a sufficient number of psychiatrists (and other physicians), psychologists, social workers, drug counselors and other mental health clinicians to provide evidence-based treatments. Training of primary care clinicians in addictions treatment, and development of clinical treatment protocols suitable for use in primary care settings, will broaden the base of addictions treatment and improve access to services. Clinical training in addictions treatment requires didactic training (through seminars, courses and reading) as well as supervised clinical experience in addictions treatment settings. The SATU faculty members have developed training programs for clinicians that are used locally (e.g., for the CMHC and Yale Department of Psychiatry trainees), regionally, nationally and internationally. The training curriculum for physicians in general practice, developed as part of our initial study of medical maintenance, served as the model for the core training curriculum that is provided across the U.S. to physicians seeking certification to prescribe buprenorphine for office-based maintenance treatment. The SATU and APT clinical programs also serve as major sites for providing hands-on, supervised clinical experience. Trainees in these programs have gone on to take leadership roles developing and running treatment and training programs and providing treatment around the country.

Conclusion

Looking back at the remarkable clinical, programmatic, teaching and research accomplishments of the SATU over the nearly forty years of its existence, it is hard to imagine that when the CMHC initially opened in 1966, reflecting the low status of addiction treatment within medicine and psychiatry, the CMHC did not include specialty services targeting addictive disorders. Since then, the recognition of addictive disorders as medical and psychiatric disorders, the development of clinical and training programs targeting addictive disorders, and the extraordinary flowering of clinical research on them have led to substantial improvements in their treatment. Nevertheless, stigma and a lack of resources continue to hinder progress in preventing and treating addictive disorders. Effective pharmacological treatments have not been established for cocaine or methamphetamine dependence. Current treatments for addictive disorders are not effective for all patients with these disorders and services for individuals with co-occurring addictive and psychiatric disorders are often not available. Finally, the majority of those experiencing addictive disorders in the U.S. and worldwide do not have access to or do not receive treatment for their addictions. We have accomplished much, and can take pride in our accomplishments, but we have far to go, and will need to increase our efforts to address the many problems that face us.

References

Anton RF, Hogan I, Jalali B, et al: Multiple family therapy and naltrexone in the treatment of opiate dependence. Drug Alcohol Depend 8:157–68, 1981

Anton RF, O'Malley SS, Ciraulo DA, et al: Combined pharmacotherapies and behavioral interventions for alcohol dependence: the COMBINE study: a randomized controlled trial. JAMA 295:2003–17, 2006

Ball SA, Maves LC, DeTeso JA, et al: Maternal attentiveness of cocaine abusers during child-based assessments. Am J Addict 6:135–43, 1997

Ball SA, Schottenfeld RS: A five-factor model of personality and addiction, psychiatric, and AIDS risk severity in pregnant and postpartum cocaine misusers. Subst Use Misuse 32:25–41, 1997

Breese GR, Chu K, Dayas CV, et al: Stress enhancement of craving during sobriety: a risk for relapse. Alcohol: Clin Exp Res 29:185–95, 2005

Carroll KM: Relapse prevention as a psychosocial treatment approach: a review of controlled clinical trials. Exp Clin Psychopharmacol 4:46–54, 1996

Carroll KM: A cognitive behavioral approach treating cocaine addiction. NIDA Therapy Manuals for Drug Addiction. NIH Publication No. 98-4308, 1998

Carroll KM, Ball SA, Nich C, et al: Motivational interviewing to improve treatment engagement and outcome in individuals seeking treatment for substance abuse: a multisite effectiveness study. Drug Alcohol Depend 81:301–12, 2006

Carroll KM, Ball SA, Nich C, et al: Targeting behavioral therapies to enhance naltrexone treatment of opioid dependence: efficacy of contingency management and significant other involvement. Arch Gen Psychiatry 58:755–61, 2001

Carroll KM, Easton CJ, Nich C, et al.: The use of contingency management and motivational/skills-building therapy to treat young adults with marijuana dependence. J Consult Clin Psych 74:955–66, 2006

Carroll KM, Fenton LR, Ball SA, et al: Efficacy of disulfiram and cognitive behavior therapy in cocaine-dependent outpatients: a randomized placebo-controlled trial. Arch Gen Psychiatry 61:264–72, 2004a

Carroll KM, Kosten TR, Rounsaville BJ: Choosing a behavioral therapy platform for pharmacotherapy of substance users. Drug Alcohol Depend 75(2):123–34, 2004b

Carroll KM, Nich C, Ball SA: Practice makes progress? Homework assignments and outcome in treatment of cocaine dependence. J Consult Clin Psychol 73(4):749–55, 2005

Carroll KM, Nich C, Ball SA, et al: One-year follow-up of disulfiram and psychotherapy for cocaine-alcohol users: sustained effects of treatment. Addiction 95:1335–49, 2000

Carroll KM, Nich C, Ball SA, et al: Treatment of cocaine and alcohol dependence with psychotherapy and disulfiram. Addiction 93:713–28, 1998

Carroll KM, Rounsaville BJ, Gawin FH: A comparative trial of psychotherapies for ambulatory cocaine abusers: relapse prevention and interpersonal psychotherapy. Am J Drug Alcohol Abuse 17(3):229–47, 1991

Carroll KM, Rounsaville BJ, Gordon LT, et al: Psychotherapy and pharmacotherapy for ambulatory cocaine abusers. Arch Gen Psychiatry 51:177–87, 1994a

Carroll KM, Rounsaville BJ, Nich C, et al: One-year follow-up of psychotherapy and pharmacotherapy for cocaine dependence. Delayed emergence of psychotherapy effects. Arch Gen Psychiatry 51:989–97, 1994b

Carroll KM, Sinha R, Nich C, et al: Contingency management to enhance naltrexone treatment of opioid dependence: a randomized clinical trial of reinforcement magnitude. Exp Clin Psychopharmacol 10:54–63, 2002

Chang G, Carroll KM, Behr HM, et al: Improving treatment outcome in pregnant opiate-dependent women. J Subst Abuse Treat 9:327–30, 1992

Charney DS, Heninger GR, Kleber HD: The combined use of clonidine and naltrexone as a rapid, safe, and effective treatment of abrupt withdrawal from methadone. Am J Psychiatry 143:831–7, 1986

Charney DS, Riordan CE, Kleber HD, et al: Clonidine and naltrexone. A safe, effective, and rapid treatment of abrupt withdrawal from methadone therapy. Arch Gen Psychiatry 39:1327–32, 1982a

Charney DS, Sternberg DE, Kleber HD, et al: The clinical use of clonidine in abrupt withdrawal from methadone. Arch Gen Psychiatry 38:1273–7, 1982b

Chawarski MC, Schottenfeld RS, Mazlan M: Heroin dependence and HIV infection in Malaysia. Drug Alcohol Depend 82:S39–S42, 2006

COMBINE Study Research Group: Testing combined pharmacotherapies and behavioral therapies in alcohol dependence: Rationale and methods. Alcohol: Clin Exp Res 27:1107–22, 2003

DeRubeis RJ, Crits-Christoph P: Empirically supported individual and group psychological treatments for adult mental disorders. J Consult Clin Psychol 66:37–52, 1998

Fiellin DA, O'Connor PG: Office-based treatment of opioid dependent patients. New Engl J Med 347:817–23, 2002

Fiellin DA, O'Connor PG, Chawarski M, et al: Methadone maintenance in primary care: a randomized controlled trial. JAMA 286:1724–31, 2001

Fiellin DA, Pantalon MV, Chawarski MC, et al: Counseling plus buprenorphine-naloxone maintenance therapy for opioid dependence. New Engl J Med 355:365–74, 2006

Fiellin DA, Pantalon MV, Pakes J, et al: Treatment of heroin dependence with buprenorphine in primary care. Am J Drug Alcohol Abuse 28:231–41, 2002

Fischman MW, Foltin RW, Nestadt G, et al: Effects of desipramine maintenance on cocaine self-administration by humans. J Pharmacol Exp Ther 253:760–70, 1990

Fox HC, Garcia M, Anderson G, et al: Gender differences in responses to stress and drug-cues in cocaine dependent individuals. Presented at The College on Problems of Drug Dependence Annual Meeting, Orlando, FL, 2005

Gawin FH, Kleber HD: Abstinence symptomatology and psychiatric diagnosis in cocaine abusers. Clinical observations. Arch Gen Psychiatry 43:107–13, 1986

Gawin FH, Kleber HD: Evolving conceptualizations of cocaine dependence. Yale J Biol Med 61:123–36, 1988

Gawin FH, Kleber HD, Byck R, et al: Desipramine facilitation of initial cocaine abstinence Arch Gen Psychiatry 46:117–21, 1989

Gawin FH, Riordan C, Kleber HD: Methylphenidate treatment of cocaine abusers without Attention Deficit Disorder: a negative report. Am J Drug Alcohol Abuse 11(3–4):193–97, 1985

Gelernter J, Kranzler H, Coccaro E, et al: D4 dopamine-receptor (DRD4) alleles and novelty seeking in substance-dependent, personality-disorder, and control subjects. Am J Human Genetics 61:1144–52, 1997

Gelernter J, Kranzler HR, Satel SL, et al: Genetic association between dopamine transporter protein alleles and cocaine-induced paranoia. Neuropsychopharmacology 11:195–200, 1994

George TP, Chawarski MC, Pakes J, et al: Disulfiram versus placebo for cocaine dependence in buprenorphine-maintained subjects: a preliminary study. Biol Psychiatry 47:1080–6, 2000a

George TP, Termine A, Sacco KA, et al.: A preliminary study of the effects of cigarette smoking on prepulse inhibition in schizophrenia: involvement of nicotinic receptor mechanisms. Schizophrenia Res 87:307–15, 2006

George TP, Vessicchio JC, Termine A, et al: A placebo-controlled study of bupropion for smoking cessation in schizophrenia. Biol Psychiatry 52:53–61, 2002

George TP, Zeidonis DM, Feingold A, et al: Nicotine transdermal patch and atypical antipsychotic medications for smoking cessation in schizophrenia. Am J Psychiatry 157:1835–42, 2000b

Gold MS, Pottash AC, Sweeney DR, et al: Opiate withdrawal using clonidine. A safe, effective, and rapid nonopiate treatment. JAMA 243: 343–6, 1980

Gold MS, Redmond DE, Jr., Kleber HD: Clonidine blocks acute opiate-withdrawal symptoms. Lancet 2:599–602, 1978

Hughes JR, Oliveto AH, Riggs R, et al: Concordance of different measures of nicotine dependence: two pilot studies. Addict Behav 29:1527–39, 2004

Hurzeler M, Gerwirtz D, Kleber H: Varying clinical contexts for administering naltrexone. NIDA Res Monogr 9:48–66, 1976

Hyman SM, Garcia M, Kemp K, et al: A gender specific psychometric analysis of the Early Trauma Inventory Short Form in cocaine dependent adults. Addict Behav 30:847–52, 2005

Irvin JE, Bowers CA, Dunn ME, et al: Efficacy of relapse prevention: a meta-analytic review. J Consult Clin Psychol 67:563–70, 1999

Jaffe AJ, Rounsaville B, Chang G, et al: Naltrexone, relapse prevention, and supportive therapy with alcoholics: an analysis of patient treatment matching. J Consult Clin Psychol 64:1044–53, 1996

Jantzen K, Ball SA, Leventhal JM, et al: Types of abuse and cocaine use in pregnant women. J Subst Abuse Treat 15:319–23, 1998

Kain ZN, Mayes LC, Pakes J, et al: Thrombocytopenia in pregnant women who use cocaine. Am J Obstet Gynecol 173:885–90, 1995

Khantzian EJ, Gawin F, Kleber HD, et al: Methylphenidate treatment of cocaine dependence: a preliminary report. J Subst Abuse Treat 1:107–12, 1984

Kleber HD: Student use of hallucinogens. J Am Coll Health 14:109–17, 1965

Kleber HD: Prolonged adverse reactions from unsupervised use of hallucinogenic drugs. J Nerv Ment Dis 144:308–19, 1967

Kleber HD: The New Haven Methadone Maintenance Program. Int J Addict 5:449–63, 1970

Kleber HD: The Drug Dependence Unit of the Connecticut Mental Health Center, in Organization and Administration of Drug Abuse Treatment Programs: National and International Edited by Cull JG, Hardy RE. Charles C. Thomas, Springfield, IL, pp 51–60, 1974

Kleber HD: Clinical aspects of the use of narcotic antagonists: the state of the art. Int J Addict 12:857–61, 1977

Kleber HD, Gawin FH: Cocaine. Drug abuse and drug dependence. APA Annual Review 5:160–85, 1986

Kleber HD, Kosten TR, Gaspari J, et al: Nontolerance to the opioid antagonism of naltrexone. Biol Psych 20:66–72, 1985a

Kleber HD, Riordan CE, Rounsaville B, et al: Clonidine in outpatient detoxification from methadone maintenance. Arch Gen Psychiatry 42:391–4, 1985b

Kleber HD, Topazian M, Gaspari J, et al: Clonidine and naltrexone in the outpatient treatment of heroin withdrawal. Am J Drug Alcohol Abuse 13:1–17, 1987

Kleber HD, Weissman MM, Rounsaville BJ, et al: Imipramine as treatment for depression in addicts. Arch Gen Psychiatry 40:649–53, 1983

Kosten TR: Clinical and research perspectives on cocaine abuse: the pharmacotherapy of cocaine abuse. NIDA Res Monogr 135:48–56, 1993

Kosten TR, Kleber HD: Strategies to improve compliance with narcotic antagonists. Am J Drug Alcohol Abuse 10:249–66, 1984

Kosten TR, Morgan CM, Falcione J, et al: Pharmacotherapy for cocaine-abusing methadone-maintained patients using amantadine or desipramine. Arch Gen Psychiatry 49:894–8, 1992

Kosten TR, Rounsaville BJ, Kosten TA, et al: Gender differences in the specificity of alcoholism transmission among the relatives of opioid addicts. J Nerv Ment Dis 179:392–400, 1991

Kosten TR, Scanley BE, Tucker KA, et al: Cue-induced brain activity changes and relapse in cocaine-dependent patients. Neuropsychopharmacology 31:644–50, 2006

Krishnan-Sarin S, Meandjiza B, O'Malley SS: Nicotine patch and naltrexone for smoking cessation: a preliminary study. Nicotine Tob Res 5:851–7, 2003

Krishnan-Sarin S, Rosen MI, O'Malley SS: Naloxone challenge in smokers: evidence for an opioid component in nicotine dependence. Arch Gen Psychiatry 56:663–8, 1999

Leshner AI: Science-based views of drug addiction and its treatment. JAMA 282:1314–6, 1999

Li CS, Kosten TR, Sinha R: Sex differences in brain activation during stress imagery in abstinent cocaine users: a functional magnetic resonance imaging study. Biol Psych 57:487–94, 2005

Luthar SS, Cushing G, Merikangas KR, et al: Multiple jeopardy: risk and protective factors among addicted mothers' offspring. Develop Psychopathol 10:117–36, 1998

Luthar SS, Cushing G, Rounsaville BJ: Gender differences among opioid abusers: pathways to disorder and profiles of psychopathology. Drug Alcohol Depend 43:179–89, 1996

Luthar SS, Suchman NE: Developmentally informed parenting interventions: the Relational Psychotherapy Mothers' Group, in Rochester Symposium on Developmental Psychopathology. Edited by Cicchetti D, Toth SL. Rochester, NY: University of Rochester Press, 271–309, 1999

Luthar SS, Suchman NE, Altomare M: Relational Psychotherapy Mother's Group: a randomized clinical trial for substance abusing mothers. Devel & Psychopath 19:243–61, 2007

Lynch WJ, Roth ME, Carroll ME: Biological basis of sex differences in drug abuse: preclinical and clinical studies. Psychopharmacology 164:121–37, 2002

Lynch WJ, Taylor JR: Sex differences in the behavioral effects of 24-h/day access to cocaine under a discrete trial procedure. Neuropsychopharmacology 29:943–51, 2004

Lynch WJ, Taylor JR: Decreased motivation following cocaine self-administration under extended access conditions: effects of sex and ovarian hormones. Neuropsychopharmacology 30:927–35, 2005a

Lynch WJ, Taylor JR: Persistent changes in motivation to self-administered cocaine following modulation of cyclic AMP-dependent protein kinase A (PKA) activity in the nucleus accumbens. Eur J Neuroscience 22:1214–20, 2005b

Malakoff ME, Mayes LC, Schottenfeld RS: Language abilities of preschool-age children living with cocaine-using mothers. Am J Addict 3:346–54, 1994

Martino S, Carroll KM, O'Malley SS, et al: Motivational interviewing with psychiatrically ill substance abusing patients. Am J Addict 9:88–91, 2000

Maude-Griffin PM, Hohenstein JM, Humfleet GL, et al: Superior efficacy of cognitive-behavioral therapy for urban crack cocaine abusers: main and matching effects. J Consult Clin Psychol 66:832–7, 1998

Moore BA, Fiellin DA, Barry D, et al.: Primary care office-based buprenorphine treatment: comparison of heroin and prescription opioid dependent patients. J Gen Int Med 22:527–30, 2007

Mayes LC, Granger RH, Frank MA, et al: Neurobehavioral profiles of neonates exposed to cocaine prenatally. Pediatrics 91:778–83, 1993

Mazlan M, Schottenfeld RS, Chawarski MC: New challenges and opportunities in managing substance abuse in Malaysia. Drug Alcohol Review 25:473–8, 2006

McKay JR, Alterman AI, Cacciola JS, et al: Continuing care for cocaine dependence: comprehensive 2-year outcomes. J Consult Clin Psychol 67:420–7, 1999

McLellan AT, Arndt IO, Metzger DS, et al: The effects of psychosocial services in substance abuse treatment. JAMA 269:1953–9, 1993

Morgenstern J, Longabaugh R: Cognitive-behavioral treatment for alcohol dependence: a review of evidence for its hypothesized mechanisms of action. Addiction 95:1475–90, 2000

MTP Research Group: Brief treatments for cannabis dependence: findings from a randomized multisite trial. J Consult Clin Psychol 72:455–66, 2004

Nich C, McCance-Katz EF, Petrakis IL, et al: Sex differences in cocaine-dependent individuals' response to disulfiram treatment. Addict Behav 29:1123–8, 2004

NIDA: Principles of drug addiction treatment: a research-based guide. Bethesda, MD, National Institutes on Drug Abuse, 1999

NIDA: Principles of Drug Addiction Treatment: A Research-Based Guide. Bethesda, MD, National Institutes on Drug Abuse, 2000

O'Brien CP: A range of research-based pharmacotherapies for addiction. Science 287:66–70, 1997

O'Connor PG, Carroll KM, Shi JM, et al: Three methods of opioid detoxification in a primary care setting: a randomized trial. Ann Intern Med 127:526–30, 1997a

O'Connor PG, Farren CK, Rounsaville BJ, et al: A preliminary investigation of the management of alcohol dependence with naltrexone by primary care providers. Am J Med 103:477–82, 1997b

O'Connor PG, Molde S, Henry S, et al: Human immunodeficiency virus infection in intravenous drug users: a model for primary care. Am J Med 93:382–6, 1992a

O'Connor PG, Oliveto AH, Shi JM, et al: A randomized trial of buprenorphine maintenance for treating heroin dependence in a primary care versus a drug treatment setting. J Gen Int Med 12(Supplement):78, 1997c

O'Connor PG, Oliveto AH, Shi JM, et al: A randomized trial of buprenorphine maintenance for heroin dependence in a primary care clinic for substance users versus a methadone clinic. Am J Med 105:100–5, 1998

O'Connor PG, Selwyn PA, Schottenfeld RS: Medical care for injection-drug users with human immunodeficiency virus infection. N Engl J Med 331:450–9, 1994

O'Connor PG, Waugh ME, Carroll KM, et al: Primary care-based ambulatory opioid detoxification: the results of a clinical trial. J Gen Int Med 10:255–60, 1995

O'Connor PG, Waugh ME, Schottenfeld RS, et al: Ambulatory opiate detoxification and primary care: a role for the primary care physician. J Gen Int Med 7:532–4, 1992b

O'Malley SS, Carroll KM: Psychotherapeutic considerations in pharmacological trials. Alcoholism: Clin Exp Res 20:17a–22a, 1996

O'Malley SS, Jaffe AJ, Chang G, et al: Six-month follow-up of naltrexone and psychotherapy for alcohol dependence. Arch Gen Psychiatry 53:217–24, 1996

O'Malley SS, Jaffe AJ, Chang G, et al: Naltrexone and coping skills therapy for alcohol dependence: a controlled study. Arch Gen Psychiatry 49:881–7, 1992

O'Malley SS, O'Connor PG, Farren C, et al: Initial and maintenance naltrexone in combination with cognitive behavior or medical model counseling. Presented at Research Society on Alcoholism, South Carolina, 1998

O'Malley SS, Rounsaville BJ, Farren C, et al: Initial and maintenance naltrexone treatment for alcohol dependence using primary care vs specialty care: a nested sequence of 3 randomized trials. Arch Int Med 163:1695–1704, 2003

Paliwal P, Hyman SM, Sinha R: Gender specific effects in the effects of child maltreatment on cocaine relapse outcomes. Presented at The College on Problems of Drug Dependence Annual Meeting, Orlando, FL, June 18–23, 2005

Pantalon MV, Fiellin DA, O'Connor PG, et al: Counseling requirements for buprenorphine maintenance in primary care: lessons learned form a preliminary study in a methadone maintenance program. Addict Disorders Treat 3:71–6, 2004

Petrakis IL, Carroll KM, Nich C, et al: Disulfiram treatment for cocaine dependence in methadone-maintained opioid addicts. Addiction 95:219–28, 2000

Petry NM, Alessi SM, Hanson T: Contingency management improves abstinence and quality of life in cocaine abusers. J Consult Clin Psych 75:307–15, 2007

Petry NM, Tedford J, Austin M, et al: Prize reinforcement contingency management for treating cocaine users: how low can we go, and with whom? Addiction 99:349–60, 2004

Pierson PS, Rapkin RM, Kleber HD: Naloxone in the treatment of the young heroin abuser. Am J Drug Alcohol Abuse 1:243–52, 1974

Project MATCH Research Group: Matching alcoholism treatments to client heterogeneity: Project MATCH posttreatment drinking outcomes. J Stud Alcohol 22:7–29, 1997

Project MATCH Research Group: Matching alcoholism treatments to client heterogeneity: treatment main effects and matching effects on drinking during treatment. J Stud Alcohol 59:631–9, 1998

Rawson RA, Huber A, McCann M, et al: A comparison of contingency management and cognitive-behavioral approaches during methadone maintenance treatment for cocaine dependence. Arch Gen Psychiatry 59:817–24, 2002

Riordan CE, Mezritz M, Slobetz F, et al: Successful detoxification from methadone maintenance. Follow-up study of 38 patients. JAMA 235:2604–7, 1976

Rounsaville BJ, Anton SF, Carroll KM, et al: Psychiatric diagnoses of treatment-seeking cocaine abusers. Arch Gen Psychiatry 48:43–51, 1991a

Rounsaville BJ, Dolinsky ZS, Babor TF, et al: Psychopathology as a predictor of treatment outcome in alcoholics. Arch Gen Psychiatry 44:505–13, 1987

Rounsaville BJ, Glazer W, Wilber CH, et al: Short-term interpersonal psychotherapy in methadone-maintained opiate addicts. Arch Gen Psychiatry 40:629–36, 1983

Rounsaville BJ, Kleber HD: Psychotherapy/counseling for opiate addicts: strategies for use in different treatment settings. Int J Addict 20:869–96, 1985a

Rounsaville BJ, Kleber HD: Untreated opiate addicts. How do they differ from those seeking treatment? Arch Gen Psychiatry 42:1072–7, 1985b

Rounsaville BJ, Kosten TR, Weissman MM, et al: Evaluating and treating depressive disorders in opiate addicts. National Institute on Drug Abuse, Treatment Research Monograph, 1985

Rounsaville BJ, Kosten TR, Weissman MM, et al: Prognostic significance of psychopathology in treated opiate addicts: a 2.5 year follow-up study. Arch Gen Psychiatry 43:739–45, 1986

Rounsaville BJ, Kosten TR, Weissman MM, et al: Psychiatric disorders in relatives of probands with opiate addiction. Arch Gen Psychiatry 48:33–42, 1991b

Rounsaville BJ, Kranzler HR, Ball S, et al: Personality disorders in substance abusers: relation to substance use. J Nerv Ment Dis 186:87–95, 1998

Rounsaville BJ, Weissman MM, Crits-Christoph K, et al: Diagnosis and symptoms of depression in opiate addicts: course and relationship to treatment outcome. Arch Gen Psychiatry 39:151–6, 1982a

Rounsaville BJ, Weissman MM, Kleber H, et al: Heterogeneity of psychiatric diagnosis in treated opiate addicts. Arch Gen Psychiatry 39:161–8, 1982b

Sacco KA, Bannon KL, George TP: Nicotinic receptor mechanisms and cognition in normal states and neuropsychiatric disorders. J Psychopharmacol 18:457–74, 2004

Sacco KA, Termine A, Seyal A, et al: Effects of cigarette smoking on spatial working memory and attentional deficits in schizophrenia: involvement of nicotinic receptor mechanisms. Arch Gen Psychiatry 62:649–59, 2005

Schottenfeld R, Carroll K, Rounsaville B: Comorbid psychiatric disorders and cocaine abuse. NIDA Res Monogr 135:31–47, 1993

Schottenfeld RS, Chawarski MC, Fiellin D: Abstinence achievement during opioid agonist maintenance treatment: when to shift gears? Presented at CPDD 67th Annual Scientific Meeting, Orlando, FL, 2005a

Schottenfeld RS, Chawarski MC, Pakes J, et al: Methadone versus buprenorphine with contingency management or performance feedback for cocaine and opioid dependence. Am J Psychiatry 162:340–9, 2005b

Schottenfeld RS, Mazlan M, Chawarski MC: Randomized, double blind comparison of drug counseling combined with buprenorphine, naltrexone or placebo for treating opioid dependence and reducing HIV risk in Malaysia. Presented at The College on Problems of Drug Dependence Annual Meeting, Scottsdale, AZ, 2006

Schottenfeld RS, Pakes JR, Oliveto A, et al: Buprenorphine versus methadone maintenance treatment for concurrent opioid dependence and cocaine abuse. Arch Gen Psychiatry 54:713–20, 1997

Schottenfeld RS, Pascale R, Sokolowski S: Matching services to needs: vocational services for substance abusers. J Subst Abuse Treat 9:3–8, 1992

Schottenfeld RS, Viscarello RR, Grossman J, et al: A comprehensive public health approach, in When Drug Addicts have Children: Reorienting Child Welfare's Response. Edited by Besharov DJ. Washington, D.C.: Child Welfare League of America, American Enterprise Institute, pp 81–90, 1994

Sholomskas DE, Carroll KM: One small step for manuals: Computer-assisted training in twelve-step facilitation. J Stud Alcohol 67:939–45, 2006

Sholomskas DE, Syracuse-Siewert G, Rounsaville BJ, et al: We don't train in vain: a dissemination trial of three strategies of training clinicians in cognitive-behavioral therapy. J Consult Clin Psychol 73(1):106–15, 2005

Sinha R, Catapano D, O'Malley S: Stress-induced craving and stress response in cocaine dependent individuals. Psychopharmacology 142:343–51, 1999

Sinha R, Fox C, Kemp K, et al: Enhanced sensitivity to stress and drug craving in abstinent cocaine-dependent individuals compared to matched control volunteers. Presented at The College on Problems of Drug Dependence Annual Meeting, Scottsdale, AZ, June 17–22, 2006

Sinha R, Fuse T, Aubin LR, et al: Psychological stress, drug-related cues and cocaine craving. Psychopharmacology 152:140–8, 2000

Sinha R, Lacadie C, Skudlarski P, et al.: Neural circuits underlying emotional stress in humans. Annals NY Acad Sci 1032:254–7, 2004

Sinha R, Lacadie C, Li C, et al: Stress-related fMRI brain activity predicts cocaine relapse outcomes. Presented at The College on Problems of Drug Dependence Annual Meeting, Orlando, FL, 2005

Sinha R, Robinson J, O'Malley S: Stress response dampening: effects of gender and family history of alcoholism and anxiety disorders. Psychopharmacology 137:311–20, 1998

Sinha R, Rounsaville BJ: Sex differences in depressed substance abusers. J Clin Psychiatry 63:616–27, 2002

Sinha R, Talih M, Malison R, et al: Hypothalamic-pituitary-adrenal axis and sympatho-adreno-medullary responses during stress-induced and drug cue-induced cocaine craving states. Psychopharmacology 170:62–72, 2003

Sullivan LE, Chawarski M, O'Connor PG, et al: The practice of office-based buprenorphine treatment of opioid dependence: is it associated with new patients entering into treatment? Drug Alcohol Depend 79:113–6, 2005

Uhlenhuth EH, Lipman RS, Covi L: Combined pharmacotherapy and psychotherapy. J Nerv Ment Dis 148:52–64, 1969

Verheul R, Kranzler HR, Poling J, et al: Co-occurrence of Axis I and Axis II disorders in substance abusers. Acta Psychiatrica Scandinavica 101:110–8, 2000

Vining E, Kosten TR, Kleber HD: Clinical utility of rapid clonidine-naltrexone detoxification for opioid abusers. Br J Addict 83:567–75, 1988

Weinberger AH, Reutenauer EL, Allen TM, et al: Reliability of the Fagerstrom Test for nicotine dependence, Minnesota Nicotine Withdrawal Scale, and Tiffany Questionnaire for smoking urges in smokers with and without schizophrenia. Drug Alcohol Depend, 86:278–82, 2007

3

Law and Psychiatry at the Connecticut Mental Health Center

Howard Zonana and Madelon Baranoski

In the 1960s, the interface between psychiatry and law mushroomed as courts defined the civil rights of psychiatric patients. At the CMHC, Yale psychiatry faculty collaborated with the Yale Law School, representing hospitalized psychiatric patients seeking discharge. That collaboration launched the Law and Psychiatry Division. Now an internationally renowned program for educating forensic psychiatrists, the Division shapes policy and legislation related to the treatment of patients with mental illness in the community, hospitals and prisons. The Division conducts forensic evaluations in criminal and civil cases, consults to the CMHC, and educates the legal and psychiatric community. The evolution of the Division has been inextricably linked to scientific, social and legal developments in mental health services, and the perception of mental illness. The Division has established programs, policy, and research in substance abuse and domestic violence, risk assessment, sex offender assessment, jail diversion, and other areas mutual to psychiatry and law.

When the Connecticut Mental Health Center (CMHC) opened in 1966, psychiatry and the law were separate disciplines with limited interaction. Medical jurisprudence in the United States at that time had been evolving from the initial adoption of procedures from England in the post-revolutionary period. Medical opinions could be solicited for legal proceedings, but it was not general practice to do so. Indeed, there were few formal structures or policies relevant to the intersection of medical and legal issues. Doctors were generally not paid to evaluate defendants and offer their expertise or opinions in legal cases. Although they could be required under subpoena to conduct appropriate evaluations in criminal procedures, they generally tried to avoid such coerced service, which was viewed by the medical profession as both beyond the scope of practice and a threat to the reputation of the physician.

Through the 1960s, the collaborative interface between law and medicine was just beginning. Medical malpractice suits (almost non-existent until 1830, but by 1900 at levels similar to those presently found) engaged physicians as expert witnesses on a case-by-case basis depending on the specialty involved in the court action. Psychiatrists offered expert opinions in cases involving the capacity of persons with psychiatric disability or advanced age to write wills, to testify, and to manage financial and

40 Years of Academic Public Psychiatry. Edited by Selby C. Jacobs and Ezra E. H. Griffith
© 2007 John Wiley & Sons, Ltd.

business affairs. The role for psychiatrists in the courts broadened as the laws for the involuntary commitment of persons to hospitals evolved to include stricter standards reliant on evidence of psychiatric illness and functional impairment. Civil commitment hearings required psychiatrists to testify as expert witnesses, selected for their medical knowledge and experience. Psychiatrists appeared more frequently as experts in the courtroom, but the specialty of forensic psychiatry had not yet been developed.

In criminal cases, the involvement of psychiatry was rare but often sensational, involving the insanity defense, which strove to reduce personal culpability because of mental illness. Then as now, the defense evoked controversy among legal and psychiatric professionals regarding the standards to be applied in the defense. The public perceived it to be a legal tactic employed by the wealthy to escape the consequences of criminal behavior. Increased psychiatric involvement in legal cases raised new ethics concerns regarding the questionable testimony of the so-called "hired gun" experts who offer opinions to agree with the side that hired them. The various controversies reinforced the concerns of the medical profession that the reputations of ethical psychiatrists were sullied by involvement in legal intrigue. Two cases illustrate the fickle application and outcome of the early insanity defenses. The first exemplifies the amorphous definition of insanity that could, because of its non-specific definition, be shaped to apply to a wide variety of circumstances. Dan Sickles, a Democratic congressman from New York, shot and killed his wife's lover, Philip Barton Key (the son of Francis Scott Key) in the park across from the White House. He pleaded temporary insanity and became the first defendant in the United States to be acquitted on this defense. The court ruled, with the help of psychiatric testimony, that the provocation of the illicit affair was sufficient to have caused a state of mind that made him legally non-responsible (in the absence of a mental illness). This ruling foreshadowed the development of what is now a defense of "extreme emotional disturbance," a form of diminished capacity that mitigates but does not negate the culpability of the defendant. But in 1859 at the time of the verdict, the popular press viewed the psychiatric testimony as purchased by a powerful defendant.

In the second case, Charles Guiteau, who shot President Garfield, proffered an insanity defense, unleashing the "battle of the experts" as psychiatrists on either side provided expert testimony addressing the defendant's capacity to understand the wrongfulness of his act. The psychiatric experts for the prosecution and the defense used the same facts of the case and the same psychiatric theory to argue passionately and definitively in support of opposing opinions—that Mr. Guiteau was either fully capable of understanding the wrongfulness of his act or entirely incapable of appreciating that his act was wrong and criminal. Throughout the trial, the experts evoked more controversy than clarity. In the aftermath of Garfield's assassination and the ensuing trial, Congress reacted with their power to the confusing proceedings and created legislation clarifying the meaning of insanity, a legal construct that demands a black—white conclusion about the convoluted, and unusually unknowable, process in a troubled mind. Guiteau's conviction and execution in 1882 seemed more the result of public outrage over the assassination than the result of any consensus regarding the degree of insanity required for criminal responsibility, a concept that remains as murky and political in 2006 as it was more than a century ago. The rare and sensational cases raised suspicion over the role of psychiatry in the courtroom and did little to shape a sub-specialty with standards and professional oversight.

It was the changing view of psychiatric illness and psychiatric patients that laid the foundation for what is now forensic psychiatry. Indeed, the story of the CMHC and the Law and Psychiatry Division is intricately tied to the changes in how the country has viewed persons with mental illness.

The development of Law and Psychiatry at the CMHC and Yale

The CMHC opened because of a dramatic shift in the care of persons with mental illness—the diagnosis of a psychiatric illness no longer meant lifetime confinement in a psychiatric institution. Although advances in psychopharmacology with the creation of new medications decreased many of the symptoms of the more severe psychotic and depressive disorders, the civil rights movement of the 1960s ended the permissive hospitalization of psychiatric patients that had existed long before the 1700s.

Through the middle ages, asylums warehoused the "undesirables" throughout Europe. The confinement included no treatment; people with mental illness and retardation and often with physical infirmities were sealed off from public view and left to die. The early hospitals for the mentally ill minimally improved their living conditions, but had no means of treating the mental disease. Restraints and isolation were common methods of control. In the early 1800s, prisons served as the new asylums; they were cheaper and not much worse than hospitals. Reforms were minimal, and patients were confined for life.

The Dorothea Dix movement in the United States, in the 1840s, brought an end to the incarceration of persons solely on the basis of mental illness by creating accessible state hospitals. This first substantial reform transferred persons with mental illness from jails and almshouses to hospitals, but the lack of effective treatment for psychiatric illnesses through the 1940s made confinement of persons with mental illness the sole and necessary choice in the public's view. Confinement was used less to treat than to ostracize patients in order to protect the comfort and safety of others. Cure was neither expected nor possible.

In the first half of the 20th century, advances in psychiatry optimistically marked the era of "curability" of mental illness. But the bright promise of cure and treatment was soon tarnished. As the numbers of persons confined in mental hospitals increased and cures were far less frequent than expected, the state hospitals became holding environments that still served the public interest of isolation rather than patient welfare.

Through the 1960s, the legal standard for commitment to a mental hospital was largely permissive: a claim of mental illness by any interested party, professional or private, was often enough to commit a person who then had the burden of proving sanity in order to gain release. In the courts the perception of insanity rather than specific psychiatric documentation of severe illness was enough to institutionalize a person for life. A notable example of the permissive commitment standards concerned

Elizabeth Packard, the wife of a minister, who in 1864 had been hospitalized for three years in a mental hospital under an Illinois statute that permitted the hospitalization of wives without any requirement that evidence of insanity be offered. Although Ms. Packard began a crusade to reform the laws of commitment, her efforts had minimal long-term impact, and commitment laws remained permissive through the mid-20th century.

Most states had statutes similar to that found in Connecticut, where commitment requirements were that a patient be "mentally ill"—broadly defined as a "mental or emotional condition that had adverse effects on the individual's behavior"—and that the person be "a fit subject for confinement." This standard indicated that the legislatures were comfortable letting physicians decide, with minimal judicial oversight, who was appropriate to be committed to a mental hospital. In Connecticut, during the 1960s, an emergency commitment certificate could be signed by a single physician and was sufficient to hold a patient for 30 days before review by a probate court. Civil commitment by the probate court could confine a patient indefinitely.

A growing number of Americans experienced lengthy hospitalizations. During the peak of psychiatric institutionalization in the mid-1950's, when the U.S. census was around 166 million (Daily Almanac, 1955, 2006), 560,000 or one in three Americans were confined in mental hospitals (Brilliant Madness, 2006). The lengthy hospitalizations of a growing number of patients in state institutions that were supported by inadequate state funding led to the state mental hospitals' being characterized as total institutions and "snake pits." The civil rights movement of the 1960s fanned the winds of change, and commitment laws became a main target for reform. The political climate emphasized the right to be different and psychiatry was accused of labeling persons as sick simply because they did not conform. Thomas Szasz, a popular theorist of the day, argued that persons with mental illness did not have actual pathology, but were merely showing a human variation and, therefore, should not be involuntarily treated or institutionalized. He argued that if they broke the law, they should be arrested and afforded the same due process as all Americans charged with crimes.

Patient's rights and the treatment of persons with psychiatric illness became a legal matter and a focus for attorneys across the country who worked toward the goal of abolishing civil commitment. There was growing professional and public consensus that the laws needed to be changed, and the time was ripe. The herculean challenge was to craft laws that simultaneously protected patients, the public and civil rights. It was this challenge that coincided with the development of forensic psychiatry at Yale.

Forensic psychiatry emerges at the CMHC

The CMHC opened in the wake of the civil rights movement of the mid-1960s, when challenges to both the substantive and procedural requirements for the civil commitment of patients with mental disorders were gaining momentum. Across the country in the growing frenzy toward new, more restrictive civil commitment legislation, psychiatry became concerned that the legal and political views were ignoring the brain disorders that resulted in altered moods and behavior. Although psychiatrists wished to have their opinions represented, psychiatry and the law seemed to speak different languages, and few psychiatrists wanted to deal with attorneys or were prepared to write legislation.

In the mid-1970s, Yale Law School students, supervised by faculty, began to represent patients at the civil commitment hearings held at the Connecticut Valley Hospital (CVH), the largest of three public mental hospitals with a census of almost 3000 patients. Howard Zonana, a new faculty member in psychiatry at the Yale School of Medicine, joined the endeavor. As a young psychiatrist and scientist, he found the law both perplexing and compelling. Unlike many of his senior physician colleagues, he was not afraid to venture into legal territory. He began to spend time at the Yale Law School, consulting with those faculty and students representing patients at civil commitment hearings. The consultation was mutually beneficial—as Zonana learned about the legal process, the lawyers were introduced to the complexity of mental illness from a psychiatric perspective.

While Zonana worked with the law students applying the laws, he appreciated the need for psychiatry to have a voice in the shaping of the laws themselves. To learn about the legislative process, he joined the small legislative committee of the Connecticut Psychiatric Society (a district branch of the American Psychiatric Association). His comfort with legal matters was obvious to the other members and he was soon asked to chair the committee. That position gave him the opportunity to review and suggest changes to the legislative drafting committee working on the new psychiatric commitment legislation. In his position as chair, he interacted directly with Eric Plaut, then Commissioner of the Connecticut State Department of Mental Health. The two psychiatrists began a fruitful collaboration that lasted until Commissioner Plaut's retirement in 1981.

Although Zonana's impact on the legislation and application of laws affecting persons with mental illness would unfold over several decades, his forays into the legal and legislative arenas had an immediate effect in the school of medicine. His enthusiasm for the role of psychiatry in the law was obvious as he shared his experiences with medical students, residents and colleagues. Although not aware of it at the time, he was sowing the seeds of the Forensic Psychiatry Fellowship.

The Forensic Psychiatry Fellowship: keystone of Law and Psychiatry

The future fellowship in forensic psychiatry began modestly as an elective training program in forensic work for second-year psychiatric residents at the CMHC in 1973–74. The program and the work on the civil commitment revisions began at about the same time. The de-institutionalization of persons with mental illness meant that communities needed new initiatives to provide services and support. Funding was available for community-oriented consultation programs. Marc Rubenstein, Attorney Lansing Crane of the Yale Law School and Zonana studied the new legislation and community initiatives and published their findings (Crane et al., 1977; Rubenstein et al., 1977). Based on their work, the team began teaching a course for second-year residents. This made Yale one of only a handful of medical schools in the country that offered any training in forensic psychiatry, which was not yet a recognized sub-specialty in psychiatry. Through 1978 psychiatry residents were offered an elective experience in legal matters in psychiatry.

In 1979 Zonana and Attorney Lansing Crane took over as core faculty and obtained a training grant from the National Institute of Mental Health (NIMH) to begin a fellowship in forensic psychiatry for psychiatrists who had completed their psychiatry residency. The newly launched fellowship required opportunities for the psychiatric fellows to practice forensic psychiatry. Coincidentally, a new statute was passed by the Connecticut legislature establishing three regional court clinics created to perform competency-to-stand-trial evaluations, court-ordered evaluation of defendants to assure their capacity to understand proceedings and participate in their defense. A demonstration program in Hartford showed that a team of a psychiatrist, psychologist and social worker was able to do these evaluations efficiently, and team members became proficient in learning both the procedures and the legal standards (Herron et al., 1983).

Zonana and Crane received state funding to develop a fourth court clinic to perform competency-to-stand-trial evaluations for New Haven and the surrounding region. This funding provided salary for two faculty and two support staff and launched the Law and Psychiatry Division of the Department of Psychiatry at Yale. Over the years, that program has grown into the present Law and Psychiatry Division, with ten faculty, six clinicians and five support staff.

The core of the Law and Psychiatry Division has remained the forensic psychiatry fellowship. To provide rich and extensive opportunities for the fellows, faculty have, over the years, developed an ongoing collaboration with a number of Yale, state and national organizations, and have cultivated myriad training program placement sites. The collaboration generates consultations and cases for fellows in the program. As the program has expanded, its scope of influence has reached beyond Connecticut to become an internationally recognized center for education and consultation in forensic psychiatry.

The partnership between Law and Psychiatry and the Yale Law School is one cornerstone of the fellowship. With an adjunct clinical faculty appointment in the Law School, Zonana co-teaches law students who are involved in practica through law school clinics. Other Law and Psychiatry faculty have joined in the teaching and supervise law students when psychiatric and psychological factors are central to their cases. The close connection with the law school has afforded residents and forensic fellows opportunities to consult to and teach law students who are representing a variety of clients, including individuals seeking asylum in the U.S., children with disabilities, persons with mental illness who face housing evictions, and prisoners with claims relating to their mental disorders (e.g., inmates raped by guards, state habeas claims, deliberate indifference to mental and physical health needs). In the law school clinics, the psychiatric fellows provide consultation in a number of different ways. They provide evaluations of clients, prepare reports and testify in court when required. They offer training in clinical interviewing techniques and consult with the law students and law school faculty regarding the meaning and content of the medical and psychiatric records relating to the client. They lecture on psychiatric diagnoses and psychotropic medications.

The consultation provides the psychiatric fellows with an extensive orientation to legal matters as they participate in law school classes that introduce them to legal theory and reasoning. The participation of psychiatric fellows in the classes also provides a perspective on how lawyers are educated and the difference between law and medicine.

As part of the collaboration with the law school, psychiatric residents and fellows also participate as experts in the Law School Trial Practice course with classes devoted to jury selection and expert witnesses in preparation for the mock trial exercise. The practice cases for the trials have involved variable criminal and civil matters including the assessments of psychological harm resulting from trauma, and the insanity defense offered to a charge of murder. In the role of "expert," residents and fellows undergo direct and cross-examination by the law students. An experienced judge or attorney, along with the faculty, reviews and critiques their testimony and the performance of the law students. Law and Psychiatry's extensive and mutually beneficial affiliation with the law school has become a model for other forensic psychiatry programs and demonstrates an effective method for integrating legal and psychiatric theory into practice.

Expansion of the fellowship in partnership with the State of Connecticut

The fellowship has expanded enrollment from one to four psychiatric fellows each year. Zonana, director of the fellowship, and Michael Norko, deputy director, oversee 20 full-and part-time faculty who teach seminars and provide clinical supervision in a variety of settings. The expansion of the fellowship was possible primarily through an affiliation with the State of Connecticut which has provided an extensive array of practice, consulting, teaching and research opportunities. The connection between Law and Psychiatry and the State of Connecticut was formalized in the late 1970s when Connecticut's Department of Mental Health (DMH, which was redesigned as the Department of Mental Health and Addiction Services [DMHAS] in 1995) agreed to fund the stipends required for the fellowship in exchange for the fellows' spending one and one-half to two days a week of direct service in a state facility. The initial agreement with the DMH allowed the program to expand from one to two fellows. Over the past 5 to 10 years, the Department of Correction (DOC) and the Department of Children and Families (DCF) have also participated in funding under the same agreement, allowing the program to expand to its current level of four fellows a year, including one child psychiatrist interested in child and adolescent forensic psychiatry. The partnership between the state and Law and Psychiatry has been mutually beneficial, serving as an important recruitment opportunity for the state. As a result of the experience in their fellowship year, many of the fellows have elected to accept employment in these state facilities following their year of forensic training. These positions have been made more attractive by the offer of a clinical faculty appointment at Yale if they continue to participate in the training program by teaching and supervising medical students, psychiatry residents and fellows.

In turn, the Law and Psychiatry Fellowship benefits from the association with the state and its many opportunities for placement. Fellows are involved in the Whiting Forensic Division, the maximum security unit of the CVH. At Whiting, patients include insanity acquittees, defendants with high bonds who were found incompetent to stand trial, and civil patients deemed too dangerous to be hospitalized in other psychiatric inpatient services. There are also step-down, medium-security units at the CVH where patients stay before being released to the community. The CVH now has a number of consulting forensic psychiatrists (CFPs)—almost all of whom are ex-fellows—who perform forensic evaluations of insanity acquittees prior to their hearings before the Psychiatric Security Review Board (PSRB), an independent administrative body that is authorized to monitor and approve of any change in status of insanity acquittees. The CFPs also do risk assessments when requested by other DMHAS-supported facilities. Fellows in training accompany a CFP on an evaluation and later have the opportunity to perform some of these evaluations independently as well. Other state facility placements have included the women's prison at York Correctional Institution, which houses 1400 pretrial and sentenced inmates (up from 300 inmates in the late 1980s), 700–900 of whom are prescribed psychotropic medication.

Within the DCF, fellows have been placed at Riverview Hospital, an inpatient children's hospital that also admits youths found incompetent to stand trial, and at the Connecticut Juvenile Training School (CJTS), a secure facility for young adolescents with charges in the juvenile courts. Opened in August 2001, CJTS is a 240-bed secure facility for adjudicated male delinquents committed to the department by the superior court for juvenile matters. The facility includes an assessment unit, parole revocation unit, special needs unit, general population buildings, and space for education, vocational and recreational programming. Upon arrival at CJTS, all youths receive a comprehensive assessment, including medical, dental, mental health, substance abuse and educational assessments. A new point-level system helps them chart their progress on a daily basis and as they move through the program. Other core programming (e.g., cognitive behavioral therapy and anger replacement training) play a critical part of each youth's treatment program. Reintegration planning and activities, including the active involvement of community service providers, occur throughout a youth's stay at the facility. All youths, upon return to the community, participate in an aftercare program that provides ongoing supervision and continuation of services in keeping with each youth's risk and needs assessment.

Fellows are also assigned to treat patients in prisons or at the maximum security treatment settings where insanity acquittees are hospitalized. Collectively, they perform extensive evaluations of approximately 40 cases a year in both civil and criminal courts (e.g., criminal responsibility, pre-sentence, malpractice, workers compensation, employment termination cases under the Americans with Disabilities Act).

In a unique placement that was first developed by Law and Psychiatry, fellows have a placement with prosecutors (state's attorneys) and with federal public defenders to gain a perspective on criminal due process and to consult with attorneys in a wide variety of cases involving mental health issues. The New Haven state's attorneys have included both Arnold Markle and Michael Dearington over a 30-year period. Mary Galvin, the state's attorney in Milford has also been teaching in the program for 25 years. These placements expose the fellows to a view of the legal system from a victim's perspective as well as to an introduction to the criminal justice system by observing plea negotiations, sentencing, the testimony of other expert witnesses, and the ways that prosecutors investigate and prepare for trial.

A placement in the federal defender's office in New Haven under the direction of Attorney Paul Thomas allows the fellows to follow criminal cases in the federal courts, which have different rules and procedures from the state courts. This placement dates to 1995, when Thomas joined the faculty of Law and Psychiatry, replacing Crane.

Fellows interested in child forensic psychiatry are placed in the prosecutor's office at the New Haven Superior Court for Juvenile Matters, under the direction of Attorney Cathy Edwards. This has permitted them to be exposed to Connecticut's juvenile justice system and detention centers. As a result of the collaboration with the juvenile system, Law and Psychiatry has performed competency-to-stand-trial evaluations for children in that system, and fellows have developed restoration programming for the DCF.

Professional contributions of fellows in Law and Psychiatry

Each year psychiatrists enter the fellowship new to the field of forensics and complete the program as beginning experts in the field. Since the program began, 55 psychiatrists will have completed the forensic fellowship as of the end of the 2006–07 academic year (see Table 3.1).

The graduates have contributed to the field of forensic psychiatry in many ways. Most have become active in the American Academy of Psychiatry and the Law (AAPL), the major organization of the sub-specialty. Founded in 1969, it has been the leading organization for the developing field. Over the past 25 years, the AAPL developed a sub-specialty board examination and later achieved formal recognition for forensic psychiatry as a sub-specialty by the American Psychiatric Association, the Accreditation Council for Graduate Medical Education and, most recently, the American Board of Psychiatry and Neurology.

Four of our faculty and fellows have been elected president of the academy: Zonana, Ezra Griffith, Roy O'Shaughnessy and Robert Phillips. Others have served as elected officers and councilors, and a number have become training directors and faculty of forensic psychiatry programs around the country.

The contributions of the fellows and the faculty have established the Yale fellowship as one of the premier programs in the country attracting psychiatrists from across the United States and Canada. The philosophy, values and contributions of the Yale program have shaped and defined the field of forensic psychiatry. That influence has come largely through the success of the forensic fellowship program.

The Law and Psychiatry Division also maintains a national reputation for excellence in the practice of forensic psychiatry. The division attracts high-profile cases through its reputation as a premier program, providing credible, respected, and expert consultation and evaluations in criminal and civil cases, policy development, and education. The division's role continues to expand through the work of its faculty and graduates and through referrals from a variety of professionals seeking advice on myriad legal and clinical questions in both criminal and civil law. The breadth and uniqueness of the referred cases contribute to the intellectual development, commitment and vitality of the division. In turn, thorough, creative and thoughtful consultation has garnered the respect of attorneys and judges, legislators and professional colleagues.

Table 3.1   Graduates of the Law and Psychiatry Forensic Psychiatry Fellowship Program by year of graduation

1980	1992	2001
Roy O'Shaughnessey	Debra Lambert DePrato	Humberto Temporini
		Michael Champion
		Vladimir Coric
1981	1993	2002
George Drinka	J. Leslie Kurt	Charles Dike
		Sabita Rahti
		Charles A. Morgan, III
1982	1994	2003
John Young	Deborah Giorgi-Guarnieri	William Campbell
	Paul Amble	Victoria Dreisbach
		Carolyn Drazinic
		Frank Fortunati
1983	1995	2004
Richard Belitsky	Todd Alford	Patricia Kelly
	Rahn Bailey	Varun Choudhary
		Sarghi Sharma
1984	1996	2005
Paula Bortnichak	Arlene Rivera-Mass	Michele Schaefer
	Karen Brody	Charles Saldanha
		Jerome Nwokike
		Theodore Mueller
1986	1997	2006
David London*	Sonya Lee	Bobby Singh
	Catherine Lewis	Vinneth Carvalho
		Curtis Cassidy
		Shaheen Darani
1987	1998	2007
Ann Hoeffer*	Teresa Stathas	Sarah Xavier
	Brenda Planck	Christine Naungayan
		Sameer Patel
		Kevin Trueblood
1987	1999	
Kenneth Appelbaum	Patrick Fox	
	Joseph Penn	
1988	2000	
Janet Williams	Paul Whitehead	
Michael Norko	Tonya Foreman	
1989		
Merrill Rotter		
1990		
Jeffrey Gottlieb		
1991		
Elaine Becher		

* Did fellowship on half-time basis over 2 years

Not all the teaching done by Law and Psychiatry occurs within the academic programs at Yale and the CMHC. Law and Psychiatry has developed an extensive repertoire of training programs related to forensic matters and mental health. Faculty, with fellow participation, have developed curricula and presentations for a variety of audiences including staff of the DMHAS, judges and attorneys, probation department, police departments, schools and other non-DMHAS mental health agencies. Reflecting the varied expertise in the department and the breadth of the discipline, topics have encompassed civil and criminal law, risk assessment, and practice and ethics matters.

Perhaps the most enduring and prestigious role that Law and Psychiatry has played in the profession has been in defining the work and setting the standards for forensic psychiatry. The leadership in the division has been involved in major legislation and policy development. Much of this work comes through the professional organizations in medicine, psychiatry and forensic psychiatry. From the inception of the AAPL in 1972, division faculty have been in leadership positions. The AAPL entered the Service and Specialty Society of the American Medical Association in 1997—with Phillips and Zonana as delegate and alternate delegate to the House of Delegates—when the organization was formally given a seat with voting privileges. The AAPL thereby gained a voice in developing the AMA's ethics guidelines and new policies that affect the subspecialty. Yale's delegation has become an integral part of the Psychiatric Caucus (comprising the American Psychiatric Association, American Academy of Child Psychiatry, Addictions and Geriatrics, and Military Psychiatry) that has shaped policies on the insanity defense, expert witnesses, interrogation of detainees by psychiatrists and review of expert testimony.

Since 1995 Zonana has served as only the second medical director in the organization's history. Ezra Griffith is editor of the *Journal of the American Academy of Psychiatry and the Law* and Michael Norko is the deputy editor. A number of Law and Psychiatry faculty serve on the editorial board of the journal. Law and Psychiatry faculty have also served on numerous committees and commissions and have received awards honoring their leadership and contributions to the specialty of forensic psychiatry.

Scholarship and research in Law and Psychiatry

Scholarship and research, hallmarks of a university department, developed in many directions in Law and Psychiatry, including formal instruction, faculty research and special programs. Under the tutelage of Ezra Griffith and Madelon Baranoski, the Seminar for Scholarship in Forensic Psychiatry guides psychiatry fellows and residents, psychology doctoral students, social work students and faculty in the exploration of the theory and practice of forensic work. Experienced lawyers, state and federal judges, and international forensic experts participate with the fellows in examining forensic constructs in theory and practice. Case studies are examined from historical, cultural and practical perspectives to engender an understanding of the complexity of forensic psychiatry as grounded in medical science but practiced in a social, cultural and legal context. Faculty participate in the seminar by directing modules focused on constructs relevant to practice and scholarship in forensic psychiatry. Alec Buchanan explores with fellows and faculty theoretical and empirical psychiatric jurisprudence, defined as the philosophy of law as it applies to the mentally disordered. He incorporates in his teaching the results of his empirical research on the assessment of "mental incapacity" in persons with mental disorders involved in both civil and criminal cases (Buchanan, 2000). Patrick Fox presents the foundation for the ethics of research on human subjects and psychiatric practice. In conjunction with a seminar on psychiatry in the public sector, he also presents the social, policy, and legislative influences on the practice and development of forensic psychiatry.

Unique to the Yale program is a formal examination of performance as a critical aspect of forensic psychiatrists' expertise. The seminar emphasizes the obligation of a forensic psychiatrist to communicate expertise with integrity and persuasion to clients, colleagues, attorneys, judges, juries and the public. The capstone of the seminar is a mock trial exercise in which fellows testify as experts on either side of a forensic case. A state judge presides as expert defense attorneys and prosecutors examine and cross-examine the fellows. In a de-briefing, faculty critique the performance of the fellows. This mock trial exercise provides a full dress rehearsal of case formulation and expert testimony.

Legal scholarship critical to forensic psychiatry is presented in the Landmark Cases Seminar. Developed by Zonana and Crane, the seminar, now taught by Zonana and Linda Lager, a Connecticut superior court judge, reviews United States Supreme Court and lower court decisions that shape laws related to civil commitment of persons with mental illness, the death penalty, the insanity defense and other forensic issues. Instruction by a judge and a psychiatrist exposes the fellows to legal thinking and to two different and sometimes divergent perspectives.

Fellows also participate in scholarship and research of their own, developing areas of interest or participating in ongoing faculty research. During the fellowship year, many psychiatrists and psychologists prepare presentations and papers for the annual meeting of the American Academy of Psychiatry and the Law.

Yochelson Visiting Professorship

The annual Yochelson Visiting Professorship and the Dr. Samuel and Kathryn Yochelson Lecture provide a unique opportunity for formally celebrating the forensic psychiatry program and promoting scholarship. The professorship and lecture are funded through an endowment by the Yochelson family. Yochelson was a Yale-educated psychologist and psychiatrist, best known as the senior author of *The Criminal Personality* (Yochelson and Samenow, 1976). The book presents research done by the authors at St. Elisabeth's Hospital in Washington, D.C., on 255 male criminals who were patients on the prisoner unit of the hospital. The authors concluded in their book that in order to reduce criminal behavior in persons with a criminal personality, interventions to change criminal thinking rather than permissive rehabilitation are required.

Through the professorship, a distinguished scholar in forensic psychiatry spends a week giving major lectures and seminars at the CMHC and the CVH. Meeting with the fellows, the scholars also describe their own career trajectories in forensic psychiatry. The scholars have included Bernard Diamond, Alan Stone, Alan Dershowitz, Paul Appelbaum, the team of Lauren Roth, Darrel Regier, Peter Reddaway and Richard

Bonnie, that consulted to the Soviet Union on forensic psychiatry in 1989; John Monahan, Joseph Bloom, Robert Simon and Pamela Taylor.

The Yochelson activities showcase Law and Psychiatry, the CMHC, Yale and the DMHAS. The visiting professorship and lectures, along with participation in the American Academy of Psychiatry and the Law, acculturate the fellows into the international community of forensic psychiatry and acquaint them with cutting-edge expertise and research.

Research in Law and Psychiatry

As part of Yale University, Law and Psychiatry is involved in advancing knowledge and practice in forensic psychiatry and psychology through research. Through federal, state and university grants, investigations have explored the characteristics and aftercare of persons acquitted of criminal offenses by reason of insanity, the epidemiology of mental illness in prisons, characteristics of persons charged with sexual offenses, the nature of psychiatric risk and risk assessment, the accuracy of eyewitness accounts, the detection of lying and malingering, methods and effects of introducing mediation in child custody proceedings, and the effects of jail diversion initiatives on criminal and psychiatric recidivism. These research projects, directed by Law and Psychiatry faculty, have resulted in changes in practice, policy development and further investigations.

In 2005, Caroline Easton received a research grant from the National Institute of Drug Abuse (NIDA) to develop and test an integrated intervention to decrease both domestic violence and addictive behaviors through individual and couples therapy. Based on results from pilot projects funded by the Donaghue Foundation and the Psychotherapy Development Center at Yale's Division of Substance Abuse, the study is testing the substance abuse-domestic violence therapy (SADV) approach, which had significantly reduced alcohol use and aggressive behavior in men arrested for domestic violence (Easton and Devine, 2001). Easton is also conducting a related clinical trial to assess the efficacy of cognitive behavioral therapy (CBT) combined with contingency management (CM) interventions for young adults who are dependent on marijuana and have criminal justice involvement (Easton et al., 2000). The results from earlier studies that utilized both CBT and CM strategies suggest that payment for compliance enhances engagement and increases the efficacy of social and therapeutic services. These studies are part of a program of research by Easton to investigate the relationship between substance use and criminal behavior (Easton, 2005) and effective interventions to interrupt the addictive and behavioral patterns.

Vladimir Coric and Zonana are investigating the neurophysiology of sexual deviance in an effort to identify diagnostic profiles that will aid in developing appropriate treatments. The long-term objective of the study involves neuron imaging to determine possible loci of pathology for (at least some of) those behaviors. In the first stages of the research, the investigators have established a laboratory to conduct penile plethysmography and Abel Screen Assessments of persons who show deviant sexual behaviors.

Charles Morgan has conducted investigations on the accuracy of recall in soldiers involved in the elite Special Forces (Morgan et al., 2004). His team has demonstrated that under stress, accuracy of facial recognition decreases in general, but is also influenced by individual stress reactions. His research is relevant to accuracy of eye-witness accounts in criminal case testimony. Morgan has also developed a program of research to investigate the detection of deception. The U.S. Department of Defense and Department of Homeland Security have funded investigations of non-invasive and reliable means of evaluating the veracity of information. In studies involving students and military personnel, Morgan and his team are investigating both physiological measures and language and word patterns that can distinguish between truthful and false statements. In 2006, Coric, in collaboration with Morgan, received a two-year grant from the Department of Defense to investigate methods of analysis to identify factors associated with false statements.

Marsha Kline Pruett and Kyle Pruett (of the Yale Child Study Center), with a five-year State of Connecticut grant from the Department of Justice, developed and evaluated a mediation program for parents involved in divorce proceedings. The intervention employs both conflict resolution and guided parenting support to foster paternal involvement in decision-making and child rearing. The preliminary evaluation indicated that courts, attorneys and parents expressed strong satisfaction with the intervention.

Rani Desai, an epidemiologist, has directed a number of studies that evaluate the effectiveness of programs for defendants with mental illness. Her research addresses one of the unintended consequences of the efforts to deinstitutionalize people with mental illness—an increase in the rate of incarceration of those with mental illness (Torrey et al., 1992). Desai, in collaboration with Baranoski, conducted a comprehensive study of all individuals arraigned in New Haven Superior Court over a five-year period. The epidemiologic evidence indicated that about 40% of those arraigned had a history of contact with the mental health system, many of them for substance abuse treatment or evaluation (Hoff et al., 1999a, 1999b).

In the late 1990s, Michael Hoge obtained a contract to provide mental health services to juvenile detention facilities throughout Connecticut. Desai, Hoge and researchers in the Court Support Services Division (the state judicial branch responsible for juvenile detention) embarked on a line of research on mental health care services in juvenile detention facilities. First, the team identified that despite a clear need for mental health services in detention, few services were offered, and an evidence base for appropriate services for this population was lacking (Desai et al., 2006). More recently the team is studying the phenomenon of disproportionate minority confinement (DMC); first finding that violence risk was not a determinant of DMC and then that mental health status did not mediate the association between race and perceived violence risk. They continue to investigate whether violence risk assessments accurately predict criminal justice recidivism (Chapman et al., 2006a, 2006b).

Paul Amble, working with attorneys and the Waterbury Mental Health Authority, is evaluating an intervention to help persons with mental illness who are determined by the probate court to need a conservator because of the severity of their mental illness. The conservator assumes control of major life decisions for the person during a specified period of time. The intervention assigns a case manager to those conserved to enhance their understanding of the process, their compliance with treatment and their access to other resources. Goals of the intervention are to promote return to independent control over life decisions such that he or she may ultimately be released from conservatorship and to facilitate communication between the mental health agency, the conservator and the client. The preliminary results of the study show that clients, probate court judges and conservators report satisfaction with the intervention. Since the intervention has been in place, more attorneys—the most common non-family conservators—are willing to serve in the role. Therefore, more clients who require the supervision of a conservator are able to be served with a shorter waiting list.

The division's impact on public psychiatry

Although the most significant impact of the Law and Psychiatry Division, like all academic institutions, will come through the education of the students, the division has had direct influence on the profession and on the delivery of psychiatric services. The relationship between the Law and Psychiatry Division and the DMHAS has been a model for an inter-dependent and mutually advantageous relationship. In general, the state has contributed to the financial support of the tripartite mission of the university (research, training and service), and Law and Psychiatry has contributed to the state's mission (delivery of quality mental health and addiction services) by providing consultation and staffing for state facilities from among its graduates.

Law and Psychiatry's contributions to DMHAS

The CMHC evolved in response to new demands posed by psychiatric clients. In the 1980s, administration of the CMHC debated, in accordance with the psychotherapy model, whether the Center could or should serve patients caught up in the criminal justice system. The argument against including persons with active criminal charges invoked the separation of legal and therapy matters: psychotherapy was for curing and managing mental illness in a protected and private relationship and legal matters were for the court. Just twenty years later, such a debate would seem frivolous. Over 50% of the CMHC clients are involved in the criminal justice system; the same is true for most public psychiatric services around the state and country. A large proportion of patients at the CVH are there as insanity acquittees or for restoration of competency to stand trial. When they are discharged to the community, their forensic involvement increases the complexity of caring for them. The question is no longer whether the CMHC should see clients with legal involvement. The new questions are more complicated: how best to help clients deal with legal problems, what principles will best guide the interface between clinical and legal domains, what skills and interventions are necessary to navigate the new terrain?

Law and Psychiatry helped the CMHC develop policy and interventions as the number of forensic clients increased and as the mission for mental health evolved to include clients who are mandated for treatment, diverted from jail, or evaluated to answer a legal question. The wisdom of the CMHC to include a division that focused on the complexities of the interface between the law and mental health has been substantially rewarded.

The contribution of Law and Psychiatry reached beyond the CMHC. Mental health services across Connecticut were faced with the changing population of clients seeking services through public psychiatry. The influence of the division has increased substantially as the proportion of state mental health services for forensic clients has grown to become the major portion of long-term services and inpatient care. A number of forensic fellowship graduates and faculty (Amble, Buchanan and Fox) have taken positions with the state as consulting forensic psychiatrists performing evaluations of insanity acquittees, risk assessments around the state and competency-to-stand-trial evaluations.

Law and Psychiatry also provides training and consultation for new state professional staff (psychiatrists, social workers and psychologists) assigned to conduct forensic assessments and evaluations. The division consults with the DMHAS and the Connecticut legislature regarding pending mental health legislation.

The position of Director of Forensic Services, Department of Mental Health was created in 1986. Since its inception the position has been staffed by members of the Yale faculty who came from the Department of Psychiatry's residency program or from our Law and Psychiatry Division. Robert Phillips became the first director of Forensic Services and was concurrently named director of Whiting Forensic Institute (now Division), the DMHAS maximum security facility. The next two directors came from positions in Law and Psychiatry. In 1989 Deborah Scott became Deputy Director of Forensic Services; she assumed the position of director in 1993. In 1994 Gail Sturges became director of Forensic Services and remained in that position through September 2006. Of note, 19 of the 51 physician graduates of the Forensic Psychiatry Fellowship program have taken positions in Connecticut's mental health, correction and child welfare systems after graduating from the program. These Law and Psychiatry psychiatrists have been well prepared for both staff and leadership roles in the state programs. Norko has served as medical director of the Whiting Forensic Division, the maximum security unit of CVH, where persons found not guilty by reason of insanity are hospitalized. Charles Dike, another program graduate, was appointed medical director of that division in 2006.

Psychiatry Security Review Board: Aftercare and supervision of insanity acquittees

On March 30, 1981, John Hinckley shot President Ronald Reagan. The failed assassination attempt shocked the world. On June 21, 1982, John Hinckley was acquitted on the grounds that he was insane. After a "battle of the experts," the jury deliberated for over three days before reaching the conclusion that the prosecution had not met its burden to prove beyond a reasonable doubt that John Hinckley was sane. The shot that nearly killed the president stunned the world, but the jury's decision had a speedy and lasting effect on insanity defense law across the country. Public outrage spurred Congress and state legislatures to tighten the laws that in the public view had clearly allowed a guilty man to escape punishment. Connecticut joined the cry for reform.

In 1983, at the request of the legislature, Connecticut appointed a law revision commission to review the insanity defense standards and procedures. The commission included Zonana and Jay Katz, both on the faculties of Yale's medical and law schools. Zonana had provided the commission with data that he had compiled about persons found not guilty by reason of insanity in Connecticut during the 1970s.

Zonana continued his investigation of Connecticut's acquittees and created a research collaboration involving post-graduate and graduate students from various departments at Yale. The team applied for a grant to study NGRI acquittees in Connecticut (Zonana et al., 1990a), established the first registry of NGRI acquittees in Connecticut and completed a descriptive study of women acquitted by NGRI defenses (Zonana et al., 1990b). In September 1985, Josephine Buchanan assumed responsibility for the development and maintenance of the registry, which she presently continues to administer, as a research associate with Law and Psychiatry.

The recommendations of the law revision commission resulted in legislation creating an administrative body to review the state's insanity acquittees, to monitor their care and to authorize the transition from maximum security to eventual return to the community for some acquittees. Only the second state—Oregon having been the first—to create such a board, Connecticut imbued the Psychiatric Security Review Board (PSRB) with broad policing powers. The PSRB oversees the care and placement of acquittees and governs the movement from maximum security units at the hospital to step-down units with progressively less security. The ultimate goal is the return of the acquittee to the community. The PSRB authorizes access to the community and approves treatment plans for acquittees on temporary leave or conditional release to the community. The PSRB has the authority to order state police to transport back to the hospital any acquittee who is non-compliant with the treatment plan. The PSRB's authority to re-hospitalize a patient represents the only outpatient commitment of persons with mental illness legislatively authorized in Connecticut. The PSRB is an independent board of governor-appointed professionals and lay members. Griffith was one of the first psychiatrists to serve on the PSRB.

Over the next twenty years, the PSRB and the CVH adopted policies that have resulted in lengthy hospitalizations and restrictive outpatient supervision. The length of confinement has led to a marked drop in the number of defendants who choose to plead insanity. Not surprisingly, given the tight supervision of these acquittees, the rate of criminal recidivism after an NGRI has been very low. The board often requests Law and Psychiatry to perform independent evaluations in challenging cases and the division has provided consultation to other states and commentary on the insanity defense based on the registry of Connecticut's insanity acquittees.

The consultation has been based on ongoing research conducted by faculty of Law and Psychiatry on insanity acquittees. Zonana's team conducted the first post-Hinckley investigation of the insanity defense in Connecticut. The exploratory study found that persons found not guilty by reason of insanity were often lost to follow-up after leaving inpatient care. The research also found that the insanity defense was not "a defense of class privilege" (a belief widely held among professionals and the public) in that the majority of persons acquitted by reason of insanity were of lower social economic status (Zonana et al., 1990c).

Other investigations by Law and Psychiatry faculty demonstrated that NGRI acquittees in Connecticut are committed to the PSRB for a significantly longer time than defendants are sentenced to incarceration after a conviction for the same types of crimes. The insanity defense in Connecticut since 1985 is used primarily for serious felonies as a "defense of last resort." Another investigation identified four phenomenological profiles of familial homicides which included psychotic killing, mercy killing, rebellion-against-authority killing and accidental killing (Lewis et al., 1998).

Coric led research on the factors related to successful integration of acquittees into the community after hospitalization. Substance abuse and personality disorders were related to a higher incidence of failure of conditional release. Tonya Warner, while a psychiatric resident with the division, conducted survival-curve research on acquittees released from commitment to the PSRB. Her findings show that although 25% are re-hospitalized in the first two years after release, less than 5% were rearrested in the first two years, and none of the acquittees in the study was charged with violent offenses (Zonana et al., 1999).

The CMHC Community Forensic Services and the Jail Diversion Program

One day in early September, Jim, a homeless man suffering from paranoid schizophrenia, goes from one empty table to the next at a local coffee shop, eating whatever customers have left behind. A woman complains to the manager who asks Jim to leave. Jim refuses, arguing that he owns the store, Yale University, and New Haven. He "fires" the manager and insults the woman. On the way out, he spits on the ground and curses in front of a mother with two young children. The manager calls the police who detain Jim right outside the shop and charge him with breach of peace, criminal trespass, risk of injury to a minor and resisting arrest. In the past Jim's arrest would trigger a series of events devoid of mental health services. Although he clearly needs treatment, he would go to jail, and the judge would order a competency-to-stand-trial evaluation as a back-door entry into treatment. He would be incarcerated until the evaluation and hearing; then he would be found not competent and be hospitalized for 76 days (on average) while being treated for his psychiatric disorder, attending classes about court proceedings, and generally getting better. At a cost of nearly $45,000, Jim would return to court, have his charges dismissed, and return homeless to the community without follow-up care.

When community mental health services and criminal justice had no formal interface, clients fell into the gap between the two systems. Criminal justice entry into psychiatric services was through a different route with different outcomes. In 1995, Law and Psychiatry took on the challenge presented by Jim and the hundreds of other persons with mental illness who are marginally connected to psychiatric services. The progressive closings during the first half of the 1990s of two of the three large state facilities, Fairfield Hills and Norwich State Hospitals, along with the downsizing of the CVH have forced persons with severe mental illness to make their own way in the community. But much of the money saved by closing the hospitals did not follow the patients to the community. Community services were already overtaxed. The lack of beds for those who need higher levels of care means that more people are now in the community who would have been long-term patients in long-term facilities. Their capacity to survive in the community without running afoul of the criminal justice system is limited; thus, many are arrested for misdemeanors or minor felonies and incarcerated. In Connecticut and elsewhere, the prisons have become the new mental hospitals by default.

Law and Psychiatry developed the New Haven Jail Diversion Program to provide psychiatric assessment, referral and follow-up for persons with severe mental illness who are arrested on minor charges (Baranoski et al., 1996). The program, one of the first three in Connecticut, addressed the problem of an increasing number of persons with mental illness entering the criminal justice system because of behaviors related to their illness, homelessness and poverty. The criminal court had limited access to treatment options except through incarceration and subsequent referral to mental health services in jail and prison or through competency evaluations that had uncertain outcomes with costly inpatient placement and inadequate referral to the community upon discharge. Incarcerating defendants more in need of treatment than punishment contributed to jail overcrowding, ineffective treatment, unsuccessful community reintegration and high criminal recidivism. Law and Psychiatry investigated the extent of the problem and demonstrated that criminal justice proceedings for defendants with serious mental illness but minor crimes provided a backdoor entrance into the mental health system for hard-to-engage clients. The sheer cost of court-accessed treatment was prohibitive and the benefits sparse. The revolving door through the courts to partial treatment and back was ineffective, inefficient and expensive.

Law and Psychiatry launched the New Haven Diversion Program to provide persons with mental illness access to services and to provide judges with alternatives for defendants whose offenses do not warrant jail. The diversion clinicians provide priority assessments and referral to defendants charged with misdemeanors. With the client's permission, a treatment plan can be offered to the court as an alternative to incarceration, sometimes as a means of having charges dismissed outright.

Although the New Haven Diversion Program was one of the initial three programs (with Hartford and Bridgeport) in Connecticut, the influence of the CMHC's Law and Psychiatry Division has shaped the policies and procedures that protect the rights of the clients as mental health patients and criminal defendants; as well, it addresses the risk of violence and criminal recidivism. The early days of the program were filled with challenges: the eager commitment to do "good" was complicated by the "partnership" between mental health and criminal justice. Faculty from Law and Psychiatry became the ad hoc consultants to the statewide program addressing issues of confidentiality, legal standing and clinical management. A new genre of legal and ethical issues arose. Challenges concerning the role and limitations of the clinicians in the court, the confidential status of information collected from the defendant and the means of protecting the defendant's right to refuse treatment required the crafting of specific policies for practice and case review.

Under the leadership of Law and Psychiatry Division faculty, the principles and goals of the program were delineated, and the New Haven program became the primary model for program development and training in the state. Since 1995, national attention to jail diversion has resulted in federally funded grants to study different approaches to diverting persons with mental illness from incarceration to treatment. In 2000, the Connecticut legislature, acknowledging the potential of the jail diversion program to reduce unnecessary incarcerations, passed a law that mandated jail diversion programs in all lower criminal courts in the state.

Shortly after the new legislation, the New Haven Diversion Program expanded to include assessments of inmates with mental illness who are returning to the community on completion of their incarcerations. As the services expanded, the division inaugurated the CMHC Community Forensic Services Program under the direction of Madelon Baranoski. The program encompasses jail diversion and liaison services to inmates who are returning to the community. Referral to treatment and community resources is aimed at reducing criminal recidivism and relapse of psychiatric illness. Based on the success of the jail liaison work in connecting prisoners returning to the community, the DMHAS obtained federal funding to establish the Connecticut Offender Reentry Program (CORP). Through that program, clinicians from the CMHC and similar agencies in Hartford and Bridgeport work with inmates before release to teach life skills and anger management and provide a connection to resources to ease transition back to the community.

The most recent initiative in the CMHC Community Forensic Services provides clinical liaison to the New Haven Police Department to help manage community crises. The faculty also provides training to the police academy on the policing of persons with special needs. The CMHC Community Forensic Program serves between 300 and 400 persons a year and has reduced incarceration for the target group by over 30%. The program serves as a training site for new jail diversion programs and has been recognized for its clinical expertise, protection of civil rights, cost-effectiveness, value to the court and direct benefit to the clients.

In 1998 Linda Frisman, an epidemiologist with the University of Connecticut, and Baranoski along with a team from the DMHAS, obtained a federal grant from the Substance Abuse and Mental Health Services Administration (SAMHSA) to investigate the impact of jail diversion on the Connecticut courts. The study was one of eight research programs in the multi-site study sponsored by SAMHSA. Defendants in Connecticut courts that had diversion services were compared to those in courts without them on selected outcome variables. Satisfaction of court personnel was also evaluated. The results indicated that defendants in courts with diversion spent less time in jail and had fewer re-arrests (Frisman et al., 2006). Court personnel—including the defense, prosecution and judges—expressed strong satisfaction with diversion services. Because of the characteristics of the people served and intensity of the treatment, diversion programs have not increased risk to the public. Rowe and Baranoski (2000) investigated the effectiveness of adding peer support to usual jail diversion and found that such services reduced the need for inpatient treatment.

The New Haven Office of Court Evaluations

In May 2005, Michael Ross, a 46-year-old Cornell University graduate convicted of eight murders of young women in New York and Connecticut, was executed in Connecticut by lethal injection. His execution, which followed a 44-year hiatus in executions in New England, came after a flurry of court hearings concerning Ross's competency to waive his right to all further appeals in his case. Subjected to a number of competency evaluations in the past concerning his capacity to participate in decisions about his sentencing, he had refused to allow his defense team to pursue further appeals that if successful would have commuted his death sentence to life in prison. Michael Norko, on the faculty of Law and Psychiatry, had evaluated Ross's competency in the past and was requested by the State of Connecticut to do so again. This time the question of competency concerned Mr. Ross's capacity to appreciate what was involved in his decision: did he have a rational understanding of the consequences of waiving his right to pursue further legal recourse, or did he have a mental illness that impaired his capacity to make an informed choice? Norko interviewed Ross, reviewed past records, and testified that Ross did have the capacity to make a rational and informed decision; that is, Ross did not suffer from a mental illness that impaired his decision making about his case.

In this and other high-profile cases, the courts have consulted with Law and Psychiatry faculty as recognized experts in the area of competency in criminal proceedings. Beyond offering expertise in high-profile cases, the Law and Psychiatry Division conducts about one-fourth of the competency evaluations ordered by the Connecticut courts.

In 1979 the newly developed Law and Psychiatry unit agreed to direct one of the four court clinics created by DMHAS to conduct court-ordered competency-to-stand-trial evaluations, write reports on those evaluations and testify at competency hearings. The new responsibility of directing the New Haven Court Clinic allowed Law and Psychiatry to add faculty, develop and refine expertise in this area, and provide rich educational opportunities for the forensic psychiatry fellows. Renamed the New Haven Office of Court Evaluations in the 1990s, the office serves eight courts in three judicial districts in central Connecticut, conducting over 200 competency evaluations a year with nearly half requiring testimony in court. It also serves as a training and consultation site for the other three DMHAS-directed offices of court evaluations.

The New Haven Office of Court Evaluations provides the psychiatric forensic fellows with unique clinical and forensic experience. Under the direction of experienced faculty members, they learn to conduct evaluations, write reports and testify in court in a variety of cases. The office of court evaluations is also a training site for forensic psychologists and social workers in graduate programs and for new social workers and psychologists assigned to the other offices of court evaluation.

Following Deborah Scott and Gail Sturges, the first directors of the clinic, both of whom left the division to become director of Forensic Services for Connecticut, Susan Devine is the current director. Under Devine's leadership, consultation to other court clinics has increased and the training of psychiatric fellows, psychology post-doctoral candidates and master-level social work students has grown in scope and organization.

Devine also directed the integration of court-ordered substance-dependence evaluations into the office when the Department of Mental Health and the entity responsible for addiction services merged to become the Department of Mental Health and Addiction Services. Different from competency evaluations, the substance-dependence evaluations—over 150 per year—provide the court with a determination as to whether a defendant was substance dependent at the time of the offense and recommend a referral for treatment when appropriate.

The third type of court-ordered evaluation provided by the office is a pre-sentencing evaluation to determine if a convicted felon has special mental health needs that require a more extensive inpatient evaluation at Whiting Forensic Division before the court sets the sentence. Although these evaluations are few, the cases are complex and require clinical and diagnostic expertise.

A relatively new development in the area of competency to stand trial involves the assessment of children and adolescents arrested on criminal charges. The criminalization of the juvenile justice system, which occurred in the 1980s, shifted the original emphasis of the system from one of advocacy and protection for children (viewing the offending child as one in need of services) to a criminal model of adjudication and punishment. Because children in Connecticut can now face trial in juvenile court, the court is obligated to ascertain their ability to understand the proceedings and assist in their defense. Although the same Connecticut statute governs assessment of competency for children and adults, the question of competency in children is complicated by developmental factors and limited treatment facilities.

Risk assessment, risk management and ethics in psychiatric care

The public perception of persons with mental illness narrowly focuses on the risk for violence. Images of Mr. Westin's shooting guards in the United States Capitol, of Mr. Ferguson's causing carnage in the Long Island railcar, of Mr. Hinckley shooting President Reagan, and of Ms. Yates drowning her five children in Texas crystallize the common misperception that all psychiatric patients will eventually become violent. These rare but tragic cases fuel the development of stigma.

Recent research indicates that persons with severe mental illnesses do pose a moderate increase in risk when they actively experience particular kinds of symptoms. Even then, the risk to the public is significantly below that posed by persons using illicit substances and those driving under the influence of alcohol. Still, the image of violence connected with mental illness persists. The deinstitutionalization of psychiatric patients has made mental illness more visible in the community. Mental health care providers feel the burden of managing risk that is often difficult to assess. In 1999, Norko and Baranoski developed a risk assessment and management curriculum for over 300 clinicians and staff of the Department of Mental Health and Addiction Services. Based on the feedback from participants, the team has expanded the curriculum into a conceptual model that reframes risk assessment and management to focus on a functional assessment of thought organization, emotional modulation and behavioral control. The model, with an exhaustive review of literature on risk assessment (Norko and Baranoski, 2005), has been presented biannually as a course at the AAPL annual meetings and was presented as a master class at the annual meeting of the Forensic Psychiatry Faculty of the Royal College of Psychiatrists in Newcastle, England in 2006.

The burgeoning increase in the number of CMHC clients with criminal justice involvement, the decline in urban neighborhoods, and the growing complexity in laws and policy governing the care of clients with mental health needs have thrust upon Law and Psychiatry an ever-increasing consultative role for the CMHC and the Department of Psychiatry in all forensic matters. As the informal consultation increased, the Center recognized the need for a formal review process. Law and Psychiatry assumed responsibility for establishing a Risk Management Committee. Under the co-leadership of Zonana and Devine, the committee functioned as a forum for reviewing high-risk cases and offering guidance and strategies to manage risk factors.

Although the Risk Management Committee was dissolved as a formal committee in 2001, Zonana and Devine continue to review high-risk cases and, in the event of a critical incident involving patient or staff, conduct a peer review to analyze the factors that contributed to the event with the goal of prevention and improved risk management.

Law and Psychiatry faculty and forensic fellows participate in individual risk assessment and management consultations for the Center. These assessments focus on the management of risk factors and strategies for enhancing clients' chances of being safely re-integrated into the community.

As the clientele of the CMHC increased in complexity, so did the roles of psychiatry, social work, nursing and psychology. The new programs, such as the Assertive Community Treatment (ACT) team, Jail Diversion, and the Outreach and Engagement team were forging ahead in uncharted therapeutic territory. Ethics questions about practice, roles and boundaries increased with the work.

In response, the CMHC Ethics Committee was formed in 1996. Drawing on Zonana's experience as a member of the Yale-New Haven Hospital Ethics Committee, the CMHC leadership charged its new committee with the mission of supporting clinicians through a review of complex ethics questions that arise in practice. Zonana served as the first chair. Since 2002 Griffith and Devine have co-chaired the committee. The committee has reviewed issues as diverse as the ethics involved in accepting novelty items like pens and calendars from drug companies to the balance between patient privacy and rights and safety in proposed policies that require clients to sign in and show identification at the CMHC entrance.

A place of excellence now and for the future

Law and Psychiatry began with one new psychiatrist curious about the nexus between law and mental health. What emerged from the initial forays into the legislative committees and the law school was a new dimension in psychiatry. What began as an interest grew into a discipline. Law and Psychiatry advanced through a multi-disciplinary faculty that attracted bright, compassionate, creative, risk-taking experts in mental health who carved a path of policy, standards and principles through uncharted territory.

Law and Psychiatry has always been a vital, productive, ever-expanding division in the CMHC but its impact reaches far beyond the Center and New Haven through the contributions of the graduates of the program. The fifty-one forensic psychiatrists educated in Law and Psychiatry now practice in 20 states and Canada; a number of them have developed or now direct forensic psychiatry programs. The significance of Law and Psychiatry can also be measured by its reputation among colleagues, perhaps the most difficult group to impress, and its invitational involvement in critical national and international debates.

Perhaps the strongest legacy of Law and Psychiatry is found within the CMHC itself. As Law and Psychiatry evolved from a small sub-specialty practice to a multifaceted program, the nature of psychiatric practice itself was also evolving. Forensic clients, once in the minority, now represent the majority of clients in public psychiatric services. Law and Psychiatry led the CMHC and the state as they adapted to the changing character of public psychiatry. But the story is far from complete. As the face of the CMHC clients continue to change, as forensic issues become more complex, Law and Psychiatry will also evolve and continue to refine its mission, advance forensic education and scholarship and contribute to policy and legislation.

Many new forensic issues confront public psychiatry now. Forensic clients with violent histories require risk assessments and management above and beyond the usual discharge planning. Clinicians must work with probation while maintaining confidentiality and a therapeutic alliance. Special populations such as sex offenders create the need for treatments despite the lack of empirical evidence that current interventions work. Relatively new treatment teams such as the ACT teams, Homeless Outreach Teams and police liaison clinicians provide treatment in the community for clients who are hard to engage, non-compliant with treatment and often have criminal records.

Three areas create special challenges and new opportunities for Law and Psychiatry and will likely represent the next major advances in the discipline of forensic psychiatry. The first concerns the assessment and treatment of persons with mental illness who are arrested for sexual offenses. Prosecution of persons for internet sex crimes is increasing as is the demand for management of persons with sexual assaults of children. The psychiatric underpinnings of sexual deviance are still speculative and assessments of risk of sexual offenses are difficult. Court-mandated treatment for sex offenders released from incarceration has placed new demands on mental health service providers at the CMHC and in the state in general (Zonana, 1977). Effective treatment has not yet been identified and the cost of inpatient confinement would overwhelm state resources. Through a task force that included Zonana, Norko and Sturges, DMHAS was successful in blocking a formal civil commitment statute for "sexual predators" who were being released from prison (after the Supreme Court declared such statutes to be constitutional in *Kansas v. Hendricks*, 521 US 346 (1997)). However, persons who have sexual deviant disorders still require monitoring, treatment and other services, including appropriate housing. Indeed, inmates with pedophiliac disorders have, on their own, contacted Law and Psychiatry asking for treatment so that they will not re-offend. Some of these people have remained hospitalized for longer than a year, because appropriate housing is difficult to find and safety of both the client and the public impossible to guarantee. The challenges of evaluating treatment, monitoring, policy development, and legislation fall within the domain of Law and Psychiatry.

A second critical challenge concerns the incorporation of culture as a central factor in forensic psychiatry. Effects of ethnicity, religion and language on intimate relationships, response to stress, manifestations of mental disorders and criminal behavior have been minimally addressed by psychiatry and law. Indeed both disciplines in America have developed from a European foundation. Globalization, the collapse of the Soviet Union and regional wars have shifted the immigration patterns to include an influx of persons from Eastern Europe, the Middle East and the Pacific Rim. A growing number of these persons have civil and criminal legal cases. Forensic psychiatry is called upon to enable successful resolution of cases when communication and understanding between the person and the legal system break down. To complete assessments accurately, to treat effectively and to work with the courts on these cases, an in-depth understanding of culture and its impact is necessary. Forensic psychiatry stands at the forefront of the cultural evolution in mental health services. Law and Psychiatry will develop initiatives to formulate relevant questions, conduct investigations to evaluate different treatment and assessment approaches, and develop curriculum and policy to assure that persons of different cultures are effectively served as consumers of both psychiatry and legal services.

The third anticipated challenge for forensic psychiatry is the incorporation of the advances in neuro-imaging and brain studies in forensic assessments and treatments. The advances in brain studies offer forensic psychiatry powerful new tools for evaluation. The challenge is to understand the new science and establish reliable and valid measures and interpretations to use in forensic assessments. Building on the developing program in the neuro-psychological investigation of sexual deviance, Law and Psychiatry will forge a collaboration with neurologists and scientists in brain imaging to incorporate the newest valid techniques in behavioral assessments.

As Law and Psychiatry evolves to meet these challenges, new dimensions based on scientific and clinical studies will emerge and shape forensic psychiatry, expert testimony, and the legal and medical interface. With all change, a critical and pervasive focus will continue to be the definition and maintenance of ethical practice in forensic psychiatry. New science, new legal decisions and growing public demand for protection from deviant behaviors create a constant pressure on forensic psychiatry to take responsibility for more complex problems. The challenge for the division and all of forensic psychiatry is to maintain its independence and identity as a medical specialty with the expertise to enlighten legal decisions. As Law and Psychiatry meets the new challenges, it will continue to grow and change. What will not change is its commitment to ethical practice, to excellence in education and scholarship, and to leadership in policy and legislation to preserve human dignity and social justice for persons with mental disorders.

References

Baranoski M, Adams L, Peterson L, et al: Court diversion: mental health and legal partnerships to serve the mentally ill offender. Discovery 60–9, Spring 1996

Brilliant Madness, A. American Experience on PBS Home, 1999–2002. Available at: http://www.pbs.org/wgbh/amex/nash/index.html. Accessed September 1, 2006

Buchanan A: Care of the Mentally Disordered Offender in the Community. London: Oxford University Press, 2000

Chapman JF, Desai RA, Falzer PF: Mental health service provision in juvenile justice facilities: pre- and postrelease psychiatric care. Child Adolesc Psychiatric Clin N Am 15:445–58, 2006a

Chapman JF, Desai RA, Falzer PR, et al: Violence risk and race in a sample of youth in juvenile detention: the potential to reduce disproportionate minority confinement. Youth Violence and Juvenile Justice 4:170–84, 2006b

Crane L, Zonana H, Wizner S: Implications of the Donaldson decision: a model for periodic review of committed patients. Hosp Community Psychiatry 28:827–33, 1977

Daily Almanac 1955. Infoplease Pearson Education, 2000–2006. Available at: http://www.infoplease.com/year/1955.html. Accessed September 1, 2006

Desai RA, Goulet JL, Robbins J, et al: Mental health care in juvenile detention facilities: a review. J Am Acad Psychiatry Law 34:204–14, 2006

Easton C, Devine S: Battered Person Syndrome. J Am Acad Psychiatry Law, 29:116–8, 2001

Easton C, Swan S, Sinha R: Prevalence of family violence in clients entering substance abuse treatment. J Subs Abuse Treat 18:23–8, 2000

Easton CJ: Substance abuse and criminality in the mentally disordered defendant. J Am Acad Psychiatry Law 33:196–8, 2005

Frisman L, Lin HJ, Sturges GE, et al: Outcomes of court-based jail diversion programs for people with co-occurring disorders. J Dual Diagnosis 2:5–26, 2006

Herron D, Zonana H, Crane L: Competence to stand trial in Connecticut: an historical overview of competence to stand trial evaluations by a clinical team. Bull Am Acad Psychiatry Law 11:261–71, 1983

Hoff RA, Baranoski MV, Buchanan J, et al: The effects of a jail diversion program on incarceration: a retrospective cohort study. J Am Acad Psychiatry Law 27:377–86, 1999a

Hoff RA, Rosenheck RA, Baranoski M, et al: Diversion from jail of detainees with substance abuse: the interaction with dual diagnosis. Am J Addict 8:201–10, 200, 1999b

Lewis ME, Scott DC, Baranoski MV, et al: Prototypes of intrafamily homicide and serious assault among insanity acquittees. J Am Acad Psychiatry Law 26:37–48, 1998

Morgan CA, III, Hazlett G, Doran A, et al: Accuracy of eyewitness memory for persons encountered during exposure to highly intense stress. Int J Law Psychiatry 27:265–79, 2004

Norko MA, Baranoski MV: The state of contemporary risk assessment research. Can J Psychiatry 50:18–26, 2005

Rowe M, Baranoski M: Mental illness, criminality, and citizenship. J Am Acad Psychiatry Law 28:262–4, 2000

Rubenstein M, Zonana H, Crane L: Civil commitment reform in Connecticut: a perspective for physicians. Conn Med 41:709–17, 1977

Torrey EF, Stiebar J, Ezekiel J, et al: Criminalizing the Seriously Mentally Ill. Washington, D.C.: Public Citizens' Health Research Group and the National Alliance for the Mentally Ill, 1992

Yochelson S, Samenow, S: The Criminal Personality, Volume I: A Profile for Change. New York: J Aronson Publishers, 1976

Zonana H: The civil commitment of sex offenders. Science 278:1248–9, 1997

Zonana H, Lewis ME, Werner T, et al: After NGRI acquittal: trajectories of recovery. Panel presentation at the 29th annual meeting of AAPL at Baltimore, MD, October 16, 1999

Zonana H, Scott DC, Getz, MA: Monitoring insanity acquittees: Connecticut's Psychiatric Security Review Board. Hosp Community Psychiatry 41:980–4, 1990

Zonana H, Wells JA, Getz MA, et al: Part I: the NGRI registry: initial analyses of data collected on Connecticut insanity acquittees. Bull Am Acad Psychiatry Law 18:115–28, 1990

Zonana HV, Bartel RL, Wells JA, et al: Part II: sex differences in persons found not guilty by reason of insanity: analysis of data from the Connecticut NGRI registry. Bull Am Acad Psychiatry Law 18:129–42, 1990

4

The neuroscience research program at the Connecticut Mental Health Center

George R. Heninger, John H. Krystal, Ronald S. Duman,
Benjamin S. Bunney, Malcolm B. Bowers, Jr. and
George K. Aghajanian

When the Connecticut Mental Health Center opened in 1966, it began a bold and distinctive experiment by combining patient care, teaching and research within a community mental health center organization. In the ensuing 40 years, the usefulness of this concept has been well documented with numerous examples of successful interactions between patient care, education, and research that have led to the creation of new and improved treatments. Research within the Neuroscience Research Program has led to a fundamental improvement in our understanding of brain function and the causes of mental illness; this in turn has led to the development of several new and more effective methods to treat patients. These new treatments are now being used to improve patient care both at the CMHC and across the nation. The Neuroscience Research Program has provided a rich training environment for individuals who have gone on to lead in the development of new service delivery, training and research enterprises both within the CMHC, and at other institutions throughout the country. The accomplishments over the past 40 years demonstrate that future support for the interaction of patient care, education and research within the CMHC will continue to be a successful method for improving the treatment of individuals with mental illness.

The Connecticut Mental Health Center (CMHC) is unique among the community-based mental health centers that emerged during the 1960s because basic and clinical neuroscience research was central to the CMHC mission from the beginning. This has proven to be a wise decision as evidenced by the contributions of that research program to the high quality of care delivered by the Center over the past 40 years. The research has provided fundamental new insights into brain physiology, helped to guide our current understanding of the biological bases of severe mental illnesses and substance abuse disorders, and has introduced important new treatments for the field. In addition, the success of the neuroscience training mission has had an enormous impact on the development of several generations of leading scientists and clinicians. These individuals have assumed leading roles within the CMHC, the Connecticut

40 Years of Academic Public Psychiatry. Edited by Selby C. Jacobs and Ezra E. H. Griffith
© 2007 John Wiley & Sons, Ltd.

Department of Mental Health and Addiction Services (DMHAS), the Yale Department of Psychiatry, universities across the United States, and the pharmaceutical industry.

Neuroscience research conducted at the CMHC has been an important contributor to the "revolution" in neuroscience that has reshaped the way that we view psychiatric illnesses. Schizophrenia, for example, was at one time seen as a functional impairment arising from abnormal communication between mother and child. Although there remains much to learn, we now know enough about the neurobiology of schizophrenia to view this illness as a disorder of the development of the brain. The understanding of the neurobiology of schizophrenia drives the testing of novel pharmacological, physiological, psychological and rehabilitative treatments for schizophrenia that could not have been anticipated without the backdrop of neuroscience research. The revolutionary idea of placing neuroscience research within the framework of a community mental health center is now coming full circle: neuroscience advances are at the center of our improved understanding of the causes of mental illness and they are helping improve the recovery of patients at the CMHC.

History

The Neuroscience Research Program that would come to be located at the CMHC when it opened in 1966 had its roots in the Yale Medical School Departments of Pharmacology and Psychiatry through the combined efforts of a pharmacologist, Nicholas Giarman, and a psychiatrist, Daniel X. Freedman. Before the discovery, during the 1950s, of the "major" tranquilizers, such as chlorpromazine, and the antidepressants, such as imipramine, there were no effective drugs for the treatment of mental illness. At the same time, the discovery of psychedelics such as LSD provided evidence that normal mental function was dependent on a delicate biochemical balance. These discoveries were the beginning of the modern era of neuropsychopharmacology. In order to improve our understanding of the neurochemistry and neuropharmacology of both normal and abnormal mental function, and to take advantage of these new therapeutic opportunities, Giarman and Freedman instituted a combined research and training program in neuropharmacology at Yale. This was titled the Biological Sciences Training Program (BSTP). This program was initiated at Yale in 1961 with a NIMH training grant. It moved to the CMHC when it opened in 1966, and it continues at the CMHC to this day.

The CMHC was designed as a community mental health center located in an academic setting where patient care, community service, professional training and research were combined. This structure was intended to stimulate research on the causes of and treatments for mental illness. It was also planned to foster the rapid dissemination of discoveries from researchers to clinicians, who would use the new knowledge to improve the care of their patients. When the neurobiologic research program was initiated, the concepts and methods embodied within the BSTP formed the core of the program. There was a combined clinical and basic science research effort. Two of the original trainees in the BSTP, George Aghajanian and Malcolm Bowers, became the first leaders of the CMHC neuroscience research program. Bowers became the director of the Clinical Neuroscience Research Unit (CNRU) located on the third floor of the Center. On the laboratory side of the third floor, Aghajanian and his colleagues (including Floyd Bloom) initiated studies on fundamental neurobiologic mechanisms by which the new antipsychotics, antidepressants and psychedelic drugs act on the brain. The original director of the neurobiologic research group was Roger McDonald. He recruited John Flynn to work in the basic science laboratories on the neurobiology of anger and aggression and George Heninger to work on the CNRU on the neurobiology of depression. By 1967, important original research findings were emerging from the CMHC Neuroscience Program (Aghajanian et al., 1967).

The central goal of the BSTP, which has continued throughout the history of the neurobiologic research program, is the translation of scientific understanding to improve clinical care. This has been primarily focused on discovering the neurobiologic abnormalities of mental illness and understanding the mechanisms of action of neuropharmacologic drugs. The origin of the BSTP within both the Pharmacology and Psychiatry Departments was critical to its success, since it facilitated the application of the solid scientific methods of neuropharmacology to clinical psychiatry.

The chronology of many of the important NIMH grants and other activities and organizations that originated from personnel and programs supported by the CMHC's neurobiologic research program are outlined in Table 4.1. It can be seen that the influence of the program extends into Child Psychiatry, which provides opportunities for early intervention. In addition, the CMHC Neuroscience Research Program has fostered research programs in schizophrenia, drug and alcohol abuse, and posttraumatic stress disorders (PTSD) at the Veterans Administration Medical Center in West Haven (VAMC). The establishment of the Research Division structure of the Department, spanning institutions, has optimized the utilization of the precious CNRU inpatient resources. All Departmental programs now have access to the CNRU to develop novel research methods and to evaluate the safety and efficacy of novel treatments in the highly controlled inpatient setting, where intensive monitoring of patients is possible. This step is often critical in the development of new treatments that can be tested in clinical settings. Because of this capacity, the CNRU played an important role in the development of methadone, naltrexone and buprenorphine, the medications now prescribed for opiate dependence and utilized at the CMHC.

The neurobiologic research program started with a small number of individuals in 1966. It has progressively expanded into a large array of programs and treatment interventions located throughout the CMHC and the Psychiatry Department. This has had a national impact as evidenced by the continual NIMH support, the many important publications and awards, and the large number of graduates of the training programs who now lead important programs in other areas of the CMHC and at other institutions across the nation.

The current academic program

Although the neurobiologic research program is centered at the CMHC, its influence extends widely throughout the Department of Psychiatry and the University. The program conducts an array of preclinical studies that investigate the neurobiology of currently utilized effective treatments. New treatments can then be done in animal

Table 4.1   Historical development of the neurobiological research program at the CMHC

1961	Origin of the Biological Sciences Research Training Program (BSTP-NIMH Training Grant)—designed to bring the power and rigor of the biological sciences to bear on the clinical problems seen in psychiatry.
1966	Opening of the Abraham Ribicoff Research Facilities at the CMHC—this included the Clinical Neuroscience Research Unit (CNRU) and Neuropharmacological Research Laboratories. Roger McDonald was the original Director.
1969	Addition of the Neurobehavioral Laboratory within the Ribicoff Facilities.
1970	John Flynn became Director of the Ribicoff Facilities.
1972	Pioneering research on the role of specific brain areas (locus coeruleus, raphe nuclei, midbrain dopamine neurons) regulating brain norepinephrine, serotonin and dopamine function, the systems targeted by our current psychiatric medications.
1973	Origin of the NIMH Program Project Grant, "Neurobiologic Basis of Major Psychiatric Disorders," Morton Reiser, Program Director—this grant has provided continual research support until the present.
1975	Clinical studies of norepinephrine, serotonin and dopamine metabolism in psychiatric patients—this led to better understanding of abnormalities in these systems in psychiatric patients.
1977	Discovery of the use of clonidine for the treatment of opiate withdrawal resulted in the awarding of a major prize from the American Psychiatric Association (APA) to the four-person research group at the Ribicoff Facilities.
1978	Origin of the NIMH Clinical Research Center Grant (CRC) in Adult and Child Psychiatry, Malcolm Bowers, Principal Investigator. George Heninger became the Director of the Ribicoff Research Facilities.
1984	Discovery of lithium augmentation in the treatment of refractory depressed patients. This continues today to be the first alternative treatment in non-responding patients.
1985	Discovery of the novel use of opiate and benzodiazepine antagonists in the treatment of opiate and benzodiazepine addiction.
1986	Origin of the NIDA Clinical Research Center on Cocaine and Opiate Addiction—many initial studies were supported by the CNRU.
1987	Establishment of the CNRU Division of Outpatient Research with the creation of the Anxiety Disorders Research Clinic to focus on disorders most commonly treated in outpatient settings. This Division is the current home for the following research clinics: Alcoholism, Cocaine Dependence, Depression, Obsessive-Compulsive Disorders (OCD), Psychosis and Women's Behavioral Health; Initiation of the Molecular Psychiatry Research Program; Addition of Basement Laboratories to the Ribicoff Research Facilities.
1988	Initiation of the Neurobiological Research Program in Psychiatry at the Veterans Affairs Medical Center (VAMC)—a major expansion of neurobiological research supported by personnel and equipment from the Ribicoff Research Facilities under the leadership of Dennis Charney.
1989	Initiation of the National Center for PTSD (Clinical Neuroscience Division), the only center of its kind supported by the Department of Veterans Affairs. This Center generated most of the current hypotheses related to the neurobiology of PTSD (noradrenergic hyperactivity, glucocorticoid receptor dysfunction, reductions in hippocampal volume as a consequence/risk factor for PTSD, NE/NPY balance in stress resilience, etc.) and it is a leader in PTSD treatment.
1989	Establishment of the Molecular Genetics Laboratories at the VA.
1990	Initiation of the Schizophrenia Biological Research Center at the VAMC (one of three nationally) and the Ribicoff Research Facilities. This Center conducted the first demonstration of dopamine hyperactivity in schizophrenia and provided the most comprehensive evaluation of the NMDA glutamate receptor deficit model of schizophrenia; Initiation of the Neuroimaging Program at the VAMC and Department of Psychiatry.

Table 4.1 *Continued*

1991	Initiation of the Alcohol Research Center at the VAMC and Ribicoff Facilities and introduction of the use of naltrexone in the treatment of alcoholism. Eric Nestler became the Director of the Ribicoff Research Facilities.
1992	Initiation of the NIDA-sponsored Basic Science Research Training Program in Drug Abuse. Initiation of the Fifteen Hospital Study of the Long-Term Effects of Clozapine on Symptoms and Health Care Costs in Schizophrenia.
1993	Initiation of the NIDA Program Project Grant, "Molecular Neurobiology of Drug Addiction," and clinical trials of novel pharmacotherapies. Opening of the Laboratory of Clinical and Molecular Neurobiology at the Yale Psychiatric Institute (YPI).
1994	Construction of the new Substance Abuse Center addition to the Ribicoff Research Facilities to house part of the Neurobiology Research Program on Drug Addiction.
1996	Establishment of the research program on the Molecular and Cellular Basis of Antidepressant Drug Action, which stimulated a national effort in this research area.
1997	Discoveries on the molecular biology of drug addiction—followed by similar research in many other research laboratories. Establishment of the Clinical Research Program on Neurodevelopmental Disorders focusing on adolescents and adults with autism and pervasive developmental disorders.
1998	Initiation of the Division of Cognitive and Clinical Neuroscience, the Department-wide program to facilitate clinical research, including the CNRU. John Krystal named Deputy Ribicoff Director for Clinical Research. Initiation of Functional Magnetic Resonance Imaging Program in Affective Disorders.
1999	Collaboration with Yale Magnetic Resonance Research Center yields first applications of magnetic resonance spectroscopy to characterize disturbances in cortical GABA levels in vivo in patients with psychiatric and addictive disorders, the first evaluations of the role of human GABA systems in the treatment of depression and anxiety, and the recovery from alcoholism.
2000	Establishment of the NIAAA Center for the Translational Neuroscience of Alcoholism. Enlargement of the Laboratory of Psychiatric Genetics. Ronald Duman became the Director of the Ribicoff Research Facilities.
2001	Initiation of the research programs in the Woman's Behavioral Gynecology Clinic.
2002	Establishment of a research program in clinical neurophysiology jointly on the CNRU and the VA.
2003	Initiation of International Studies on the Genetics of Drug Addiction.
2004	Discovery of the role of genetics in childhood abuse which causes mental illness later in life and depression which is a worldwide public health problem.
2005	Initiation of the Neuroproteomics Program in collaboration with other University Departments.

models. At the clinical level, studies are conducted to identify the neurobiological abnormalities in patients and to evaluate new treatments. There are studies on the mechanism of action of antipsychotic treatments, antidepressant treatments, antianxiety treatments and treatments for drug abuse. In these studies, investigators utilize a variety of methods: preclinical studies of animals with genetic vulnerability toward behaviors thought to represent animal models of psychiatric illness. Clinical studies involve patients with a variety of psychiatric diagnoses. These studies extend from basic molecular investigations into the regulation of neurotransmission all the way up to more complex behavioral models in animals and studies of human illness.

Preclinical laboratory research studies

Depression is ranked among the top four disorders producing the highest burden of disease (years lost to illness), and current treatments are still only partly effective. Since stress is known to be a major factor involved in precipitating most forms of mental illness, especially depression, a major research program has been undertaken to understand better the roll of stress in depression. The preclinical laboratory of Ronald Duman was one of the first to demonstrate that stress, in addition to producing depressive symptoms, impairs the expression of neurotrophic factors and reduces neurogenesis in the hippocampus. Specifically, brain-derived neurotrophic factor (BDNF) and neurogenesis are decreased by stress and this can be prevented by antidepressant treatment (Duman et al., 2001). This has lead to a major new theory of depression, which involves stress-induced decreases in BDNF function, which leads to a failure in the maintenance of healthy brain function and results in the symptoms of depression. The stress-induced decrease in BDNF in the hippocampus has been related to the reduced generation of new neurons in this area, which has important implications for the role of stress in impairing learning, memory and neuronal plasticity.

In laboratories within the Ribicoff Facilities, Angus Nairn, David Russell, Ralph DiLeone and Patrick Allen all have active and productive research programs on the intra-cellular molecular biology of addictive drugs and drugs used for treatment in psychiatry. These studies are providing a more fundamental understanding of the intricate genetic, cellular and molecular mechanisms involved in drug action, and help provide insight into the possible cellular and molecular abnormalities involved in producing illness in patients.

Since drugs used in the treatment of patients change neurotransmitter function, studies in the neurophysiology laboratories are investigating the detailed effects of drugs on the transmitters serotonin, glutamate, GABA, acetylcholine and peptides that are involved in neuronal function. In these studies, it is possible to identify the molecular and pharmacologic action of drugs used in psychiatry and to understand better the neuronal circuits operating in learning, memory and other important brain functions. Aghajanian's laboratory has described the role of the serotonin system and the glutamatergic system in the action of psychotomimetic drugs and drugs used to treat schizophrenia (Aghajanian and Marek, 2000). Meenakshi Alreja's laboratory has discovered a new and important role of the GABA system in the hippocampus for the function of learning and memory (Alreja et al., 2000).

Investigations of drug addiction are being conducted that include studies describing the molecular events that underlie repeated drug administration that leads to dependence. Changes have been observed in gene regulation that can be the basis for the long-term effects that end in addiction. In addition, many of the receptor and genetic vulnerabilities to drug addiction have been studied. This includes studies of nicotine by Marina Picciotto where she has been able to describe the molecular actions of nicotine that lead to addiction (Picciotto, 2003). Neurocognitive and behavioral studies by Jane Taylor have described the influence of impaired cortical function on decision-making relative to addiction since there is evidence from human studies that impaired judgment is involved in drug addiction. The effects on decision-making of chronic administration of drugs of abuse such as cocaine and amphetamine have been studied.

It has been found that repeated use of stimulants impairs executive function mediated by the frontal lobes, and this appears to be similar to the impaired judgment observed in addicted humans. As an extension of these ideas, studies have been conducted with cocaine in rats that are directly related to dual diagnosis in schizophrenia (Chambers and Taylor, 2004).

Two new faculty at the Ribicoff Research Facilities include Arthur Simen, who leads a program on the molecular genetics of depression, and Arie Kaffman, who studies molecular determinants of the vulnerability or resilience to the effects of early life stresses. Both of these laboratories use the most modern methods of molecular biology and genetics to investigate these important areas. By understanding the molecular mechanisms involved in producing illness it will be possible to develop improved methods of treatment and prevention.

Clinical research studies

An outline of the current CNRU organizational structure is provided in Figure 4.1. As can be seen from the outline, the three missions of the CNRU are integrated into its organizational structure. Robert Malison directs the CNRU. The Inpatient Division is the principal teaching and clinical arm of the CNRU. Under the direction of Vladimir Coric it plays an important role in the training of medical students and psychiatric residents in the context of caring for inpatients participating in CNRU research studies. The Outpatient Research Clinics have focused clinical research missions related to particular psychiatric and substance abuse disorders. They often conduct both inpatient and outpatient research. Therefore, these clinics work closely with the Inpatient Unit.

The educational mission is extremely important to the CNRU. Under the leadership of Malison and Neill Epperson, the CNRU is involved in clinical training, as noted earlier. It is a core resource for clinical research training within the Department. Under the leadership of Ralitza Guerguieva, the Biostatistics Program on the CNRU has evolved from a pure "service core" of the CNRU to an active research program that is jointly supported by the Section of Biostatistics in the School of Epidemiology and Public Health. This Program is developing novel methods for analyzing clinical research data while applying methods to CNRU studies.

Alcoholism research clinic

Alcoholism research at CMHC was initiated by Stephanie O'Malley, and Bruce Rounsaville. In 1992, they published one of two studies that led to the approval of naltrexone for the pharmacotherapy of alcoholism. In 1991, an Alcohol Research Center also was established at the VA under the leadership of John Krystal. These programs converged in 2000 with the establishment of the NIAAA Center for the Translational Neuroscience of Alcoholism and the CNRU Alcoholism Research Clinic, under the direction of Krystal. This center provided the first human evidence that the blockade of glutamate receptors contributed to human ethanol intoxication. Using MRS, PET and psychopharmacology, this center described disturbances in

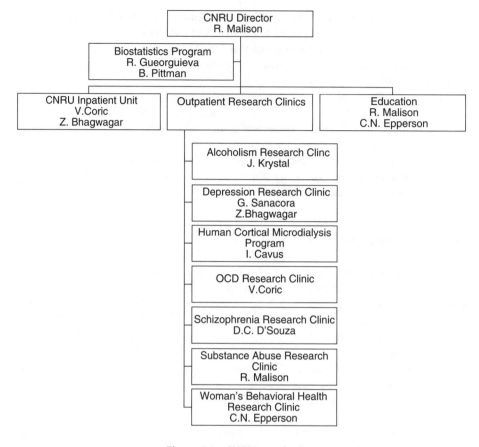

Figure 4.1   *CNRU organization*

glutamatergic, GABAergic and dopaminergic neurotransmission associated with alcohol dependence and the vulnerability to alcoholism. Building on these insights, this clinic is testing novel glutamatergic approaches to the pharmacotherapy of alcoholism.

Depression research clinic

The Depression Research Clinic was founded in 1987 under the leadership of Pedro Delgado. This clinic was revitalized under the leadership of Gerard Sanacora in 1997. In collaboration with the Yale Magnetic Resonance Research Center, the clinic first found deficits in cortical GABA levels and increases in cortical glutamate levels associated with subgroups of depressed patients using MRS imaging (Sanacora et al., 2004). Sanacora also found that some treatments (serotonin uptake inhibiting antidepressant, electroconvulsive therapy) but not cognitive-behavioral therapy, increased cortical GABA levels and normalized them in patients with GABA level deficits (Sanacora et al., 2006). At the VA, Berman, Charney and Krystal showed that a glutamate receptor blocker had antidepressant effects. Sanacora is extending this research and high-lighting the efficacy of drugs that reduce glutamate release or increase its uptake (elimination) from the synapse. His work highlights a novel focus on correcting cel-lular disturbances associated with depression, particularly abnormal interplay of the glutamate nerve cells and their supporting cells (glia).

Human cortical microdialysis program

In 1998, Walid Abi-Saab and Krystal established a novel collaboration with the Depart-ment of Neurosurgery to lead the component of their epilepsy research involving the on-line release of neurochemicals as patients underwent evaluation for epilepsy surgery. Idil Cavus assumed the leadership of this program following the departure of Abi-Saab in 2001. This program has identified changes in cortical neurotransmission associated with hypoglycemia. Paralleling the research in the Depression Research Clinic, this clinic is describing how disturbances in the interplay of nerve cells and glia associated with epilepsy influence neurotransmission. This program is also evaluating the anti-convulsant effects of local low-frequency brain stimulation in this patient group.

OCD research clinic

The Obsessive-Compulsive Disorder (OCD) Research Clinic was established in 1986 under the leadership of Wayne Goodman. This clinic conducted one of the first rigor-ous studies that demonstrated the advantage of selective serotonin reuptake inhibiting (SSRI) antidepressant medications over a tricylic antidepressant that blocked nore-pinephrine uptake. Christopher McDougle, the next leader of this clinic, showed that antipsychotic medications enhanced the response to SSRIs in OCD patients. Vladimir Coric assumed the leadership of the clinic in 2001. Under his leadership, the clinic is exploring two novel treatments aimed at reducing glutamate hyperactivity in OCD patients who failed to respond to prior available treatments: riluzole and N-acetyl-cysteine (Coric et al., 2005).

Schizophrenia research clinic

Although schizophrenia had been initially a major CNRU focus, the CNRU Outpatient Schizophrenia Clinic was not established until 1998, under the leadership of Abi-Saab and Krystal. The clinic has probed aspects of the neurobiology of schizophrenia and tested a number of medications that have since been approved for the treatment of this disorder. In particular, they found behavioral and fMRI evidence that deficits in glutamate receptor function may disinhibit this system (Krystal et al., 2005). In col-laboration with the Institute of Psychiatry in London, they also provided the first in vivo evidence of reductions in NMDA glutamate receptor density in schizophrenia. As a result, they pioneered the evaluation of a glutamate release-inhibiting anticon-vulsant agent, lamotrigine, as an adjunct to the treatment of schizophrenia. They are also testing an NMDA receptor-facilitating agent, D-serine, for a similar purpose.

Ralph Hoffman initiated studies on the CNRU that first suggested and later demonstrated that low-frequency transcranial magnetic stimulation (rTMS) suppressed hallucinations in patients who had not responded to any prior treatment for these symptoms.

Following the departure of Abi-Saab, Deepak Cyril D'Souza assumed the leadership of this clinic. D'Souza has been probing disturbances in the endocannabinoid system, the "body's own marijuana," that may be associated with schizophrenia (D'Souza et al., 2005). These studies may help to explain why marijuana smoking appears to be a contributing factor to the onset of symptoms in a subgroup of adolescents who develop schizophrenia.

Substance abuse research clinic

As noted earlier, the CNRU has a long history of substance abuse research, led at various times by Mark Gold, Dennis Charney and Krystal. Building on this history, Malison established the Substance Abuse Research Clinic on the CNRU. Using SPECT, his work described long-lasting increases in the dopamine transporter in cocaine-dependent individuals. More recently, he established a laboratory-based cocaine self-administration method that is producing exciting new information about genetic and pharmacologic mechanisms controlling cocaine self-administration (Sughondhabirom et al., 2005). With Joel Gelernter, Director of the Department's Division of Human Genetics, Malison leads a novel international collaboration based in Thailand that studies the genetic basis of substance abuse.

Women's behavioral health research clinic

Under the leadership of Epperson, the CNRU began to address psychiatric disorders that emerge in relation to the reproductive health, i.e., late luteal phase dysphoric disorder (LLDD, also known as premenstrual syndrome or PMS), post-partum depression and mood disorders of the menopause. A major achievement of this research program, in collaboration with the Yale MRRC, was the first description of menstrual cycle-related changes in brain chemistry using MRS in healthy women (Epperson et al., 2002). She also studied disturbances in the cycle-related changes in women with LLDD, as well as the impact of smoking on cyclical changes in cortical GABA levels. Epperson, in collaboration with Linda Mayes and George Anderson of the Yale Child Study Center, has also studied the impact upon the development of infants of maternal antidepressant consumption during pregnancy.

Teaching and training

All of the above activities in both the preclinical and clinical areas involve a great deal of scholarship activity. The research findings are published in leading scientific journals in the fields of psychiatry, pharmacology, neuroscience and psychology, and also outstanding general scientific journals such as *The Proceedings of the National Academy of Science, Nature, Science* and medical journals including the *New England Journal of Medicine*, the *Journal of the American Medical Association*, *Lancet* and the *Archives of General Psychiatry*. The faculty have written, edited or contributed to a number of books, and they are very active in national societies and national scientific meetings.

The faculty of the Ribicoff Research Facilities are currently very active in teaching and training. A major course for first year medical students—Biologic Basis of Behavior—is taught by faculty from the Ribicoff Facilities. Faculty also participate in second year medical teaching. The third and fourth medical year students rotate through the CNRU to receive training in psychiatry.

One of the major educational endeavors is the training of psychiatric residents. Every four to six months, residents rotate through the CNRU for their psychiatric training. This has led to a steady stream of trainees who have gone on both within the CMHC and the Department of Psychiatry and also outside of Yale to assume major leadership positions.

In the preclinical area, there is a very active training program with predoctoral and postdoctoral students. The faculty are involved in the Interdepartmental Neuroscience Training Program at Yale and also have other individual postdoctoral fellows working in their laboratories. Thus, the educational efforts of the neurobiologic research group are considerable, and there has been a constant flow of productive graduates.

Contributions to the field

Over the past 40 years of its existence, the Ribicoff Research Facilities have been one of the top neurobiologic research organizations in psychiatry in the world. This contribution could be viewed from several perspectives. In 2000, ISI-Thomson, the organization that evaluates the impact of research, reported that Yale University was the third most highly cited psychiatric institution in the world based on 7888 citations of research papers that appeared between 1990 and 1998. They highlighted the contributions of the CMHC to the Yale University score for good reason: six of the 22 most highly cited authors in psychiatry were based at one time on the CNRU (see http://www.sciencewatch.com/may-june2000/sw_may-june2000_page2.htm).

Preclinical research laboratory contributions

The Ribicoff Research Facility scientists played an important role in characterizing the functional regulation of specific monoamine-containing cells in the brainstem and midbrain. Aghajanian characterized mechanisms controlling the noradrenergic nucleus locus coeruleus and the serotonergic raphe nuclei. This work laid the foundation for treatments for opiate withdrawal, depression, anxiety disorders and attention deficit disorder. Benjamin Bunney, Robert Roth and Malcolm Bowers focused on the regulation of dopamine systems. Their work and that of their trainees, such as Ariel Deutch and Bita Moghaddam, provided insights into antipsychotic medications, particularly mechanisms that might distinguish the second generation antipsychotic medications from the older "typical" neuroleptics. This has helped lead the way for the development of the new "atypical" antipsychotic drugs in wide use today.

Many of the important findings have been in the area of drug abuse. In contrast to the popular view that addiction is simply a lack of will power, it has been possible to demonstrate with animal models that repeat drug exposure results in fundamental changes in brain structure and function. The vulnerability to addiction can be related to genetic variations in laboratory animals and many of the cellular and molecular pathways involved in addiction have been identified. At the behavioral level, a cause of addiction has been discovered where repeated drug abuse alters executive function so that it leads to bad decisions. This is a major contribution to our understanding of the neurobiology of drug addiction. It shows how repeated drug use progressively alters brain function, making the individual more likely to continue repeated drug administration. This demonstrates the nature of drug addiction as an illness, and it has major implications for the design of new treatments to treat addiction, such as the use of cognitive-behavioral therapy to change attitudes and drug seeking.

One of the major discoveries was the use of clonidine in the treatment of opiate addiction. This illustrates how understanding drug actions in basic research can lead to the development of new treatments. It was discovered in laboratory animal studies that clonidine acted on specific receptors involved in norepinephrine transmission in the brain. The receptors involved acted to turn off noradrenergic neuro transmission. Since opiate withdrawal involved excessive noradrenergic transmission, the use of clonidine to inhibit the excessive transmission turned out to be an effective treatment. The use of clonidine in the treatment of opiate withdrawal is a widespread treatment today. An additional discovery was that the use of an opiate antagonist such as naloxone plus clonidine could shorten the duration of withdrawal symptoms during the treatment of opiate withdrawal (Charney et al., 1982). Initial studies with opiate antagonists preceded the now widespread use of opiate antagonists in other situations such as the treatment of alcoholism with naltrexone.

The discovery that the effects of stress on neurotrophins can be reversed by antidepressant treatment has opened up a new line of investigation into the causes and treatment of depression. Depression is highly comorbid with many other illnesses, such as heart disease, stroke, neurodegenerative disorders, diabetes and inflammatory disorders. Previously there was no clear explanation of why this occurred. Now the Neurotrophic Hypothesis of Depression provides opportunities for investigations of the mechanism by which these other medical conditions increase the rate of depression (Duman, 2004). It is thought that these other conditions stimulate stress pathways that decrease brain neurotrophic function which can lead to reduced neurogenesis and reduced neuroplasticity. In addition, there is evidence from laboratory animal studies that factors in blood acting on endothelial cells may be an important mechanism involved in depression (Newton and Duman, 2004; Newton et al., 2003). This is leading to major breakthroughs in the field.

Clinical research contributions

The CNRU has been very successful in achieving the most important outcomes: new treatments for psychiatric illnesses. These advances are summarized in Table 4.2. Although not presented in detail, CNRU investigators not only introduced medications, but they conducted research on how to use these medications optimally in the

Table 4.2 Contributions of the CNRU to new treatments in psychiatry

---

- First use of methadone in the treatment of opiate addiction in Connecticut
- First use of lithium in the State of Connecticut
- First use of several "second generation" antipsychotic medications in Connecticut
- Discovery of clonidine to treat opiate withdrawal
- Discovery of lithium to augment antidepressant drug treatments
- Discovery of the first "rapid detoxification" strategy for opiate dependence (clonidine/naloxone-naltrexone)
- First use of fluvoxamine, a selective serotonin uptake inhibitor (SSRI) in the treatment of OCD and in panic disorder
- First evaluation of combination of a benzodiazepine and a SSRI in the treatment of panic disorder
- Discovery of the antidepressant and antiobsessional properties of drugs that block or reduce glutamate effects
- Discovery of the application of transcranial magnetic stimulation (TMS) to treat hallucinations that fail to respond to antipsychotic medications
- First evaluation of glutamate-facilitating agents in combination with cognitive rehabilitation to reduce the cognitive impairments of schizophrenia
- First evaluation of cognitive-behavioral treatment (CBT) to improve outcomes after electroconvulsive treatment (ECT) for depression
- First evaluation of phosphodiesterase inhibition treatment for depression
- First demonstration of the utility of second generation antipsychotic medications in the treatment of autism and related developmental disorders in adults

---

treatment of patients. Also, as in the case of treatments for panic disorder, faculty contributed reports on the treatment of individual patients or conducted long-term follow-up studies on the effectiveness of medication treatments.

CNRU investigators have been leaders in the implementation of unique research technologies that translate basic science findings to novel clinical insights. For example, CNRU investigators were the first group to measure cortical GABA levels non-invasively using magnetic resonance spectroscopy in alcohol dependence, depression, panic disorder and schizophrenia. Also, the CNRU was among the first to describe alterations in receptor levels in depression, cocaine dependence, alcoholism and schizophrenia using novel non-invasive (PET/SPECT) receptor imaging techniques. This unit also developed the standard evaluation tool for evaluating Obsessive-Compulsive Disorder, and the Yale-Brown Obsession and Compulsion Scale (YBOCS). The CNRU faculty at the VA contributed to the standard assessment tool for posttraumatic stress disorder, the Clinician Administered PTSD Scale (CAPS), and the most commonly used scale for measuring state-related changes in dissociation symptoms, the Clinician-Administered Dissociation States Scale (CADSS).

From another perspective, the investment by the State of Connecticut in the Ribicoff Research Facilities is paying off handsomely with respect to bringing federal grant support and pharmaceutical industry investment to Connecticut. In 2004, Yale received the third highest level of NIH funding of any department of psychiatry in the country. If one adds the more than 10 million dollars in research support coming to the Department of Veterans Affairs, it is likely that Yale would rank higher still. Connecticut pharmaceutical companies, particularly Pfizer and Bristol-Myers-Squibb, collaborate with CNRU faculty on basic and clinical research projects. In 2004, Pfizer established a Clinical Research Center across the street from the CMHC to take advantage of potential synergies with the Ribicoff Research Facilities and other Yale faculty. Scientists John Tallman, and Dorothy Gallagher, moved on from the Ribicoff Research Laboratories in the late 1980s to create Neurogen, a biotechnology company that continues to develop new treatments for neuropsychiatric disorders. Thus, the State of Connecticut's investment in CMHC research is producing an even greater stimulation of the Connecticut economy.

The Ribicoff Research Laboratories and the CNRU also have been extremely successful in training future leaders in psychiatry and neuroscience. The CNRU training programs have been a local and national resource, providing a generation of leaders of American psychiatry and the pharmaceutical industry, many of whom are listed in Table 4.3:

Contributions to public sector psychiatry

The Ribicoff Research Facilities make a direct contribution to the public sector by improving the treatment of patients with mental illness. The causes of mental illness include both genetic and other developmental neurobiologic risk factors that interact with the personal and social environmental risk factors that lead to development of illness. There are clear differences between individuals in their sensitivity to the environmental risk factors that increase vulnerability to mental illness. The important practical consequence of understanding these interactions is that it shows how mental illness can be prevented and treated on many different levels. Epidemiological and clinical research can help identify the personal and environmental risk factors that increase the probability of disease. The neurobiologic research can help identify the genetic factors and neurobiologic mechanisms that increase vulnerability to disease. By combining both approaches, mental illness can be more effectively treated and prevented. In addition, by understanding the mechanisms by which currently effective treatments work, it will be possible to use this knowledge to develop improved treatments for future use. It is the improved knowledge and development of new treatments that constitute the major contributions of the neurobiologic research program of the Ribicoff Research Facilities to the public sector.

In addition to the publication, dissemination, and application of the new knowledge and treatments, the program makes a major contribution by training individuals who go on to lead additional programs at the CMHC, the Department of Psychiatry and other institutions throughout the country. Table 4.4 lists individuals who trained or were faculty in the Ribicoff Facilities and are now leading major research and service programs at the CMHC and in the Department of Psychiatry.

A major contribution of the Neurobiological Research Program has been its active and effective contribution to the Biological-Psychological-Social model of mental illness at the CMHC. At the biological level, the basic preclinical research and the neurobiologically oriented clinical research have made major progress in identifying the neurobiological abnormalities in patients with mental illness and developing new pharmacologic treatments. At the psychological level, there have been studies of the interaction of pharmacological treatments with behavioral treatments such as

Table 4.3 Selected individuals who emerged from the CNRU to achieve leadership roles at other academic departments and the pharmaceutical industry

Person	Current Role
Amit Anand, MD	Professor, Indiana University
Anissa Abi-Dargham, MD	Professor, Columbia University
Walid Abi-Saab, MD	Senior Director, Abbot Laboratories
Robert Berman, MD	Senior Director, Bristol-Myers Squibb
Alan Breier, MD	Vice President & Chief Medical Officer, Lilly Pharmaceuticals
J. Douglas Bremner, MD	Professor of Psychiatry and Nuclear Medicine and Director of PET Imaging, Emory University
Dennis Charney, MD	Dean for Academic & Scientific Affairs, Mt. Sinai School of Medicine
Pedro Delgado, MD	Chairman of Psychiatry, University of Texas (San Antonio)
Tony George, MD	Director of the Division of Substance Abuse, University of Toronto
Earl Giller, MD	Senior Director, Maranis Pharmaceuticals
Andrew Goddard, MD	Professor of Psychiatry, Indiana University
Wayne Goodman, MD	Chairman of Psychiatry, University of Florida (Gainesville)
Robert Innis, MD	Director, Molecular Imaging Branch, NIMH IRP
Kenneth Kendler, MD	Professor of Psychiatry and Genetics, Medical College of Virginia
James Kennedy, MD	Professor of Psychiatry and Genetics, University of Toronto
Thomas Kosten, MD	Professor of Psychiatry, Baylor University
David Kupfer, MD	Chairman of Psychiatry, University of Pittsburgh
Jaakko Lappalainen, MD	Senior Director of Molecular Genetics, AstraZeneca
Marc Laruelle, MD	Vice President, Glaxo-SmithKline and Professor of Psychiatry, Imperial College of Medicine (London)
James Leckman, MD	Professor, Child Study Center, Yale University
Julio Licinio, MD	Professor of Psychiatry, University of California
Gerard Marek, MD	Senior Research Fellow, Lilly Pharmaceuticals
Christopher McDougle, MD	Chairman of Psychiatry, Indiana University
Eric Nestler, MD	Chairman of Psychiatry, University of Texas Southwestern Medical Center (Dallas)
David Pickar, MD	Chief Scientific Officer, Gabriel Pharmaceuticals
David Rubinow, MD	Chairman of Psychiatry, University of North Carolina (Chapel Hill)
Lawrence Price, MD	Vice Chairman of Psychiatry, Brown University
John Seibyl, MD	Chief Scientific Officer, Molecular Neuroimaging
Alan Swann, MD	Vice Chairman of Psychiatry, University of Texas (Houston)
Flora Vaccarino, MD	Associate Professor, Yale Child Study Center, Yale University

Cognitive-Behavioral Therapy (CBT). These and other studies, including some of the preclinical studies, have helped identify some of the relationships between the biological factors and the psychological-behavioral factors in mental illness. For example, how repeated cocaine exposure alters the basic neurobiologic processes supporting judgment—which can help explain why addicts continue to make poor decisions in their daily lives. At the social level, the research programs help identify the important social factors involved in producing illness. An example is the finding that child abuse interacts with a particular genetic make-up in individuals who later develop depression (Kaufman et al., 2006). The research has helped develop and educate practitioners

Table 4.4 Prior trainees and faculty of the Ribicoff research facilities who now lead research and science programs at the CMHC and department of psychiatry

Individuals	Independent Program
John Krystal	Deputy Chair for Research Department of Psychiatry
	Director Schizophrenia Research Center VAMC
	Director National PTSD Research Center VAMC
	Director Alcoholism Research Program VAMC
Scott Woods	Director Service Delivery Research Program CMHC
	Director Schizophrenia Early Intervention Program CMHC
Eugene Redmond	Director Cell Transplant Program for Parkinson's Disease Department of Psychiatry
Bruce Wexler	Director Schizophrenia Cognitive Remediation Program CMHC
Robert Malison	Director CNRU at CMHC
Marc Potenza	Director Gambling Addiction and Treatment Program CMHC
Malcolm Bowers	Director Inpatient Unit and Partial Hospitalization Program Department of Psychiatry
Zoran Zimolo	Director Depression Metabolic Disorders Program VAMC

at the CMHC to the view that mental illness results from the combination of neuro-biologic vulnerabilities that interact with psychological injury stemming from social factors. This model then provides many opportunities for treatment intervention at either the biological, psychological or social levels. Combined treatment directed at addressing problems on all three levels is most effective.

Future developments

Future developments can also be best understood from the Biological-Psychological-Social perspective. This allows a deeper understanding of the issues and helps reconcile what could appear to be conflicting points of view. This can be illustrated by examining the evolution of current treatments for patients at the CMHC. Prior to the early 1960s when effective pharmacologic treatments for severe mental illness became available, patients were housed in the three large custodial mental health institutions in the state. Subsequently, the use of pharmacological treatments that helped control the most florid symptoms allowed for the development of psychosocial treatment systems that in turn facilitated deinstitutionalization of a majority of patients. Currently, the control of symptoms by effective pharmacotherapy now allows patients to benefit from psychosocial interventions, including individual and group psychotherapy and rehabilitation. If the pharmacotherapy were discontinued, a majority of patients would have a symptomatic relapse and the psychosocial treatments would fail. Conversely, if patients were only given medication without the necessary psychosocial therapy and support they would not be able to maintain an independent existence outside the institution. This illustrates how problems at the social, psychological and biological levels must all be effectively addressed to insure optimal therapeutic effectiveness. In the future it will be necessary to combine more efficiently different forms of treatment in order to obtain optimal success.

Future neurobiological progress and the care of patients

The current molecular-genetic revolution changing the practice of medicine will also affect psychiatry. The sequencing of the human genome and other advances in molecular biology has now ushered in the era of molecular medicine. It is increasingly possible to identify genes that lead to disease, and the elucidation of the molecular and cellular mechanisms involved provide new opportunities for the development of more specific and effective treatments (e.g., the molecular basis of specific treatments that target some cancers). In psychiatry this is on the near horizon. For example, it has been found that individuals with a particular mutation in the gene for the serotonin transporter are much more vulnerable to the effects of childhood abuse and stress in producing depression (Caspi et al., 2003). Individuals with a gene variant of a dopamine-metabolizing enzyme are much more vulnerable to developing a schizophreniform psychosis if they have used cannabis (Caspi et al., 2005). These two instances illustrate that we will be able to use genetic methods to identify individuals with increased vulnerability to developing illness. However, there will need to be psychological and social interventions in the lives of the individuals with the vulnerability genes in order to reduce the probability of illness (e.g., the reduction of stress or abstinence from cannabis). This illustrates how the neurobiological factors that confer vulnerability to illness will need to be dealt with at the psychological and social levels if effective progress in prevention and treatment is to be made.

Another important area where neurobiological research will make a major contribution in the future is drug abuse. In the research facilities it has been possible to develop animal models where self administration of drugs of abuse leads to addiction. This has allowed investigators to identify the biochemical pathways involved and to evaluate possible new treatments. Through these types of investigations it will be possible to develop new drugs that can attenuate reinforcement and withdrawal (Picciotto et al., 2005). Just as with the treatment of other types of mental illness, a combination of drug treatment with cognitive, behavioral and psychosocial treatment will be required to achieve optimal results.

Summary

The original concept of combining service, teaching and research at the CMHC has been validated by the significant progress that has been made over the past 40 years. The inclusion of neurobiological research in an environment of service and education has been mutually beneficial. The immediate needs of patients have helped focus the research efforts so that the program has been able to develop new and more effective treatments. This has led to major advances in the quality of care delivered at the CMHC and at other institutions. The associated training programs have produced a successive stream of outstanding graduates who have gone on to lead new treatment, research and educational programs at the CMHC, the Department of Psychiatry and at other institutions across the nation. Thus, the tripartite formula of service, teaching and research at the CMHC has been a successful recipe for 40 years of progress.

References

Aghajanian GK, Marek GJ: Serotonin model of schizophrenia: emerging role of glutamate mechanisms. Brain Res Rev 31:302–12, 2000

Aghajanian GK, Rosecrans JA, Sheard MH: Serotonin release in the forebrain by stimulation of midbrain raphe. Science 156:402–3, 1967

Alreja M, Wu M, Liu W, et al.: Muscarinic tone sustains impulse flow in the septohippocampal GABA but not cholinergic pathway: implications for learning and memory. J Neuroscience 20:8103–10, 2000

Caspi A, Moffitt TE, Cannon M, et al.: Moderation of the effect of adolescent-onset cannabis use on adult psychosis by a functional polymorphism in the catechol-O-methyltransferase gene: longitudinal evidence of a gene X environment interaction. Biol Psychiatry 57:1117–27, 2005

Caspi A, Sugden K, Moffitt TE, et al.: Influence of life stress on depression: moderation by a polymorphism in the 5-HTT gene. Science 301:386–9, 2003

Chambers RA, Taylor JR: Animal modeling dual diagnosis schizophrenia: sensitization to cocaine in rats with neonatal ventral hippocampal lesions. Biol Psychiatry 56:308–16, 2004

Charney DS, Riordan CE, Kleber HD, et al.: Clonidine and naltrexone: a safe, effective, and rapid treatment of abrupt withdrawal from methadone therapy. Arch Gen Psychiatry 39:1327–32, 1982

Coric V, Taskiran S, Pittenger C, et al.: Riluzole augmentation in treatment-resistant obsessive-compulsive disorder: an open-label trial. Biol Psychiatry 58:424–8, 2005

D'Souza DC, Abi-Saab WM, Madonick S, et al.: Delta-9-tetrahydrocannabinol effects in schizophrenia: implications for cognition, psychosis, and addiction. Biol Psychiatry 57:594–608, 2005

Duman RS: Role of neurotrophic factors in the etiology and treatment of mood disorders. NeuroMolecular Med 5:11–25, 2004

Duman RS, Nakagawa S, Malberg J: Regulation of adult neurogenesis by antidepressant treatment. Neuropsychopharmacology 25:836–44, 2001

Epperson CN, Haga K, Mason GF, et al.: Cortical gamma-aminobutyric acid levels across the menstrual cycle in healthy women and those with premenstrual dysphoric disorder: a proton magnetic resonance spectroscopy study. Arch Gen Psychiatry 59:851–8, 2002

Kaufman J, Yang BZ, Douglas-Palumberi H, et al.: Brain-derived neurotrophic factor-5-HTTLPR gene interactions and environmental modifiers of depression in children. Biol Psychiatry 59:673–80, 2006

Krystal JH, Perry EB, Jr., Gueorguieva R, et al.: Comparative and interactive human psychopharmacologic effects of ketamine and amphetamine: implications for glutamatergic and dopaminergic model psychoses and cognitive function. Arch Gen Psychiatry 62:985–94, 2005

Newton SS, Collier EF, Hunsberger J, et al.: Gene profile of electroconvulsive seizures: induction of neurotrophic and angiogenic factors. J Neurosci 23:10841–51, 2003

Newton SS, Duman RS: Regulation of neurogenesis and angiogenesis in depression. Current Neurovascular Research 1:261–7, 2004

Picciotto MR: Nicotine as a modulator of behavior: beyond the inverted U. Trends Pharmacological Sci 24:493–99, 2003

Picciotto MR, Hawes JJ, Brunzell DH, et al.: Galanin can attenuate opiate reinforcement and withdrawal. Neuropeptides 39:313–15, 2005

Sanacora G, Fenton LR, Masula MK, et al.: Cortical gamma-aminobutyric acid concentrations in depressed patients receiving cognitive behavioral therapy. Biol Psychiatry 59:284–6, 2006

Sanacora G, Gueorguieva R, Epperson CN, et al.: Subtype-specific alterations of gamma-aminobutyric acid and glutamate in patients with major depression. Arch Gen Psychiatry 61: 705–13, 2004

Sughondhabirom A, Jain D, Gueorguieva R, et al.: A paradigm to investigate the self-regulation of cocaine administration in humans. Psychopharmacology 180:435–46, 2005

5

Psychiatric epidemiology, services research, prevention and public health

Selby C. Jacobs, David L. Snow, Rani Desai and Gary Tischler

Chapter 5 traces the history of studies starting in the 1970s that addressed questions of central interest to the community mental health movement. Public psychiatrists and their colleagues at the Connecticut Mental Health Center carried out studies of early detection, community development and services utilization. By the early 1980s, formal programs in prevention, psychosocial and descriptive epidemiology, and services research had crystallized. All three domains, forming the basic science of public health practice, made signal contributions to the field of public psychiatry over the next 25 years, helping to guide development at the Center. The chapter highlights a population perspective on the development and organization of services as well as the impact of psychiatric public health on patient care. Finally, the chapter reviews key challenges in the future of public psychiatry and how preventive, epidemiologic, and services research might help understand them and meet them.

At the dedication of the Connecticut Mental Health Center (CMHC) on October 1, 1966, Frederick Redlich identified three "specific academic tasks" through which the Center could make important and badly needed contributions (Redlich, 1968). They were epidemiological study, evaluation of the effects of mental health efforts, and educational innovation. The first two set a course for the academic programs described in this chapter, and the third task was integrated into virtually all the activities of the Center. Redlich was the Chairman of the Department of Psychiatry at the Yale University School of Medicine and a co-author of the study *Social Class and Mental Illness (1958)* that observed high rates of schizophrenic illness in the lowest socio-economic class (Hollingshead and Redlich, 1958). As well, he was one of the original developers of the Connecticut Mental Health Center concept, in collaboration with Connecticut Governor Abraham Ribicoff.

Redlich's view of the core academic tasks of the CMHC resonates with the uses of epidemiology put forth by Morris in his classic book and elaborated upon by Henderson three decades later (Henderson, 1996; Morris, 1964). The uses included (1) the documentation of secular trends of disease; (2) the description and estimates of the distribution of diseases in populations and communities; (3) the completion of

40 Years of Academic Public Psychiatry. Edited by Selby C. Jacobs and Ezra E. H. Griffith
© 2007 John Wiley & Sons, Ltd.

the clinical picture, as in providing age and sex variation in disease occurrence; (4) the computation of risks of disease or relapse; (5) the identification of new syndromes; (6) the search for causes through investigation of risk factors; (7) the evaluation of services, now referred to as services research; and (8) the evaluation of preventive interventions. The pages that follow describe how the academic programs of the CMHC have contributed significantly to public psychiatry in all these ways. They also demonstrate the extent to which the course of action set by Redlich has been realized over the past 40 years.

The origin of academic programs

In his remarks, Redlich also heralded the development of the Center's Hill-West Haven Division. One of 675 centers funded through the Community Mental Health Centers Act of 1963, the Division was viewed by Redlich as a "vivid demonstration of Yale's commitment to the community." It also served, initially, as the catalyst for the prevention and public health programs as well as epidemiological and services research at the Center. As a federally funded mental health center, the Division was the only component of the CMHC designed to provide comprehensive mental health services to a geographically defined catchment area. The Hill neighborhood of New Haven and the city of West Haven made up the service area. Poor income, unemployment, low educational level, substandard housing and overcrowding were characteristic of the Hill. African Americans constituted one-third of the total population. Approximately one-half of the Spanish-speaking inhabitants of New Haven resided in the neighborhood. West Haven, geographically contiguous to the Hill, was a predominantly lower-middle class, less diverse, working class town heavily dependent upon New Haven-based agencies for social and health care services.

The service model of the Hill-West Haven Division held that service to a community represented a working alliance between consumer and provider. The goals of the alliance were: (1) to seek out and modify features of the social, economic and institutional environment harmful to mental health, through research, primary and secondary prevention, and social action; (2) to support individuals in their efforts to deal with mental illness and emotional disorders, through comprehensive clinical services, characterized by ease of access and continuity of care; and (3) to develop an effective community mental health manpower base, through training residents of the service area to work as paraprofessionals in all aspects of the Division's operations. Thus, consumer participation, social action, clinical care, prevention, consultation, research and training were each viewed as critical to the Division's mission.

In the late 1960s, under the leadership of Max Pepper, Leo Fichtenbaum, William Ryan and, subsequently, Claudwell Thomas, the emphasis of the Division's research was on (1) elucidating the philosophy of service, (2) recounting the nature of its prevention and clinical programs, and (3) evaluating their impact. Social psychologist Ryan articulated the conceptual underpinnings of the Division's primary prevention programs (Ryan, 1967, 1969, 1971). Postulating an inextricable link between power, pathology and prevention, the programs made extensive use of community organization and social action techniques that empowered individuals to act on their own behalf and, through these efforts, change circumstances known either to be corollaries of mental illness or inimical to mental health. A second empowerment strategy was built upon an educational platform designed by Kermit Nash. It took the form of a graded job development program in concert with a degree equivalency program that provided career mobility in the allied health professional field. The third strategy involved actively engaging community members in the governance of the Division. One can envision that this was no mean task, given that the Division was a federally funded center within a cooperative venture of the State of Connecticut and Yale University. The process and problems involved in attempting to achieve a viable balance among the oft-competing interests of a community board, government agencies and the academy were described and analyzed (Tischler et al., 1975a; Wellington and Tischler, 1972).

To a greater extent than ever before, NIMH regulations (U.S. DHEW, 1971) asserted that the new CMHC program was to incorporate both prevention and treatment approaches. The public health model of primary, secondary, and tertiary prevention strongly influenced the formulation of federal policy and the guidelines for implementation of the new CMHC programs. Through 1978, the impetus for the development of community-based prevention and early intervention programs fell to the Hill-West Haven Division's satellite programs overseen by Rachel Robinson, with the satellite in West Haven headed by David Snow and that in the Hill neighborhood, by Robert Washington. In addition to providing outpatient clinical services, these settings committed substantial resources to the development of programs in prevention, consultation and related training. A primary task involved building relationships with groups and organizations in the community. A product of these activities was the design and piloting a range of preventive and consultative interventions. In 1978, as the specter of block grant funding for community mental health loomed at the federal level, a decision was made to identify prevention and mental health consultation as a Center-wide, not merely Hill-West Haven, responsibility. With that goal, The Consultation Center was established as a Division of the CMHC with Snow as its Director. This reorganization formed the basis for the continuing evolution of the Center's academic program in prevention and public health.

The descriptive and anecdotal studies that characterized the early academic activities of the Hill-West Haven Division were complemented by methodologically innovative and policy-relevant investigations of a central feature of the federal program, catchmenting. A comparison of the demographic characteristics of admissions during a twelve-month period to catchmented versus non-catchmented service delivery system was done. It indicated significantly greater service utilization by socially disadvantaged groups of the catchmented service, an outcome consistent with the goal of the federal program (Tischler et al., 1972b). To determine whether the result was a function of catchmenting, two demographically comparable areas were constructed and matched on a group of environmental variables highly correlated with service utilization. One was drawn from the area served by the catchmented program. The other was drawn from the area served by the non-catchmented program (Tischler et al., 1972a). Admissions to the two programs were then compared. Although the overall volume of service provided by the catchmented program remained significantly higher, demographic differences in the patient populations no longer achieved significance. From this, it was concluded that attention to the ecology of a service area coupled with assigned provider responsibility for its residents was an effective means for achieving greater accessibility and equity in the allocation of services. Further support for the view that the accessibility and responsiveness of a service program is a corollary of a catchment-orientation was derived from a third study (Goldblatt et al., 1975). Intake was briefer, more patients were recommended for treatment, more treatment time per clinician was available, waiting lists were shorter and more patients started treatment on the catchmented as compared to the non-catchmented service. Other studies of the catchment demonstrated that factors other than psychological impairment, including age, disadvantaged social status, and familial or social disorganization were powerful mediators of service allocation (Tischler et al., 1975b, 1975c). This body of research highlighted the utility of population-based research for clarifying crucial issues concerning underserved populations and the value of ecological analysis as an experimental and planning tool.

Another CMHC program affording a platform for psychosocial, epidemiological research in the early 1970s was the Depression Research Unit led by Gerald Klerman. One of Klerman's colleagues, Eugene Paykel, pursued groundbreaking studies of psychosocial stressors and their roles in the onset of major depression (Paykel et al., 1969, 1971). He also collaborated in similar studies of first episode, schizophrenic illness with Selby Jacobs (Jacobs and Myers, 1976; Jacobs et al., 1974). These studies, using newly developed structured scales for assessing and estimating the severity of recent life experience, provided evidence that psychosocial stressors were related to the onset of both illnesses. In the case of major depression, losses and threats to autonomy were related to illness in a distal and formative manner. In the case of schizophrenic illness, the salient events were failed developmental milestones such as starting college or legal troubles and related to illness onset as precipitating events. This line of research resurfaced later in the 1990s, when Carolyn Mazure, Martha Bruce and Jacobs studied recent life experience in relation to the onset of major depressive illness, including the interaction with cognitive personality style (Mazure et al., 2000). In these retrospective, case-controlled studies, individuals with autonomous personality styles were more vulnerable to events threatening their independence and individuals with rejection sensitivity were more vulnerable to losses and interpersonal conflict. Taken together, these studies emphasized the importance of the environment and significant life stressors in the occurrence of psychiatric illnesses and provided background for later studies of early intervention in psychosis.

It was the Psychiatric Utilization and Review Project (PURE), which provided a bridge between the social epidemiology of Redlich and Hollingshead of the 1950s and the descriptive epidemiology of the Epidemiologic Catchment Area (ECA) Study of the 1980s. The PURE Project grew from Klerman's interest in promoting evaluative studies and the State of Connecticut's efforts to upgrade data systems for the Department of Mental Health. Three prior experiences facilitated the project. Donald Riedel and his colleagues had already developed a basic utilization review program for general hospitals. Also, the long history of collaborative research among the Departments of Psychiatry, Sociology, and Public Health provided a foundation. Finally, the pioneering efforts of the CMHC and the Rockland Research Institute in implementing an automated psychiatric information system made the Center an ideal setting for evaluating the potential cost and effectiveness of a mental health utilization review program (Levine, 1975; Riedel et al., 1972). The project's criterion-oriented approach provided procedures for developing guidelines to evaluate individual cases by diagnosis that were the harbinger of today's expert consensus and guideline methodologies (Tischler and Riedel, 1973).

A utilization review system was developed to facilitate patient care evaluation and many aspects of program evaluation. The scheme included several features: a data system, mechanisms for selecting charts for review, guidelines for evaluating the quality of care, indications/methods for conducting supplementary epidemiological, and follow-up studies (Goldblatt et al., 1973; Henisz et al., 1974; Tischler, 1975). Efforts were undertaken to evaluate the efficiency of case-selection mechanisms (Henisz et al., 1974), to develop methodologies for establishing length of stay norms (Weiner, 1975), to screen patients being considered for hospitalization (Flynn and Henisz, 1975) and to assay the validity of normative criteria (Kirstein et al., 1975a, 1975b). Also included was a process for evaluating the adequacy, appropriateness and effectiveness of case-oriented consultations that was then applied to assess community service programs for children (Cytrynbaum, 1974; Cytrynbaum et al., 1975; Tischler, 1976). A comprehensive model for evaluating the availability, accessibility, appropriateness, adequacy and acceptability of psychiatric care with examples of its application was put forth by Riedel et al. (1974); Tischler and Astrachan (1982) expanded upon the model by providing an exposition of the topic from a "why" and "how to" perspective, while demonstrating the impact of societal, organizational and procedural factors upon quality assurance activities.

Academic programs and public sector practice

By the late 1970s, three major areas of academic inquiry with relation to public health and prevention emerged at the CMHC. They were epidemiological research, mental health services research and prevention research. These academic programs have made substantive contributions to psychiatry in the public sector.

Psychiatric epidemiology

The New Haven studies of the 1950s and 1960s provided significant epidemiological data on impairment rates and their key socio-cultural corollaries. The dimensional measure of impairment used in these studies, however, did not generate rates for specific disorders. A crucial community study conducted by Weissman and Myers in 1975 demonstrated that reliable clinical diagnoses and prevalence estimates could be generated using a structured diagnostic interview and research diagnostic criteria (Weissman and Myers, 1977; Weissman et al., 1978). The scope of these studies was broadened by the NIMH-sponsored ECA Study of the 1980s. New Haven was one of five sites selected for a study that heralded a major shift in paradigms from dimensional measures of psychological distress to a categorical, diagnostic approach. The existence of structured criteria for diagnoses and a study design that drew samples from five ecologically distinct sites allowed investigators to establish firmer point and period prevalence estimates for most of the major psychiatric disorders. Weissman and associates were able to expand upon their previous work (Leaf et al., 1986b; Weissman et al., 1984, 1986, 1988). Their studies of the age- and sex-specific prevalence of affective disorders affirmed female gender as a risk factor for Major Depressive Disorder (MDD). The highest rates of MDD were found among the youngest cohort. Additional risk factors for major depression included living alone, marital separation/divorce and difficulties in spousal relationships. Cross-site analyses revealed mean rates for bipolar disorder ranging from 0.7/100 at two weeks to a lifetime mean rate of 1.2/100 and rates of major depression ranging from 1.5/100 (two weeks) to 4.4/100 (lifetime). The cross-site means for dysthymia, a chronic condition, was 3.1/100. The study documented an even higher rate among women.

Other findings by the group included a six-month prevalence rate for cognitive impairment among the elderly of 3.4% (Holzer et al., 1984; Weissman et al., 1985). The rate of severe cognitive impairment did not increase until after age 79. Among those 80 years and older, cognitive impairments were more common in women than in men. A population prevalence rate of 1% was found for schizophrenic disorder (Myers et al., 1984). This rate was consistent with those reported in the United States/ United Kingdom cross-national study and suggested that the longstanding hypothesis of higher rates of schizophrenia in the United States as opposed to other cultures was not sustainable. Indeed, the prevalence rate of 1% has now been observed around the world, an observation leading to a shift in thinking about the biologic causes and risk factors for schizophrenia, while crystallizing interest in psychosocial risk factors, such as migrant status in dense urban centers.

In the late 1970s and 1980s, Adrian Ostfeld and Stanislav Kasl, both at the School of Epidemiology and Public Health, and Selby Jacobs at the Connecticut Mental Health Center began studies of the general and mental health consequences of bereavement (Hays et al., 1994; Jacobs, 1993). Bereavement was chosen for study as a single and severe stressor. These studies confirmed that bereavement, which figured prominently in life event schedules mentioned earlier, was a severe psychosocial stressor with a wide range of health consequences. Of particular interest to psychiatry, loss was associated with a higher risk of major depression, anxiety disorders and pathologic forms of grief. In 1996, Holly Prigerson began to lead analyses of data from this study and other sources. These analyses indicated that pathologic grief, a clinical concept stemming from Freud's original paper on mourning and melancholia, was indeed independent of depressions and anxiety disorders and occurred commonly after loss (Prigerson et al., 1996). Eventually, Prigerson and colleagues completed studies to evaluate consensus diagnostic criteria (Prigerson et al., 1996, 1999). Their work resulted in the imminent publication of the first empirically tested, consensus criteria for a new diagnostic entity named Prolonged Grief Disorder, which may be incorporated into the next *Diagnostic and Statistical Manual* (DSM). The utility of these diagnostic criteria for Prolonged Grief Disorder has been documented in multiple countries and cultures. Also, the availability of criteria has stimulated both new studies of the occurrence of Prolonged Grief Disorder after disasters and studies of treatment interventions. Among the treatment interventions are studies of selective serotonin reuptake inhibitors and specific, cognitive behavioral therapies.

In the early 1990s, stemming from the ECA Study, Kathleen Merikangas organized a Genetic Epidemiology Research Unit. On this unit, she carried out studies on the familial aggregation of substance use disorders (Merikangas et al., 1998). In addition, her group examined mechanisms of psychiatric co-morbidity associated with substance use disorders. The major findings of this work demonstrated the familial aggregation of substance use disorders. For example, relatives of probands with substance use disorders had an eight-fold, increased risk of having a substance use disorder. Genetic factors operated similarly in men and women. The observations of psychiatric co-morbidity echoed one of the major findings of the National Co-morbidity Study about the high rate of co-morbidity among all psychiatric disorders. This is especially true for antisocial personality disorders, bipolar disorder, mood disorders, anxiety disorders and substance abuse. This study was a harbinger of a major shift observed in the clinical population of individuals applying for treatment at the CMHC. Whereas, in the 1980s, the modal patient who registered for care was seriously mentally ill with little, diagnosed or treated substance abuse, by the late 1990s, co-morbidity of mental illness and substance abuse, and the treatment of these co-occurring disorders, was the norm.

With the re-surfacing of state lotteries in 1964 and the rapid expansion of legalized gambling venues in recent decades came concern about the potential deleterious effects of excessive gambling (Shaffer and Hall, 2001). Two events have shaped research at the CMHC on gambling. First, the state of Connecticut became home to the two largest casinos in the world, attracting regular visitors from across the eastern seaboard and generating millions of dollars in revenue every month. Second, the DSM officially entered Pathological Gambling (PG) as a disorder that described symptoms of excessive gambling and gambling-related problems. A gambling clinic was established at the CMHC and led by Marc Potenza. This clinic has served as the basis for a number of psychopharmacology studies exploring effective ways to treat PG. In addition, in collaboration with Rani Desai and others, Potenza embarked on studies exploring the epidemiology, risk factors, and health and mental health consequences of PG. These studies have explored this disorder across the lifespan (examining adolescents, adults and older adults separately), gender, psychiatric co-morbidity groups and levels of gambling (for example, exploring the health correlates of recreational gambling which falls below criteria for PG). As a result, these studies have identified distinct gender differences in patterns of gambling and patterns of gambling-related problems (Potenza et al., 2002). For example, the phenomenon of telescoping is seen among women gamblers, in a pattern similar to that seen for alcohol use: while women start gambling later in life than men, they also have shorter courses than men of the development of gambling addictions (Desai et al., 2005). The gambling research group has also found a high risk of PG among people with mental illness, and vice versa. The studies also observed large age differences in the health correlates of both PG and recreational gambling (Desai et al., 2005). Curiously, elders who engage in recreational gambling report better physical and mental health than non-gamblers, which may be a function of their ability to get out (Desai et al., 2004).

One of the unintended consequences of the efforts to deinstitutionalize people with mental illness was that increasing numbers found themselves incarcerated or otherwise involved with the criminal justice system (Torrey et al., 1992). This has both placed a burden on the criminal justice system to find ways to care for and house people with mental illness, but also has led to increasing efforts to find alternatives to incarceration where possible. Since the mid-1990s at the CMHC, there have been a number of research efforts to explore the burden of mental illness in criminal justice populations; to determine the effectiveness of diversion strategies; and to establish an evidence base for mental health care practices in juvenile detention facilities. Desai, in collaboration with Madelon Baranoski and the Division of Law and Psychiatry at the CMHC, conducted a comprehensive study of all those individuals arraigned in New Haven Superior Court over a five-year period. With this sample, they identified what proportion of detainees had contact with the CMHC or other state mental health facilities. Among all those with a history of mental illness, they then compared those who received specialized jail diversion services to those who did not receive such services. The services research aspect of this study will be discussed later. However, the epidemiologic evidence indicated that about 40% of those arraigned had a history of contact with the mental health system, many of them for substance abuse treatment or evaluation (Hoff et al., 1999a, 1999b).

In the late 1990s, Richard Schottenfeld conducted an epidemiologic survey of 186 juveniles in detention called the Substance Abuse and Need for Treatment Assessment (SANTA) study. This study assessed the prevalence of substance use and abuse as well as histories of substance abuse and mental health treatment among detainees. The results showed that a third of detainees met diagnostic criteria for one or more substance abuse disorders. However, less than a quarter had ever received any treatment, and only about a third of those who met criteria perceived a need for treatment. The factor most strongly associated with a perceived need for treatment was the presence of co-morbid psychiatric symptoms, highlighting the important issue of co-morbidity in this vulnerable population (Goulet et al., 2003).

In summary, the ECA Study (as well as the National Co-morbidity Study) of the 1980s and 1990s provided the first reasonably accurate data on the distribution of psychiatric disorders in the community. A better understanding of the true occurrence of mental and substance use disorders facilitated the planning and implementation of services for a community, usually in the circumstances of limited resources. To complete the circle, services research, discussed next, evaluates the operating services after implementation. Also, the ECA Study affirmed female gender as an important risk factor in major depression. The NCS and studies of the co-morbidity of substance abuse disorders, supplemented by the genetic epidemiology of substance abuse, have been instrumental in defining the co-morbidity of mental illness and addiction as a central premise in clinical practice. Further, studies of gambling and mental illness among homeless and prison populations, have established the high prevalence of these problems. Knowledge of the role of psychosocial stress in the onset of depression and schizophrenia facilitated clinical recognition of incipient symptoms for early intervention. Better understanding of the clinical complications of bereavement improved disaster readiness, making preventive and early interventions more effective and specific. In an application of epidemiologic science, clinical epidemiology is progressively the foundation for evidence-based medicine programs in the clinics of the CMHC.

Services research

Just as the ECA Study stimulated research on the prevalence of mental illness in the community, it provided the platform for the mental health services research of Leaf, Bruce, Holzer and Tischler. Analyses of the relationship among clinical status, population characteristics, personal attitudes and service use helped further understanding of the discrepancy between high rates of disorder coupled with low rates of service utilization (Bruce et al., 1992; Leaf and Bruce, 1987; Leaf et al., 1985, 1986a, 1987, 1988; Tischler et al., 1988). The picture that emerged suggested that the signs, symptoms and behaviors associated with mental illness are critical factors in the quest for care. There are others. Some are predisposing factors such as age, sex or marital status. Other predisposing factors reflect cultural conditioning or social structure. The predisposing factors are but one element in the service use equation. Enabling factors are at work as well by determining the availability and accessibility of services. Some reflect attitudes toward mental illness services and the acceptability of seeking professional help. Other enabling factors include personal and economic resources, public policy, administrative procedures and treatment practices. It is the interaction between the predisposing and enabling factors that ultimately determines the use of services.

In the early 1990s, Robert Rosenheck, who pioneered mental health services research in the VA system, expanded his interest into the state-funded public sector as well. These efforts were concentrated in two large primary data collection studies, the ACCESS project (1994–1999) (Randolph et al., 2002) and the Connecticut Outcomes Study (COS, 1996–1999) (Desai et al., 2005). The Access project was an ambitious multi-site study that addressed the fragmentation of public sector services for homeless people with mental illness. Each of 18 sites across the country, one of which was located at the CMHC with Michael Hoge as the co-investigator, was randomized to receive either funding specifically to increase integration of mental health, social service and medical care across systems, or to provide care as usual to homeless people with serious mental illness. Participants were followed for up to a year to determine the effects of these services on clinical and social outcomes. The initial randomized study found that the extra funds to encourage integration did not appear to translate into improved clinical outcomes (Rosenheck et al., 1998).

The data collected during the ACCESS study led to a great increase in our understanding of the risks associated with homelessness. The data also documented those factors associated with better clinical outcomes. For example, one analysis found very high rates of suicidal ideation and suicide attempts among homeless people with serious mental illness. Also, the highest risk for suicidal ideation was among those who had been recently discharged from an inpatient program. These observations led to concern about potential dumping of patients before they had adequate housing and before psychiatric symptoms had stabilized (Desai et al., 2003). Another analysis found that those homeless clients who had recently come into contact with the criminal justice system were more likely to have childhood histories of conduct disorder, illegal behavior, unstable childhoods and a history of child abuse. This analysis suggested that the oft-cited phenomenon of the criminalization of mental illness might be overstated. However, it also highlighted the long-term effects of adverse environmental and developmental conditions such as poverty, abuse, and neglect that increase the risk for later mental illness and housing instability (Desai et al., 2000).

The COS study, conducted by Desai and Rosenheck, was funded by the VA and was designed to compare the VA system of care for people with serious mental illness with the state-funded, public system in the same geographic catchment area. This was of interest to mental health services researchers because although the two systems treat a similar demographic profile of patients (i.e., largely low income clients, many on public disability), they are organized very differently. The VA is a vertical, federally funded and integrated system where a medical model prevails. The state systems are locally funded, not well integrated into the public sector medical systems, and reha-bilitation oriented. Here, although there were some small differences between VA patients and non-VA patients in demographics and in the focus of available mental health services, there did not appear to be much difference in clinical outcomes (Desai et al., 2005).

The negative results from the ACCESS project and COS contradicted prevailing ideas that integration of services was desirable to render the public mental health system more effective and improve clinical outcomes for vulnerable patients. On the other hand, it is important not to expand this conclusion unduly. For example, another study at the CMHC, conducted by Jeanne Steiner, found dramatic results concerning the routine medical preventive care received by women who were patients at the CMHC. This was also observed for women with mental illness treated at primary care clinics. The women at the CMHC, particularly those with histories of trauma, were far less likely to receive routine gynecologic care. One implication of this study was that mental health facilities might benefit from primary care services located in the same location. Therefore integration of psychiatric and medical services might offer benefit.

In the early 1990s, William Sledge and Jack Tebes completed a study of crisis respite care as an alternative to traditional hospitalization for the target population served by the Center. Crisis respite care included placement in a residential program with 24-hour supervision and partial hospitalization services, both coordinated together. Sledge and Tebes demonstrated that for non-acutely suicidal patients in crisis, crisis respite is an effective alternative to inpatient care. They and their colleagues also carried out cost analyses, documenting the lower cost of crisis respite as an alternative to the hospital. This study broke ground in demonstrating the effectiveness of crisis respite care. It led to a progressive development of alternatives to hospital care. It ultimately contributed to the development of multiple levels of care and algorithms for moving patients among them as a strategy for reducing costs.

In the past 10 years, Scott Woods, heading a program on medication effectiveness, has studied the cost-effectiveness of both new antidepressants and new antipsychotic drugs. The results raise questions about the value of the newer drugs. The much higher costs of the newer drugs do not appear justified by efficacy that is clearly superior to old-line treatments. He has noted a bias in industry-sponsored research. Thus, the same drug performs better when studied by its sponsor than when the study is paid for by a competitor or by an independent group. This pattern, of course, raises questions about some of the claims of superiority from studies carried out by pharmaceutical companies. He has demonstrated that racial and ethnic minority groups at the CMHC are prescribed atypical antipsychotic drugs at the same rate as others. Depot antipsychotic drugs are disproportionately prescribed for African Americans. Also, Woods and Diaz have shown better adherence to antipsychotic medications by Latinos when they are prescribed once daily as opposed to divided dosing. Most recently, Woods' studies supplement the conclusions of the Clinical Antipsychotic Trials of Intervention Effectiveness (CATIE) study by demonstrating that the risk of Tardive Dyskinesia from atypical antipsychotic drugs does not materially differ from that of the traditional antipsychotics, such as perphenazine. Together with the CATIE find-ings, his studies undermine the claims that the newer, more expensive drugs offer more than "me-too" advantages.

In the late 1990s, Michael Hoge, the Director of Yale Behavioral Health and Director of Services at the Center, obtained a contract to provide mental health services to juvenile detention facilities throughout Connecticut. Rani Desai, with Hoge as well as researchers in the Court Support Services Division, which is the state judicial branch responsible for juvenile detention, embarked on a line of research on mental health care services in detention facilities. First, the group wrote a review paper on the state of mental health care in detention. They concluded that despite a clear need for such services, there were few services offered. Also, no evidence base existed for what might be appropriate in this population (Desai et al., 2006). More recently, the group has begun to focus on disproportionate minority confinement (DMC), first finding that violence risk was not a determinant of DMC. Then they observed that mental health status did not mediate the association between race and perceived violence risk. Finally, they examined whether violence risk assessments were accurate predictors of criminal justice outcomes such as recidivism (Chapman et al., 2006). The research group has plans to expand its inquiries to include decision-making by judges, police officers and probation/parole officers. In addition they will test mental health interventions in detention populations in order to clarify pathways to treatment.

In summary, services research has addressed several key questions in public sector practice. The range of observations starts with demonstration of the value of catch-menting as a strategy for more accessible and more effective treatment and preventive services. Also, services research explored the complex discrepancy between clinical diagnosis and service use. In addition, services research at the Center has assessed the value of system integration, both within mental health and between mental health and medicine, and found no added value beyond routine clinical coordination. Studies of medication effectiveness have challenged pharmaceutical companies' claims about the efficacy of new generation drugs. These studies question the value of high cost, atypical antipsychotic drugs, echoing the controversy now raging as a result of the CATIE study about the value of expensive, atypical drugs. Services research also has helped to define the epidemiology of mental disorders in criminal justice populations.

Prevention and public health

Prevention science represents a further elaboration and alternative to the public health model of primary, secondary and tertiary prevention. Prevention science more clearly differentiates prevention from treatment and rehabilitation. It leads to the continuing scientific development of prevention and public health. There is a continued emphasis on modifying individual and environmental risk and protective factors as a means of reducing the incidence of psychiatric and substance abuse disorders. Prevention science identifies three types of primary prevention activities: universal, selective and indicated (Gordon, 1987; NIMH, 1996). Universal interventions target the general public or entire population groups regardless of risk status. Selective interventions target individuals or population subgroups whose risk of developing the disorder is higher than average due to individual or environmental factors. Indicated interventions target high-risk individuals with detectable signs of the disorder, but who do not meet criteria for a psychiatric diagnosis (NIMH, 1996). Risk reduction and the enhancement of protective factors are the primary emphases of interventions in prevention science

(Kellam et al., 1999; NIMH, 1996). Thus, prevention now represents one end of a continuum of interventions that includes behavioral health treatment and extends to rehabilitation and recovery.

Beginning in the 1980s and continuing to the present, Snow, Kelin Gersick, Katherine Grady and Tebes established a program of research on school-based interventions to prevent adolescent substance abuse. The primary focus of this work was on the impact of a social-cognitive intervention to prevent substance abuse in middle school and high school. This intervention was found to be effective in preventing substance abuse among adolescents from sixth through tenth grades. Maintenance of these effects persisted at one- and two-year follow-up (Snow et al., 1992). In addition, intervention was maximally effective for at-risk children from single-parent households (Snow et al., 1997). The success of the randomized trial in the greater New Haven area prompted an extensive dissemination effort to over 200 schools in the Northeast and nationally. Dissemination led to later research in the 1990s by Tebes, Matthew Chinman and Grady that incorporated positive youth development principles into the intervention. The intervention was later expanded into after-school settings (Caplan et al., 1992; Tebes et al., 2001a). The most recent incarnation of the original school-based prevention research was developed by Tebes and his colleagues. They conducted the first successful school-based, randomized trial of mentoring on the prevention of substance abuse and problem behaviors among at-risk urban youth (DuBois et al., in press). Other extensive school-based prevention research conducted over the past several years by Nadia Ward and her colleagues has involved the evaluation of the impact of school-based affective and character education programs on several outcomes. These include academic achievement, problem behaviors, and substance abuse among urban middle school and high school students throughout Connecticut (Ward, 2006).

In the late 1980s, Snow and colleagues initiated the development and testing of a workplace preventive intervention in an effort to reach large segments of the adult population. The aim was to prevent or reduce psychological symptoms of depression, anxiety and somatic complaints, and alcohol and other drug use. Two randomized, controlled trials of the intervention with varying control conditions were conducted over the next several years. Based on a risk and protective factor model, the intervention was shown to have significant effects in reducing work and family stressors and work–family conflict. Other outcomes noted were increased social support from supervisors and co-workers, enhanced active behavioral, cognitive and social support coping, decreased avoidance coping strategies, and reduced alcohol consumption and psychological symptoms as compared to control conditions (Snow and Kline, 1995; Snow et al., 2002). In a review of published findings and based on replication of effects, the intervention was designated as an Evidence-Based Program by the Center for Substance Abuse Prevention through the National Registry of Effective Programs (NREP). It is listed by the Substance Abuse and Mental Health Services Administration (SAMHSA) as a Model Prevention Program. The intervention is now in the stage of active, national dissemination.

In the 1990s, Tebes and his colleagues began to focus on the promotion of resilience among vulnerable populations and the identification of resilience processes among at-risk groups. Tebes and Joy Kaufman have examined resilience among children of parents with serious mental illnesses, children of "sandwiched-generation" care-giving women, and urban poor adolescents. In one early study that involved mothers (who were CMHC outpatients) and their children, they found that children's mental health outcomes were related to parenting and other family psychosocial processes. These included family stress, even after accounting for parental psychopathology and psychiatric functioning (Tebes et al., 2001b, 2005b). The centrality of familial and other supportive relational processes to child resilience also was demonstrated in other research with non-patient populations involved in community-based preventive interventions.

A research program on family violence prevention has involved a series of investigations of risk and protective factors for women and men's psychiatric symptoms, substance abuse and other health outcomes in the context of intimate partner violence. Two initial studies by Suzanne Swan, Snow and Tami Sullivan, involved the identification of precursors, correlates and outcomes of women's use of violence (Sullivan et al., 2005; Swan and Snow, 2002, 2003). These included childhood traumatization, maladaptive coping strategies, motivations for violent behavior, depression, Post-Traumatic Stress Disorder and substance abuse. A third study assessed the relationships among coping strategies and substance abuse and men's use of physical and psychological abuse toward their female partners. Among other findings, this study showed that avoidance coping and problem drinking independently predicted greater use of both physical and psychological abuse (Snow et al., 2006). These risk and protective factor studies are ongoing. They will provide the basis for designing and testing the efficacy of interventions aimed at preventing intimate partner violence. Not the least of the implications of this research is the development of a knowledge base to interrupt the cycle of violence, where childhood experiences are passed from generation to generation. This destructive cycle suggests approaches not only to reduce violence among adults, but to prevent child abuse and the witnessing of violence by children. Both these experiences are risk factors for mental illness, substance use and other problem behaviors in adulthood.

Kathleen Sikkema and colleagues, over the past five years, have developed a research program to evaluate cognitive-behavioral group interventions to improve adaptive coping with HIV infection and life stressors among women living in public housing. To date, two randomized, controlled trials have been completed. One was a study of a 12-session intervention with bereavement in a sample of 268 HIV positives who had lost a loved one to AIDS. The study demonstrated reduced psychiatric distress and enhanced quality of life in participants who received the intervention as compared to a treatment on request control condition (Sikkema et al., 2005). In addition, a strong gender effect emerged, with women showing significantly more improvement than men. In a second trial of a 16-session intervention in a sample of HIV positives who experienced sexual abuse as a child or adolescent, preliminary analyses show those in the coping intervention reported greater decreases in psychiatric distress than a waitlist control condition (Sikkema et al., 2007). As the intervention model in these studies based on coping theory is proving effective across multiple samples of participants who have experienced diverse stressors, dissemination of the interventions to practice settings is under consideration.

In the early 1990s, Tebes and Kaufman began large-scale, statewide evaluations of behavioral health systems of care in Connecticut and Rhode Island. These evaluations emphasized the establishment of partnerships with key community stakeholders, such as consumers and service recipients, parents and other family members, community providers, school personnel, law enforcement officers and state department staff. The partnerships ensure that the evaluation represents the views of individuals who are likely to be impacted by the service innovation and its evaluation. This "stakeholder-based" approach to evaluation has been widely adopted across the country and has been used with considerable success in subsequent evaluations in a number of states. Most of these evaluations have emphasized the use of data to inform the development of public policy. This aim is the explicit purpose of the Rhode Island Data Analytic Center, one of only three sites nationally that was funded to build data analytic and research capacity in the field of child welfare. One innovative example of this research was a study of the development of a statewide children's behavioral health system of care over an eight-year period and its impact on systems outcomes (Tebes et al., 2005a).

In the mid-1990s, Thomas McGlashan, Woods, Tandy Miller, Larry Davidson and others established the PRIME Research Clinic for prodromal schizophrenia. The primary aim of the PRIME clinic, now directed by Woods and based at the CMHC, is to investigate methods of preventing the development of schizophrenia by focusing on indicated prevention in patients showing early or "prodromal" signs. Results to date have demonstrated that the prodrome can be described, diagnosed, and assessed with reliability and validity (Miller et al., 2002; Woods et al., 2001). PRIME's clinical trial suggested that antipsychotic medication can effectively treat prodromal symptoms (McGlashan et al., 2003) and possibly prevent or delay the development of schizophrenia (Woods et al., 2003). Unfortunately, these benefits occur at considerable cost in adverse, metabolic side effects. New studies with alternative medications are underway. In a related development, Woods, Vinod Srihari, Cenk Tek and others, are developing a clinic for early intervention in first episode psychosis (the STEP clinic), with an eye to the secondary prevention goals of reducing the severity and chronicity of psychotic illness. If prevention of chronicity by early intervention is conclusively demonstrated, this approach will likely offer very substantial cost-effectiveness advantages.

Stemming from the IOM report, *Crossing the Quality Chasm*, and related to but not officially part of the national movement led by the Institute for Healthcare Improvement to save the lives of 100,000 patients in the year before July 2006, the CMHC currently is developing a suicide awareness and prevention program for the purpose of reducing deaths from suicide among registered patients. We are engaged in a systematic chart review of all suicides since 2003 and will apply a failure mode effects analysis. Then, the goal is to stabilize or reduce the number of deaths from suicide over an annual period in reference to our baseline data (e.g., 11 suicides in 2003). We intend to pursue this goal through routine and systematic screening of patients using the PHQ-9, mobilization of the clinical programs as well as families and the community, use of a chronic disease model promulgated by the Institute for Health Care Improvement, and development of effective teamwork.

In summary, the contribution to public psychiatry of the academic program in prevention occurs in several ways. First, within The Consultation Center and other sectors of the CMHC, efforts are made to integrate research, training and service, and to create a dynamic interrelationship between prevention research and service. Second, inherent in the development of effective preventive interventions is that this process is undertaken in close collaboration with a range of public sector partners in the community. And third, initiatives are under way to disseminate science-based preventive interventions, not only within the immediate service area, but also to other communities throughout the state and nationally. Within this process, prevention programs at the CMHC have made several contributions to public sector practice. They include school-based prevention of adolescent substance use; evaluation of workplace interventions to reduce work and family stressors, enhance effective coping and social support, and reduce psychological symptoms and alcohol abuse; studies of resilience among children of parents with serious mental illness and other high-risk families; studies of risk and protective factors for psychiatric symptoms in the circumstances of intimate partner violence; testing of cognitive behavioral interventions for women in public housing coping with AIDS, as well as those who have suffered loss or prior trauma; statewide evaluations of preventive and community services; early intervention in psychosis; and, in the early stages of development, suicide awareness and prevention. The Consultation Center (TCC) has carried out an academic program in prevention research and training for nearly 30 years. The contributions of TCC were recognized in 1990 when David Snow, Director, and The Consultation Center as an organization received the Henry V. McNeil Award from the Division of Community Psychology of the American Psychological Association for outstanding achievement and innovation in the field of community psychology.

Education

Redlich's vision for the CMHC included the challenge of innovative education to develop new cadres of mental health professionals, who would root their practice in evidence, challenge traditional professional boundaries and develop advanced specialized skills, consistent with the multiple roles of professionals in modern community-based practice. Over the years, the Center has made educational innovations in public psychiatry, usually with an interdisciplinary approach at multiple levels. Examples are the development of more highly skilled paraprofessionals as well as specialized residency education in public psychiatry.

In addition, special educational endeavors were linked to each of the academic programs in epidemiology, services research and prevention. Originally these educational programs were supported out of stipends. As federal support for clinical education was cut during the 1970s and as cost-shifting from clinical services budgets to education became progressively untenable during the 1980s, Tischler, Snow, Wexler and colleagues in the programs described above pursued federal funding for specialized research education. These included education in mental health services research, prevention and chronic mental illness. Through these educational programs, the CMHC sustains its academic program elements. The academic programs contribute to maintenance of a balanced evidenced-based array of services in our public institution. Also, these educational programs prepare new generations of clinical and investigative professionals for public psychiatry, many of whom follow careers in Connecticut.

New directions and future developments

Given the rapidly changing circumstances of health and mental health care, the academic agenda is both long and challenging (Insel and Fenton, 2005). It is an agenda that emphasizes the importance of research and development as part of an overall strategy for promoting knowledge-based change through demonstration projects and prevention research. Also part of the agenda is evaluation of change in the nature and distribution of mental illness and patterns of utilization through epidemiologic and health services research.

Epidemiology

One of the most fascinating questions confronting 21st century America is the health and mental health impact of growing class distinctions, wealth discrepancies and ethnic diversification. Cultural differences in illness and health-seeking behaviors, the stress attendant on changes in social status, and discrepancies in the character and frequency of certain life events are important factors affecting the true and treated prevalence of illness. We now have better tools for reliably establishing incidence and prevalence rates of particular disorders. Reuniting approaches from the biological, clinical sciences and social sciences could significantly enrich our understanding of the causes and course of contemporary mental illnesses.

Risk factor studies, incorporating personal, genetic and neuro-biologic variables, hold promise of elaborating the contribution of the environment to the occurrence of disease for both established syndromes as well as new syndromes. Studies defining the syndrome of Prolonged Grief Disorder can include measures of vasopressin and oxytocin as well as brain imaging data. Investigations are needed of risk factors and mechanisms through the longitudinal study of cohort differences in age of onset of depressive disorder. The study of gender differences in major depressive disorder is another current challenge. Also, studies of the effect of urban environments on migrants who develop schizophrenic illness hold promise for providing a useful bridge between descriptive and social epidemiology. Similarly, studies clarifying the role of social inequality and marginalization in causing depressive disorders and substance abuse would be a powerful avenue of inquiry for addressing the issue of reducing disparities in health care outcomes.

In a somewhat different vein, the question of mental illness and trans-institutionalization is a fertile field for descriptive epidemiology. The criminalization of substance abuse over the past twenty years has resulted in the majority of prisoners' experiencing substantial problems with addictions and with co-occurring disorders. In this regard, we need a better understanding of the incidence, prevalence and treated prevalence of mental illness in prisons, detention centers and post-incarceration populations. There is a pressing need to elucidate the natural history of co-occurring addictive and mental illness co-morbidity. We also need to understand better the transitions from sub-clinical states to full syndromes, using improved strategies for dating onset of illnesses. These studies would improve early detection, access to care, and usefully drive the system of care toward further integration of mental health and addiction services.

With an emphasis on community care, studies of the natural versus treated course of severe mental illness are also an important, but neglected area of inquiry. It is one thing to espouse a course of clinical action, but quite another to determine what the unexpected side effects might be. Additionally, clinical and natural history studies of chronic mental illness and recovery are essential to our assisting patients during periods when they are not acutely ill. But perhaps one of the most useful areas of study from an epidemiological perspective would be a Framingham-like longitudinal study that followed a cohort of school-age children through their life span to explore the relationship between childhood and adult mental health and disorder.

As part of a descriptive agenda, it is also crucial to understand the occurrence of newly defined syndromes in different populations and circumstances. The changing course of society, as reflected in ethnic diversity and growing class distinctions, is continually introducing new challenges to mental health. Examples are "new" addictions such as gambling as well as exacerbations of the mental health effects of life experiences such as bereavement and large-scale natural disasters. Basic epidemiologic principles can still be used to monitor changes in the mental health impact of both common and unusual large-scale environmental life stressors.

Further, the expansion of diagnostic usage into new arenas raises important questions about the advantages and disadvantages of placing behavior or behavioral problems under a medical model rather than regarding them as a social problem. The advent of criteria-based diagnostic systems has enhanced diagnostic reliability. However, it does not address the issue of diagnostic validity. For example, studies of the attitudes of acutely bereaved individuals and their families to receiving a diagnostic label and seeing a mental health professional can help address reservations about the potential stigmatization of a diagnostic label. In this instance, needless to say, effectiveness studies documenting benefit could counterbalance the potential risk associated with labeling.

Services research

The pace of change in the system of care continues unabated. As psychiatry pursues a patient centered, patient safety and quality agenda, an integrative approach using "desktop" computer support and disease management and chronic disease models of practice can elevate the overall quality of care to new levels. Through refinement of existing and development of new institutional performance measures for public consumption, health service researchers can also contribute to a coherent and policy-relevant approach to institutional performance evaluation. Examples already exist in the veterans' health care system.

To the extent that economic and cost control strategies emphasize acute care, the impact of change on long-term care, relapse prevention, psychosocial and vocational rehabilitation, and community supports such as supported housing requires careful scrutiny. Evaluative studies and demonstration projects on disease management and chronic disease models for organizing and delivering care would help address this challenge. Ecologic models that consider social variables such as urban density or migration as risk factors in mental illness would also contribute. In addition, new methodology in economic analysis can assist systems in determining the optimal mix of services to make available. The aim would be to ensure both that clients in acute phases of illness are appropriately cared for, but also that clients who are stabilized and attempting to live the best quality of life possible with a chronic mental illness have the support they need to remain stable.

Perhaps the most crucial topic for services researchers will be the impact of the fundamental changes that the Medicaid and Medicare programs are undergoing. With Medicaid, states have been given enormous authority to reconfigure benefits, charge premiums and raise co-payments for health care and prescription drugs. It is a system where health care providers can deny services and pharmacists can refuse to fill prescriptions when recipients do not make a required co-payment. We know that a prescription cap can seriously impact the use of psychotropic drugs and acute mental health care by schizophrenic patients (Soumerai et al., 1994). A similar set of issues exists in relation to Medicare, given the newly imposed structure of the managed prescription benefit. How formularies are constructed or modified, the different co-payment options available, and variability in terms of basic cost are all factors that can significantly alter the course of an illness.

Evaluation of strategies for allocating resources and reducing the burden of disease from psychiatric disorders in the community are of critical importance. The burden of disease metric is important because mortality from psychiatric disorders, while not negligible from suicide and other co-occurring natural causes, is small by comparison with other diseases. When disability is factored into the burden of disease equation, psychiatric disorders emerge as a substantial public health problem. The concept of burden of disease is and will grow as an essential tool for arguing for resources for the treatment and rehabilitation of psychiatric disorders.

Effectiveness studies also have a role to play in relation to third-party claims of the impact of particular treatments on mental health care outcomes. For example, studies of the effectiveness of atypical antipsychotic drugs can clarify questions concerning cost and efficacy raised by recent studies that dispute the marketing claims of large pharmaceutical firms.

Equally important, there is a need to substantiate the impact of recovery programs, given the claims for their effectiveness by activists and advocates. Absent data in support of the initiative, the potential benefits of the movement may fall victim to the next budget crisis or ideological revolution. The fate of new ideological movements in psychiatric services often has been to be discarded even though they had never been tested.

Prevention

The New Freedom Commission emphasized that limited resources are allocated to preventing acute and chronic illness, while the costs of psychiatric disability are large and growing rapidly. The commissioners encouraged more attention to the front end of disorders on the assumption that the costs of prevention will be less than those for cure or rehabilitation. Furthermore, the National Mental Health Council Workgroup on Mental Disorders Prevention Research recently made several recommendations to strengthen the empirical base of prevention through development of data from scientific studies of risk factors and preventive interventions in populations (NMHC

Workgroup, 1998). They also broaden the framework of preventive interventions to include relapse prevention and prevention of disabilities, development of population intervention strategies, evaluations of the cost and effectiveness of preventive interventions, and translation of evidence into practice. Also, the Surgeon General recently issued a national call to action on suicide prevention (DHHS, 2001).

To meet these challenges, a major future direction for prevention is to further the development of a comprehensive research program that encompasses all phases of prevention science. These include (1) the pre-intervention phase (problem analyses using descriptive and risk/protective factor research); (2) the intervention phase, testing the effectiveness and cost of universal, selective and indicated approaches; and (3) the diffusion or going-to-scale phase, when proven interventions are disseminated and need maintenance. New pre-intervention studies using epidemiological and risk and protective factor models are needed and are under way in many areas. Among these are studies of stress and coping, resilience, family violence, caregiver burden, HIV/AIDS, suicide, compulsive gambling, substance abuse, and serious psychiatric disorders across various populations and settings. These studies are essential to identifying those factors that play the most central role in the onset and/or progression of behavioral health disorders and problem behaviors. Established risk factors then become the target of change in the design of preventive interventions.

Rigorous efficacy and effectiveness trials are necessary to provide a basis for preventive interventions. For example, workplace prevention trials, aimed at promoting employee health and preventing illness, would be useful for testing a systems-level intervention. There are also indications for testing an intervention targeting working caregivers, a group who are at high risk for negative health outcomes and who are providing care to an older family. Preventive interventions with kinship care families such as elders and their caregivers need development and evaluation. The interventions would aim to prevent depression and other affective disorders, substance abuse, and physical health problems and to assess the effects of health promotion interventions for individuals at risk. Building on a solid base of pre-intervention research that now has been established over a period of years, studies testing the efficacy of different program models in preventing intimate partner violence, dating violence, and the abuse of children would be useful. Research on the prevention of HIV/AIDS could test preventive interventions aimed at better addressing barriers to risk reduction among HIV-positive individuals that occur due to severe mental illness, substance abuse and childhood sexual abuse.

Initial work in the areas of suicide prevention, relapse prevention and the prevention of homelessness needs to be expanded. Effectiveness studies evaluating the impact of critical incident stress management as a component of disaster readiness plans are needed to measure the impact of preventive interventions on the clinical complications of disasters and trauma. Research on interventions to prevent the onset or early intervention for major psychiatric disorders such as schizophrenia or depression could lead to fundamental contributions early in the course of disorders. For preventive psychiatry at present, the question of what protects the healthy 50% of monozygotic twins where one of the pair has schizophrenic illness is a most interesting one. And finally, attention could be given to the development of interventions that address the important areas of co-morbidity and disability prevention.

Conclusion

American society is on the cusp of major changes in the financing, organization, and delivery of health and mental health care. It is an era where the values of the marketplace and the world of commerce have become the catalysts of change. Corporate principles now dominate where public policy once ruled. Much of what was identified as social goods is now regarded as commodities. In a world where public sector agencies are looked upon as market entities, one can only anticipate a profound redefinition of the social contract that previously governed the organization, financing and delivery of care. There is nothing intrinsically wrong in wanting to limit cost, to increase efficiency or to enhance accountability. But they should not be regarded as ends in themselves. Past research and evaluation have demonstrated that the effects of change are frequently complex, often inconsistent, at times paradoxical, but usually measurable and always enlightening. Can a system governed by corporate principles achieve the oft-stated goals of availability, accessibility, equity, excellence of care and prevention? Will the burgeoning of information technology serve to standardize care with success measured primarily in terms of productivity increments, dollar savings and profitability and, only secondarily, in terms of clinical status, burden or well-being? Is it a system of care attentive to or neglectful of the many individuals who live at the margins? Who among the mentally ill are the served, the underserved, the unserved and the inappropriately served? These are but a few of the fundamental questions that we believe epidemiological and health services research can and should address.

Epidemiology, services research and prevention are the basic sciences of public health. While epidemiologic and health services research can do much to document and evaluate a problem and our response to it, there remains the difficult but crucial task of the prevention of mental disorder. We must remain committed to translating preventive science into practice through implementing balanced academic and clinical programs. All three of these academic disciplines, assuming adequate investment, can help in systematically and objectively addressing the population, system, and preventive questions facing modern mental health care. In so doing, they can make vital contributions to progress in public psychiatry.

References

Bruce ML, Tischler GL, Leaf PJ: The relationship of usual source of health care to the prevalence of psychiatric disorder and the utilization of ambulatory mental health services in the United States, in Primary Health Care and Psychiatric Epidemiology. Edited by Cooper B, Eastwood R. New York: Tavistock/Routledge, 1992

Caplan M, Weissberg RP, Grober JS, et al: Social competence promotion with inner-city and suburban young adolescents: effects on school adjustment and alcohol use. J Consult Clin Psychol 60:56–63, 1992

Chapman JF, Desai RA, Falzer P: Mental health service provision in juvenile justice facilities: pre- and postrelease psychiatric care. Child Adolesc Psychiatr Clin N Am 15:445–58, 2006

Cytrynbaum S: The application of the criteria-oriented approach to the review of indirect service activities in a community mental health center, in Patient Care Evaluation in Mental

Health Programs. Edited by Riedel DC, Tischler GL, Myers JK. Cambridge, MA: Ballinger Publishing Company, 1974

Cytrynbaum S, Snow DL, Phillips EV, et al: Program analysis and community mental health services for children, in Mental Health in Children. Edited by Sankar DVS. Westbury, NY: PJD Publications, 1975

Department of Health and Human Services National Strategy for Suicide Prevention: Goals and Objectives for Action. Rockville, Maryland, USDHHS, Public Health Service, 2001

Desai RA, Dausey DJ, Rosenheck RA: A comparison of service delivery by the Department of Veterans Affairs and state providers: the role of academic affiliation. Adm Policy Ment Health 32:267–83, 2005

Desai RA, Goulet JL, Robbins J, et al: Mental health care in juvenile detention facilities: a review. J Am Acad Psychiatry Law 34:204–14, 2006

Desai RA, Lam J, Rosenheck RA: Childhood risk factors for criminal justice involvement in a sample of homeless people with serious mental illness. J Nerv Ment Dis 188:324–32, 2000

Desai RA, Liu-Mares W, Dausey DJ, et al: Suicidal ideation and suicide attempts in a sample of homeless people with mental illness. J Nerv Ment Dis 191:365–71, 2003

Desai RA, Maciejewski PK, Dausey DJ, et al: Health correlates of recreational gambling in older adults. Am J Psychiatry 161:1672–9, 2004

Desai RA, Maciejewski PK, Pantalon MV, et al: Gender differences among recreational gamblers: the association with alcohol use. Psychol Addict Behav, in press

DuBois D, Doolittle F, Yates BT, et al: Research methodology and youth mentoring. J Community Psychol, 34:657–76, 2006

Flynn HR, Henisz JE: Criteria for psychiatric hospitalization: experience with a checklist for chart review. Am J Psychiatry 132:847–50, 1975

Goldblatt PB, Berberian R, Goldberg B, et al: Catchmenting and the delivery of mental health services. Arch Gen Psychiatry 28:478–82, 1975

Goldblatt PB, Brauer L, Garrison V, et al: A chart review checklist for utilization review in a community mental health center. Hosp Community Psychiatry 24:753–6, 1973

Gordon R: An operational classification of disease prevention, in Preventing Mental Disorders: A research perspective. Edited by Steinberg J, Silverman M. Rockville, MD: Alcohol, Drug Abuse, and Mental Health Administration, DHHS Publication No. ADM 87-1492, pp 20–6, 1987

Goulet JL, Desai RA, Schottenfeld R: Perceived addiction treatment need among juvenile detainees. Presented at the NIMH Conference on Addictions in Adolescence, Washington, DC, 2003

Hays JC, Kasl SV, Jacobs SC: The course of psychological distress following threatened and actual conjugal bereavement. Psychol Med 24:917–27, 1994

Henderson AS: The present state of psychiatric epidemiology. Aust NZ J Psychiatry 30:99–119, 1996

Henisz JE, Goldblatt PR, Flynn HR, et al: A comparison of three approaches to patient care appraisal based on chart review. Am J Psychiatry 131:1142–4, 1974

Hoff RA, Rosenheck RA, Baranoski MV, et al: Diversion from jail of detainees with substance abuse: the interaction with dual diagnosis. Am J Addict 8:201–10, 1999a

Hoff RA, Rosenheck RA, Materko M, et al: Mental illness as a predictor of satisfaction with inpatient care at Veterans Affairs hospitals. Psychiatr Serv 50:680–5, 1999b

Hollingshead AB, Redlich FC: Social Class and Mental Illness: A Community Study. New York: John Wiley & Sons, 1958

Holzer CE, Tischler GL, Leaf PJ, et al: An epidemiologic assessment of cognitive impairment in a community population, in Research in Community and Mental Health. Edited by Greenley JR. Greenwich, CT: JAI Press, 1984

Insel T, Fenton W: Psychiatric epidemiology: it's not just about counting any more. Arch Gen Psychiatry 62:590–2, 2005

Jacobs SC: Pathologic Grief: Maladaptation to Loss. Washington, DC: American Psychiatric Press, 1993

Jacobs SC, Myers JK: Recent life events and acute schizophrenic psychosis: a controlled study. J Nerv Ment Dis 162:75–87, 1976

Jacobs SC, Prusoff BA, Paykel ES: Recent life events in schizophrenia and depression. Psychological Medicine 4:444–53, 1974

Kellam SG, Koretz D, Moscicki EK: Core elements of developmental epidemiologically-based prevention research. Am J Community Psychol 27:463–82, 1999

Kirstein L, Prusoff B, Weissman MM, et al: Utilization review and suicide attempters: a comparison of explicit criteria and clinical practice. Am J Psychiatry 132:22–7, 1975a

Kirstein L, Weissman MM, Prusoff B: Utilization review and suicide attempters: exploring discrepancies between experts' criteria and clinical practice. J Nerv Ment Dis 160:49–56, 1975b

Leaf PJ, Bruce MM: Gender differences the use of mental health-related services: A re-examination. J Health Soc Behav 28:171–83, 1987

Leaf PJ, Bruce MM, Tischler GL: The differential effect of attitudes on the use of mental health services. Soc Psychiatry 21:187–92, 1986a

Leaf PJ, Bruce MM, Tischler GL, et al: Contact with health professionals for the treatment of psychiatric and emotional problems. Med Care 23:1322–37, 1985

Leaf PJ, Bruce MM, Tischler GL, et al: Factors affecting the utilization of specialty and general medical mental health services. Med Care 26:9–26, 1988

Leaf PJ, Bruce MM, Tischler GL, et al: The relationship between demographic factors and attitudes towards mental health services. J Community Psychol 15:255–84, 1987

Leaf PJ, Weissman MM, Myers JK, et al: Psychosocial risk and correlates of major depression in one United States urban community, in Mental Disorder in the Community: Progress and Challenge. Edited by Barrett J, Rose R. New York: Guilford Press, 1986b

Levine MS: Support system for the Multi-State Information System, in Safeguarding Psychiatric Privacy: Computer Systems and Their Uses. Edited by Laska EM, Bank R. New York: John Wiley & Sons, 1975

Mazure CM, Bruce ML, Maciejewski PK, et al: Adverse life events and cognitive personality characteristics in the prediction of major depression and antidepressant response. Am J Psychiatry 157:896–903, 2000

McGlashan TH, Zipursky RB, Perkins D, et al: The PRIME North America randomized double-blind clinical trial of olanzapine vs. placebo in patients at risk of being prodromally symptomatic for psychosis: I. study rationale and design. Schizophr Res 61:7–18, 2003

Merikangas KR, Stolar M, Stevens D, et al: Familial transmission of substance use disorders. Arch Gen Psychiatry 55:973–9, 1998

Miller TJ, McGlashan TH, Rosen JL, et al: Prospective diagnosis of the prodrome of schizophrenia: preliminary evidence of interrater reliability and predictive validity using the Structured Interview for Prodromal States (SIPS). Am J Psychiatry 159:863–5, 2002

Morris JN: Uses of Epidemiology. Baltimore, MD: Williams and Wilkins, 1964

Myers JK, Weissman MM, Tischler GL, et al: Six month prevalence of psychiatric disorders in three communities. Arch Gen Psychiatry 41:959–67, 1984

National Advisory Mental Health Council Workgroup on Mental Disorders Prevention Research: Priorities for prevention research at NIMH. NIH Publication No. 98-4321, 1998

National Institute of Mental Health: A report to the National Advisory Mental Health Council. NIH Publication No. 96-4093, 1996

Paykel ES, Myers JK, Dienelt MN, et al: Life events and depression: a controlled study. Arch Gen Psychiatry 21:753–60, 1969

Paykel ES, Prusoff BA, Uhlenhuth EH: Scaling of life events. Arch Gen Psychiatry 25:340–7, 1971

Potenza MN, Maciejewski PK, Desai RA, et al: Characteristics of gamblers: health measures and gender differences. Drug Alcohol Depend 66(suppl.1): S141, 2002

Prigerson HG, Bierhals AJ, Kasl SV, et al: Complicated grief as a disorder distinct from bereavement-related depression and anxiety: a replication study. Am J Psychiatry 153:1484–6, 1996

Prigerson HG, Shear MK, Jacobs SC, et al: Consensus criteria for traumatic grief: a preliminary empirical test. Br J Psychiatry 174:67–73, 1999

Randolph F, Blasinsky M, Morrissey JP, et al: Overview of the ACCESS Program: access to community care and effective services and supports. Psychiatr Serv 53:945–8, 2002

Redlich FC: The University and Community Mental Health. New Haven: Yale University Press, 1968

Riedel D, Brenner MH, Brauer L, et al: Psychiatric utilization review as patient care evaluation. Am J Public Health 62:1222–8, 1972

Riedel DC, Tischler GL, Myers JK: Patient Care Evaluation in Mental Health Programs. Cambridge, MA: Ballinger Publishing Company, 1974

Rosenheck R, Morrissey J, Lam J, et al: Service system integration, access to services, and housing outcomes in a program for homeless persons with severe mental illness. Am J Public Health 88:1610–5, 1998

Ryan W: Blaming the Victim. New York: Vintage Books, 1971

Ryan W: Distress in the Cities. Cleveland: Case Western Reserve University Press, 1969

Ryan W: Preventive services in the social context: power, pathology, and prevention, in Preventive Services in Mental Health Programs. Edited by Bloom BL, Puck DP. Boulder, CO: Western Interstate Commission for Higher Education, 1967

Shaffer HJ, Hall MN: Updating and refining prevalence estimates of disordered gambling behavior in the United States and Canada. Can J Public Health 92:168–72, 2001

Sikkema KJ, Hansen NB, Kochman A, et al: Outcomes from a group intervention for coping with HIV/AIDS and childhood sexual abuse: reductions in traumatic stress. AIDS Behav 11, 46–60, 2007

Sikkema KJ, Hansen NB, Meade CS, et al: Improvements in health-related quality of life following a group intervention for coping with AIDS-bereavement among HIV-infected men and women. Qual Life Res 14:991–1005, 2005

Snow DL, Kline ML: Preventive interventions in the workplace to reduce negative psychiatric consequences of work and family stress: does stress cause psychiatric illness? Edited by Mazure CM. Washington, DC: American Psychiatric Press, pp 221–70, 1995

Snow DL, Sullivan T, Swan SC, et al: The role of coping and problem drinking in men's abuse of female partners: test of a path model. Violence Vict 21:267–85, 2006

Snow DL, Swan SC, Wilton L: A workplace coping skills intervention to prevent alcohol abuse, in Preventing Workplace Substance Abuse: Beyond Drug Testing to Wellness. Edited by Bennett J, Lehman WEK. Washington, DC: American Psychological Association, pp 57–96, 2002

Snow DL, Tebes JK, Arthur MW, et al: Two-year follow-up of a social-cognitive intervention to prevent substance use. J Drug Educ 22:103–16, 1992

Snow DL, Tebes JK, Ayers TS: Impact of two social-cognitive interventions to prevent adolescent substance use: test of an amenability to treatment model. J Drug Educ 27:1–17, 1997

Soumerai SB, McLaughlan TJ, Ross-Degnan D, et al: Effects of limiting Medicaid drug reimbursement benefits on the use of psychotropic agents and acute mental health services by patients with schizophrenia. New Engl J Med 331:651–5, 1994

Sullivan T, Meese K, Swan S, Mazure C, et al: Precursors and correlates of women's violence: child abuse, traumatization, victimization of women, avoidance coping, and psychological symptoms. Psychol Women Q 29:290–301, 2005

Swan SC, Snow DL: A typology of women's use of violence in intimate relationships. Violence Against Women 8:286–319, 2002

Swan SC, Snow DL: Behavioral and psychological differences among abused women who use violence in intimate relationships. Violence Against Women 9:75–109, 2003

Tebes JK, Bowler S, Shah S, et al: Service access and service system development in a children's behavioral health system of care. Eval Program Plan 28:151–60, 2005a

Tebes JK, Chinman MJ, Shepard J: Positive Youth Development Collaborative and Evaluation. SAMHSA 1 KD1 SP09280, Rockville, MD, 2001a

Tebes JK, Connell CM, Ross E, et al: Convergence of sibling risk among children of parents with serious mental disorders. J Child Family Studies 14:29–41, 2005b

Tebes JK, Kaufman JS, Racusin GR, et al: Resilience and family psychosocial processes among children of parents with serious mental disorders. J Child Family Studies 10:115–36, 2001b

Tischler GL: Developing information systems to facilitate quality assessment in mental health, in Evaluation and Mental Health Services. Edited by Markson EW, Allen D. Lexington, MA: Heath &and Company, 1976

Tischler GL: The use of MSIS in program evaluation, in Safeguarding Psychiatric Privacy: Computer Systems and Their Uses. Edited by Laska E, Bank R. New York: Wiley and Sons, 1975

Tischler GL, Aries E, Cytrynbaum S, et al: The catchment area concept, in Progress in Community Psychiatry. Edited by Bellak L, Barten H. New York: Brunner/Mazel, 1975a

Tischler GL, Astrachan BM: Quality Assurance in Mental Health, Washington, DC, U.S. Govt. Printing Office, 1982

Tischler GL, Henisz J, Myers J: Catchmenting and the use of mental health services. Arch Gen Psychiatry 27:389–92, 1972a

Tischler GL, Henisz J, Myers J, et al: The impact of catchmenting. Adm Ment Health 1:22–9, 1972b

Tischler GL, Henisz JE, Myers JK, et al: The utilization of mental health services. I. Patienthood and the prevalence of symptomatology in the community. Arch Gen Psychiatry 32:411–5, 1975b

Tischler GL, Henisz JE, Myers JK, et al: The utilization of mental health services. II. Mediators of service allocation. Arch Gen Psychiatry 32:416–8, 1975c

Tischler GL, Leaf PJ, Holzer CE: The relationship between the need for services and the utilization of services, in Needs Assessment: Its Future. Edited by Goldsmith H, Lin E, Bell RA,

Jackson D. DHHS Pub. No. (ADM) 88-1550, Washington, DC: U.S. Govt. Printing Office, 1988

Tischler GL, Riedel D: A criterion approach to patient care evaluation. Am J Psychiatry 130:913–6, 1973

Torrey E, Steiber J, Ezekiel J, et al: Criminalizing the seriously mentally ill: the abuse of jails as mental hospitals. Washington, DC, Public Citizen's Health Research Group and the National Alliance for the Mentally Ill, 1992

U.S. Department of Health, Education, and Welfare (DHEW). NIMH, community mental health center program, operating handbook. Part 1: Policy and standards manual. Washington, DC: National Institute of Mental Health, September 1, 1971

Ward NL: Improving equity and access for low-income and minority youth into institutions of higher education. Urban Education Review, 41:50–70, 2006

Weiner OD. The use of MSIS for utilization review, in Safeguarding Psychiatric Privacy: Computer Systems and Their Uses. Edited by Kaska EM, Bank R. New York: John Wiley & Sons, 1975

Weissman MM, Leaf PJ, Holzer CE, et al: Epidemiology of depression: an update of sex differences in rates. J Affective Disorders 7:179–88, 1984

Weissman MM, Leaf PJ, Tischler GL: Affective disorders in five United States communities. Psychol Med 18:141–53, 1988

Weissman MM, Myers JK: Affective Disorders in a US urban community: the use of Research Diagnostic Criteria in an epidemiologic survey. Arch Gen Psychiatry 1304–11, 1977

Weissman MM, Myers JK, Harding PS: Psychiatric disorders in a US urban community: 1975–1976. Am J Psychiatry 135:459–62, 1978

Weissman MM, Myers JK, Tischler GL, et al: Psychiatric disorders (DSM-III) and cognitive impairment among the elderly in a USA urban community. Acta Psychiatr Scand 71:366–79, 1985

Wellington SW, Tischler GL: Community mental health: why the benign neglect? Yale J Law & Social Action 3:78–86, 1972

Woods SW, Breier A, Zipursky RB, et al: Randomized trial of olanzapine vs. placebo in the symptomatic acute treatment of patients meeting criteria for the schizophrenia prodrome. Biol Psychiatry 54:453–64, 2003

Woods SW, Miller TJ, Davidson L, et al: Estimated yield of early detection of prodromal or first episode patients by screening first degree relatives of schizophrenic patients. Schizophr Res 52:21–7, 2001

6

Ethnicity, mental health care disparities and culturally competent care at the Connecticut Mental Health Center

Howard C. Blue, Luis Añez, Manuel Paris, Dietra Hawkins and Robert Page

The Community Mental Health Centers Construction Act of 1963 promised the creation of a system of care that would better meet the needs of the mentally ill and provide responsive care to the socially, culturally and economically disadvantaged. Those promises remain unrealized, and there is substantial evidence of significant disparities in the delivery of quality mental health care to ethnic minorities and other socially disadvantaged groups. This chapter examines the history and intent of the CMHCC Act of 1963, factors associated with disparities in mental health care, and the potential of cultural competency paradigms to address the fundamental issues of disparity in mental health care.

When the Community Mental Health Centers Construction (CMHCC) Act of 1963 was signed into law, it represented the culmination of more than a century of effort to recognize the needs of the mentally ill, to destigmatize psychiatric illness, and to provide better quality and more humane treatment to those challenged with the disruptive effects of a mental illness (Cutler et al., 2003). At the time, President Kennedy proposed the development of a national mental health program rooted in comprehensive community care aimed at upgrading mental health services and placing mental health treatment into the mainstream of American medicine. This vision of mainstreaming mental health treatment occurred in the broader sociopolitical context of a thriving civil rights movement aimed at social parity for black Americans and, by extension, the recognition of the basic human rights of all people. The CMHCC Act of 1963 "signified the beginning of a national attempt at responsive service delivery to the socially, culturally, and economically disadvantaged" (Cheung and Snowden, 1990), with its emphasis on the provision of care to those without economic means. The Act represented a new hope for people dealing with psychiatric illness and led ultimately to a shift of psychiatric care from distant asylums to local communities. This "third psychiatric revolution" (Rochefort, 1984) produced a reduction in the

40 Years of Academic Public Psychiatry. Edited by Selby C. Jacobs and Ezra E. H. Griffith
© 2007 John Wiley & Sons, Ltd.

census of state and county mental health hospitals and provided seed money for the development of hundreds of federally funded community mental health centers nationwide. The Connecticut Mental Health Center (CMHC) emerged during this era and went on to establish itself as an institution with a strong tripartite mission of carrying out research, clinical service, and the education and training of mental health professionals.

While there has been tremendous advancement in the treatment and care of the mentally ill since 1963, there is also evidence of persistent failure to reach some of the most vulnerable and socially disadvantaged. In this chapter we shall review health and mental health care disparities and examine contributing factors. We shall also address the issue of cultural competency, which many see to be a potential mechanism for addressing health care disparities, and discuss examples of the CMHC's efforts to address the needs of at risk populations and to provide care that is culturally responsive and relevant.

The impact of deinstitutionalization

Over the past forty years or more, there have been considerable changes in how to deliver care to local communities most effectively, including the development of lead mental health agencies with the responsibility to monitor fiscal, quality and other dimensions of delivering care in defined geographic regions. The reductions in state and county psychiatric hospital rolls led to what has been termed deinstitutionalization, which Talbott (1979) has labeled a "misnomer." In 1955 state hospitals had a daily average census of nearly 600,000 patients; in 1990 that average daily census had been reduced to about 92,000.

In pressing for the passage of the CMHCC Act, President Kennedy believed that primary prevention and the reduction of the census in state hospitals could be achieved through community mental health centers. In his speech, *The Dream*, Kennedy contended that community-based prevention efforts were especially important in the area of mental illness if institutionalization of the mentally ill was to be reduced and halted. He believed that establishing community mental health centers would be more economically sound than maintaining large state psychiatric facilities. Moreover, he argued that primary prevention efforts would reduce the onset of mental illness and the necessity for long-term institutional care. Isaac and Armat (1990) noted that Kennedy advanced a belief that the major problem at that time was existing institutional care of patients rather than disease itself. Reduction of hospital populations became a prime objective of the CMHHC legislation; however, there was considerable lack of emphasis on where these institutionalized patients would live after discharge. Discharge from hospitals was fueled further by passage in 1962 of Aid to the Permanently and Totally Disabled Act (a precursor to SSI), which made mentally ill individuals eligible for federal benefits to pay for rent and basic needs. Few foresaw subsequent problems such as housing and employment discrimination as impediments to the integration of these patients into local communities. Notably, as deinstitutionalization rates climbed, the proportion of seriously mentally ill patients treated in community mental health centers declined (Isaac and Armat, 1990), and it became clearer that community mental health centers were focusing on the so-called "worried well."

In fact, in 1975, it was noted that few community mental health centers were in compliance with the National Institute of Mental Health's (NIMH) original 1964 guidelines that five essential services should be provided by community mental health centers: inpatient services, partial hospitalization, outpatient services, emergency services, and consultation and education services. Some 50% of community mental health services had no psychiatric beds, and few had any emergency services. Only about 6% had day treatment, and almost all were poorly staffed (Torrey, 1988). As the gaps in the mental health care system became more evident and evidence mounted that community mental health centers were not meeting the needs of deinstitutionalized patients, a Task Force on Deinstitutionalization was established in 1977 by the Secretary of the Department of Health, Education, and Welfare. The work of this task force led to the development of the Community Support Program which was designed to provide services for psychiatric patients with persistent and severe disabilities. The allocation of funds focused on the persistently and severely mentally ill led to a reduction in services to those with less serious mental health difficulties. Some argue that the 1963 CMHCC Act was never intended to establish a national counseling service but rather to fund a program to substitute for state hospitals in caring for the seriously mentally ill (those with psychotic disorders and unrelenting affective disorders). This view was shortsighted given the propensity for some non-psychotic disorders (Depressive Disorders, Panic Disorder, PTSD) to develop chronic courses if untreated.

Deinstitutionalization has proven to be an immense challenge for local communities that were not prepared with adequate resources to handle the needs of patients who were discharged from often long-term confinement in inpatient facilities. Some have used the term "trans-institutionalization" (PBS, Frontline, 2005) to reflect the reality that many patients previously housed and treated in state and county hospitals simply moved into the criminal justice system, nursing homes and homeless shelters where they received poor or inadequate care. Deinstitutionalization, in many ways, revealed the fragmentary nature of the American mental health system; a state of affairs that still receives commentary today. The effects of inadequate preparation for the discharge of multitudes of patients from institutional care altered the intent of the CMHCC Act in its vision of mainstreaming mental health care and providing care to the socially, culturally and economically disadvantaged. With limited resources and an immense mission, local mental health care agencies have had to focus more on the provision of care to those with so-called serious mental illnesses rather than on uninsured community populations dealing with less serious but still troubling emotional and psychological disturbances. Despite promising growth in the number of mental health centers during Johnson's presidency, the Nixon administration did not look favorably on them and impounded funds appropriated for mental health programs. Although funds were later released, the Nixon administration had clearly stated its disapproval of governmental mental health initiatives. Subsequent legislation to restore momentum to the flagging community mental health center movement was crushed by a veto from President Ford. By the time a more sympathetic Carter administration assumed office, economic problems were so serious that additional appropriations for mental health were constrained. Still, at the end of Carter's term, 691 mental health centers continued to receive federal assistance. With the Omnibus Budget and Reconciliation Act of 1981, however, the Reagan administration collapsed all mental health funding into a block grant available to states for any mental health services they deemed fundable. As a result, the designation of centers in direct receipt of federal funds ceased in 1981 (Karger and Stoesz, 1994). This has created problems of access which have now become a source of considerable concern as this country grapples with ways to improve the mental health care system and to address the immense unmet mental health needs of our communities.

More and more evidence has accumulated that offers a sober assessment of where we are 40 years later in this community mental health movement. It has been estimated that only one-third of patients with a psychiatric disorder get treated (Robins and Regier, 1991) and that ethnic minorities fare even worse. The Freedom Initiative authorized by President George W. Bush in 2001, and chaired by former Connecticut Mental Health Commissioner, Michael Hogan, noted in its findings in 2003 that there were still "unmet needs" and that "many barriers impeded care for people with mental illnesses" (President's New Freedom Commission on Mental Health, 2003). The commission also concluded that "the mental health system has not kept pace with the diverse needs of racial and ethnic minorities, often under-serving them or inappropriately serving them." Census projections suggest that ethnic minority groups will constitute 40% of the American population by 2025 and about 47% by 2050 (U.S. Census Bureau, 2001). This will have a major impact on our health care system and poses great challenges to understanding further and correcting the current discrepancies in health care status and outcomes between white Americans and ethnic minority Americans.

Health care disparities

The literature on health care disparities between whites and other racial/ethnic minority groups is extensive and expanding. While this chapter is concerned mainly with the mental health system, examining ethnic disparities in the general medicine arena and conceptualizations about factors related to the use of health care systems is quite instructive. Much is not known, but it is clear that the issue of discrepancies in the utilization of health care services and health care outcomes are much more complex than simple comparisons across ethnic and racial boundaries. Health care utilization involves individual choices as well as interaction effects such as engagement and cultural communication nuances. While American society has the capacity to develop institutions that can be more accessible and available, the use of health care is ultimately a personal decision.

Several landmark reports and task forces have chronicled racial and ethnic disparities in health care. The Secretary of Health and Human Services formed a Task Force on Black and Minority Health in 1984 to investigate the health problems of various ethnic and racial groups in the United States. The Task Force issued a report in 1985 which noted that there were considerable disparities between white Americans and other racial and ethnic minority groups for several health conditions. Several subsequent studies also documented relative health disadvantages of a number of racial and ethnic populations (Mayberry et al., 2000). The National Center for Health Statistics (1996) noted higher rates for coronary heart disease, breast cancer and diabetes in African Americans, and found higher infant mortality rates among African Americans, Native Americans and Native Alaskans, and higher rates of uncontrolled hypertension in Mexican Americans. Hispanics and blacks were more likely to be uninsured or to be publicly insured than whites, and Hispanics were twice as likely as whites to lack a usual source of care. Asian and Hispanic adults had more problems accessing specialty care. Overall emergency room usage to receive both routine and emergency care was higher among ethnic minority patients. A search of the literature on racial and ethnic disparities in health care, covering 1984–1994 and restricted to articles, commentaries, and letters in the *New England Journal of Medicine* and the *Journal of the American Medical Association*, revealed alarming fractures in health services along racial lines. African Americans, according to the review, are less likely than their white counterparts to receive renal transplants, receive hip or total knee replacements, and undergo gastrointestinal endoscopy, among other procedures, but are more likely to undergo hysterectomy and amputation of the lower limb. Perhaps most consistent—and most disturbing—are the repeated findings that African Americans with ischemic heart disease, even those enrolled in Medicare or fee-care systems, are much less likely to undergo angiography, angioplasty, or coronary-artery bypass grafting. In studies of the Veterans Affairs system, for example, blacks were 33% less likely to undergo angioplasty, and 54% less likely to undergo CABG than their white counterparts (Geiger, 1996). The Surgeon General's 2001 report again ushered these issues to the forefront of our social consciousness.

Other researchers have used regression-based analyses and attempted to understand the contributions that insurance status, income level and other individual characteristics may have on these disparities. Using 20 years of data, Weinick et al. (2000) examined changes in access and use over time. Their data showed that the proportion of Americans without a source of usual care changed very little between 1977 and 1996. Blacks and Hispanics were considerably more likely to lack a source of usual care; the changes were small for blacks but considerably larger for Hispanics. The study also showed that improving equality of income and health insurance coverage status among ethnic groups can result in a substantial reduction in disparities in access and use but would not eliminate disparities. These authors issued cautions about the interpretation of their data and noted that they could not attribute the disparities to access problems alone. They also pointed out that there are few data on normative utilization rates, thus using white utilization rates as the optimal benchmark may lead to false conclusions. Their work, however, pointed to a number of factors that need further clarification and study including a fuller assessment of non-financial barriers to access, determination of the effect of cultural and linguistic competence among health care providers and institutions, geographic distribution of health care providers, the role of intentional and unintentional discrimination within the health care system, and perceptions of discrimination within the health care system on the part of ethnic minorities. Disparities may also be linked to such non-financial phenomena as levels of illness and differential patterns of symptom expression in health risk behaviors, in health beliefs, in health preferences and health seeking traditions, and in health decisions (e.g., greater refusal of certain procedures). The level of aggressiveness in pursuing treatment may differ based on cultural nuances.

Lillie-Blanton et al. (2000) examined perceptions and experiences of patients with the health care system. They found the majority of Americans were unaware of health care disparities such as higher rates of infant mortality and lower life expectancy among African Americans or that Latinos are less likely to have health insurance than whites. There were striking differences by race on the question of whether the health care system treated people equally, with most minority Americans perceiving that they get lower quality of care than whites. Most white patients held contrary opinions. Overall it appeared that more minority Americans were concerned about cost rather than any perceived racial barriers.

Andersen and Newman (1973) proposed a model to explain access and use of health services which depends upon characteristics of the individual, society and the health care system. In this model, various predisposing, enabling, and need factors interact and influence decisions to seek and use health services. Predisposing factors include such characteristics as age, illness history, gender, race/ethnicity, marital status, education, occupation, and attitudes, beliefs, and values concerning health and illness. Enabling factors include income, health insurance status, cost of care, and the availability of health care institutions and providers for needed care. In the Andersen and Newman model the perception of illness and level of disability caused by an illness interact with predisposing and enabling factors to determine use of health care services. In order for a person to proceed with seeking out and using health services, the person must perceive that a problem exists, believe that the problem is severe enough to warrant professional intervention, and believe there is a solution to the problem. Failure to recognize that there is a problem will not lead to use. Thus the perception of need appears to be the critical step toward use of both general and mental health care services.

Mental health care disparities

The U.S. Surgeon General in his report (United States Public Health Services, 1999) described persistent disparities between whites and non-whites with regard to mental health outcomes. Studies have generally found that African Americans are over-represented in mental hospitals relative to their proportion in the population and that Hispanics and Asian Americans are under-represented (Cheung and Snowden, 1990; Lindsey and Paul, 1989; Sue and Sue, 1977). The Epidemiologic Catchment Area Study (Robins and Regier, 1991) established minimal differences in the rates of mental illness in ethnic minorities, with the exception of phobias in blacks. The ECA and National Co-morbidity Study (NCS) found that approximately one-third of all respondents who needed care actually received it; the rate for African Americans has been found to be substantially lower than the rate for whites (Wang et al., 2002). When seeking care, most African Americans relied on public sector programs for care. The NCS found that only 16% of African Americans with a mood disorder used mental health services for treatment. Many questions abound as to why so many of those in need of treatment fail to get it and why this is reflected disproportionately among ethnic minorities. What are the barriers? Are the underutilization patterns related to mistrust and fear of treatment, different cultural ideas about illness and health, lack of knowledge, differences in help-seeking behavior, issues of language, differences in communication patterns, racism, financial barriers, or discrimination by individual providers and institutions? It is likely that many of these factors may be involved, and along with personal characteristics, shape health care decisions and subsequent outcomes.

Financial concern, such as the lack of insurance, has been viewed as a significant barrier to psychiatric care for ethnic minorities with some 25% of African Americans being uninsured (Brown et al., 2000). Notably blacks are 1.5 times more likely than whites to be uninsured. However, Padgett at al. (1995) found that providing insurance with more generous benefits does not increase psychiatric treatment-seeking as much among African Americans as among whites. It appears that attitudes toward mental health care represent a substantial barrier to care. Stigma and lack of support in seeking care as well as fear of the mental health care system represent profound impediments. Sussman et al. (1987) found that African Americans who feared mental health care were 2.5 times greater than the proportion of whites. Leaf et al. (1987) found that most people are positively disposed toward use of mental health services. Their study found that attitudes regarding the use of mental health services were affected by age, gender, race, education and income. In general, they noted that differences in attitudes toward use of mental health services lay in the direction toward inhibition of utilization by those most at risk. Data from the NCS examined reasons that patients did not seek care. Using data from 1992, Kessler et al. (2001) found that about 6.2% of respondents met criteria for a serious mental illness in the year prior to their interviews and only 40% of those surveyed received treatment. It was noted that younger individuals and those living in non-rural residences were most likely to have unmet needs. When queried about the reasons for not seeking treatment, most respondents who did not receive treatment reported that they did not feel they had an emotional problem requiring care. Among those respondents who recognized a need for treatment but did not seek it, 52% noted situational barriers (inconvenience); 46% noted financial barriers as reasons for not seeking care. About 72% of respondents who failed to seek treatment and 56% of respondents who dropped out of treatment cited a desire to solve the problem on their own as a reason for their decision. Those not seeking care also reported a belief that the problem would simply get better without treatment. Lack of perceived need, lack of knowledge about where to get help, and inconvenience were also prominent reasons. The respondents who dropped out of treatment cited inconvenience and a wish to solve their own problem as primary reasons. A desire for self-efficacy appears to be a critically important determinant of underutilization and is consistent with the Andersen and Newman model that emphasizes beliefs about health and illness as key determinants of health services utilization.

Diala et al. (2000), analyzing data from the second part of the NCS, examined differences in attitudes between whites and African Americans toward seeking professional mental health care and utilizing mental health services. They found, somewhat surprisingly, that prior to the use of mental health services African Americans tended to have more positive attitudes than whites toward seeking treatment. However, after using mental health services the attitudes of African Americans were found to be less positive than whites. It appeared that something did happen during the interface with the system of care that rendered African Americans less willing to seek further care.

A person's awareness of an illness and its available treatments plays a critical role in health care utilization. Lack of knowledge and information about emotional disorders and their care appear to be greater among African Americans (Zylstra and Steitz,

1999). Cooper-Patrick et al. (1997) noted that stigma and spirituality affect the willingness of blacks to seek help. Religious beliefs that place the locus of control in a deity and external to the person may inhibit the person from seeking care from non-secular sources.

Ethnic and cultural factors are important to take into account because of the possibility of "interethnic differences in the distribution of cases and service utilization patterns, diagnostic and medication issues, and development of culturally relevant treatment modalities" (Snowden and Holschuh, 1992, p. 282). There is some evidence that ethnic/racial matching of patient and treater may be beneficial, but the results have not been consistent. Most researchers believe that therapist–client racial similarity alone is not related to therapy outcome (Sue, 1988); however, some evidence suggests that racial matching reduces risk of premature termination (Sue et al., 1991). There are findings that ethnic congruity between patient and provider as well as the proportion of other minorities in a treatment program can affect mental health service utilization rates, with less use of emergency services and less dropout from treatment (Snowden et al., 1995). It appears that ethnic/racial congruity between client and provider may be most useful in the least acculturated and most isolated individuals such as recent immigrants and refugees (Atkinson et al., 1986, 1989). For patients desiring ethnic/racial matching with their providers, the prospects are rather slim. Holzer and Goldsmith (1998) showed that only 2% of psychiatrists, 2% of psychologists and 4% of psychiatric social workers self-identified as African American. The percentages are smaller for other ethnic minorities. If ethnic/racial congruity in treatment is a desired goal and has a potential to decrease disparities, then institutions may have to step up efforts to recruit and retain ethnic minorities in the mental health care disciplines.

There are differential routes to care between whites and ethnic minorities. Minority patients are more likely to receive emergency room care for psychiatric concerns and are more likely to enter mental health treatment through coercion or legal mandate (Hu et al., 1991; Takeuchi and Cheung, 1998). African Americans and ethnic minorities are also more likely to go to a primary care physician than a psychiatrist (Pingitore et al., 2001), often with somatic complaints.

Once in treatment, ethnic minorities, especially African Americans, are more likely to be given more stigmatizing diagnoses and to experience high dropout rates (Sue and Sue, 1977). Atdjian and Vega (2005) noted that disparities exist in both access and the quality of mental health care for racial and ethnic minority groups in the United States. They commented on problems of access and underutilization as well as problems with treatment engagement and retention, inappropriate medication, misdiagnosis, inadequate detection and under-referral from primary care doctors, and lack of effective communication. The latter is a fundamental tenet of good care in any system.

The ethnic/racial disparities gap in health care, including mental health care, will require considerable effort to close. It appears that breaking down financial barriers will be key to this effort; however, many other changes must occur including how organizations recruit and retain diverse staff and how they train their non-ethnic staff to work with diverse populations. It is clear that personal factors such as one's own perception of need and one's own belief system shape use of health and mental health services. It is equally clear that systems can do a good deal to create an environment where minority patients feel their traditions, ways of expressing distress, and needs will be met with understanding and respect, and where professionals are self-reflective enough to know where their biases lie. These are the basic tenets of culturally competent care.

Categorical services—the Hispanic Clinic

As noted previously, census projections indicate that ethnic minorities will comprise nearly 47% of the nation's population by 2050. It will be imperative for organizations providing health care to be able to provide care that is relevant to the needs and cultural expectations of recipients of its services. While there has been much national attention to cultural competency over the past decade, its principles are not new. Researchers and providers have long noted disparities in care and created programs to address these needs at local levels through the creative development of outreach and culturally specific programming. Nearly 35 years ago, the CMHC established the Hispanic Clinic, which focused on treating Puerto Rican clients because of their high dropout rates and under-utilization of treatment services (Table 6.1).

Abad et al. (1974) noted that the Hispanic Clinic was developed to "provide special services recognizing unique linguistic, socioeconomic, and cultural dimensions" of this population and to deliver care that was "relevant to their needs, expectations, and cultural patterns" (p. 585). In developing the clinic, staff actively sought the support of key community groups and leaders because it was believed that collaboration with the indigenous power structure, including clergy and political leaders, was critical in order to establish legitimacy as an entity interested in providing care rather than expanding a research base for Yale University. At the time the Hispanic Clinic was established, the Latino population of New Haven represented about 4% of the total population, primarily of Puerto Rican origin. In comparison, the 2000 census indicated that the Latino population of New Haven was around 21%. The proposal leading to the establishment of the Hispanic Clinic noted a plan to provide a comprehensive array of services delivered by bilingual and bi-cultural staff.

The Hispanic Clinic began operation in March 1972 and was scheduled initially to operate for one afternoon per week; however, the level of demand necessitated modification, shortly after operations started, to a walk-in clinic that operated five days per week. The clinic was operated initially from the central CMHC building at Park Street. Over several years, its growth necessitated more space, and the clinic moved from Park Street to Congress Avenue and finally to its present-day location at Long Wharf.

According to Abad et al. (1974), the first proposal for the Hispanic Clinic contained the following recommendations. These included (1) provision of direct services by

Table 6.1   New Haven population (Source: U.S. Census Bureau, Census 1970, 1980, 1990, 2000)

Year	Total population	% White	% Black	% Hispanic
1970	137,707	72.6	26.3	3.6
1980	126,109	62.1	31.9	8.0
1990	130,474	53.9	36.1	13.2
2000	126,626	43.5	37.4	21.4

bilingual staff in a walk-in type clinic; (2) employment of more bilingual professionals and paraprofessionals within the larger organization of CMHC; (3) provision of health education services to the Spanish-speaking community; (4) development of ties with the Puerto Rican religious community; (5) collaboration with indigenous faith healers; (6) provision of in-service training on cultural matters to paraprofessionals; and (7) service as liaisons to local emergency rooms and hospitals. The ideals embodied in these principles are consistent with our current notions of cultural competency and with the original intent of the CMHCC Act of 1963, including taking action to develop a system of care specific to a particular population of people not adequately served by the existing system. Originally, the Hispanic Clinic focused primarily on the Puerto Rican population. However, changing demographics have necessitated approaches reflecting intra-group cultural variations distinct from language alone.

Currently, the Hispanic Clinic of the CMHC recognizes the significant challenge of providing culturally and linguistically competent behavioral health services to Connecticut's fastest growing minority population. An increasing Latino presence and a rising number of unmet behavioral health needs have prompted the clinic to seek the development of a Regional Latino Behavioral Health System for South-Central Connecticut that would work in partnership with a variety of other agencies within the region now serving large numbers of Latino clients, including monolingual clients living in suburban areas who cannot now be served by the Hispanic Clinic due to limitations on its capacity. Other agencies within the region report similar difficulties. For example, a nearby community health center, which reports serving a 70% Latino population, estimates that 28% of those clients are in need of behavioral health and substance use services. However, owing to the limited number of bilingual and bicultural behavioral health professionals, and to the increasing number of clients in need of services, the CMHC is restricted in the scope of services it can provide.

Current census figures estimate the national Latino population at 40 million, or 14.2% of the total U.S. population. It is expected that by the year 2030, the Latino population will total more than 73 million, and comprise an estimated 20% of the population. Connecticut demographics reflect national trends as recent census figures indicate that the Latino population has increased from approximately 320,000 in 2000, to a current estimate that surpasses 371,000 (U.S. Census Bureau, 2004, 2005).

These rising numbers are significant, given the population's increased vulnerability factors (i.e., acculturation difficulties, language barriers, poverty, psychosocial stressors). These factors lead to higher levels of distress, which in turn may cause, or exacerbate, substance use disorders and psychiatric illness (Ruiz, 1997). The literature demonstrates that Latinos have lower mental health utilization rates with less than 1 in 11 persons in need contacting mental health care specialists. Those who do seek care have higher treatment dropout rates than the general population (Salazar and Valdez, 2000; U.S. Department of Health and Human Services, 2001). Further, data suggest that these low service utilization and high dropout patterns may be linked to a lack of congruence between the values that permeate traditional mental health care services and the values of the Latino culture. Thus, researchers have recommended the development of culturally and linguistically appropriate therapeutic interventions to help reduce bias in diagnosis and treatment, and to increase overall treatment adherence and efficacy (Alarcon, 1995; Bernal and Scharron-del-Rio, 2001; Rogler, 1996; Rogler et al., 1987).

Given the population explosion of ethnic and racial minorities, the recruitment and retention of culturally diverse and culturally competent individuals into the behavioral health workforce have increased in national importance. Thus, efforts to enhance the overall core cultural competencies of future behavioral health providers are increasingly present at various points of professional training and development. Securing culturally diverse personnel has been a major obstacle toward creating a stable behavioral health service system for monolingual Latino clients. The current strategy proposes to build on the recruitment and retention efforts of the Hispanic Clinic and other Yale-affiliated programs in order to train and foster permanent placement of bilingual and bicultural behavioral health professionals throughout the system. As an example, through the effective use of nationally recognized and recommended practices, the Psychology Pre- and Post-Doctoral Latino track at the Hispanic Clinic of the CMHC has exhibited success in recruiting and retaining bilingual and bicultural clinical psychologists in the University system. In line with national recommendations, Latino psychologists in training at the Hispanic Clinic are offered opportunities for mentorship, practica placements with monolingual adult populations and coursework on cultural competency. Since 1999, the Latino track has recruited and/or retained fourteen clinical psychologists (ranging from pre-doctoral fellow to Associate Professor) within the Department of Psychiatry. Additionally, each year, between 12 and 15 bilingual and bicultural doctoral students apply to the pre-doctoral internship program for one slot at the Hispanic Clinic; this highlights not only a growing pool of professionals, but also a pressing need for resources to accommodate incoming students with the potential to address Connecticut's workforce needs after completion of their training. Moreover, the clinic has a Latino Social Work Track in which graduate students can complete an internship placement. Since 2000, the Social Work Track has recruited and/or retained eight social workers from such universities as Fordham, the University of Connecticut and Southern Connecticut State University.

In an effort to provide culturally competent services, behavioral health care organizations in South-Central Connecticut report the offering of translated materials, access to interpreter services, and when available, the employment of bilingual and bicultural staff. Despite their attempts, however, current population needs far exceed available agency resources and staff. Thus, the formation of an organized service system that will regularly monitor Latino population growth, track service need and availability, develop strategic planning to meet Latino needs, guide resource acquisition and allocation, and monitor actual service delivery is critical to meeting the behavioral health needs of monolingual Latino residents in South-Central Connecticut. The pursuit of developing a Regional Latino Behavioral Health System is consistent with the philosophy of cultural competency.

The community mental health movement and the Hill-West Haven Division

The Hispanic Clinic represents a prime example of the CMHC's attempts to address the needs of an ethnically diverse clinical and community population. However, it is not the only example. In 1970 New Haven was astir with activism and activists' challenges to existing paradigms of power and justice. A national spotlight was shining on New Haven as Bobby Seale, Chairman and Co-founder of the Black Panther Party, and a dozen co-defendants were set to go on trial. On the eve of that trial more than 12,000 people assembled on the New Haven Green to protest Seale's arrest and decry myriad social inequities. The rally in support of Seale and his co-defendants had been initiated by members of the Chicago Seven. In the month prior to that May Day rally, students at Yale University had voted to demonstrate in solidarity with protesters who believed that Seale and his co-defendants could not get a fair trial in the American justice system. Indeed the actions of the students led to an unprecedented shortening of the academic term by Yale President, Kingman Brewster. Antiwar activists, civil rights activists, local activists, and students from near and afar all came to New Haven. Revolutionaries of all stripes pressed for change within the political system. Black activists pressed for greater social and political parity for minority communities. Antiwar activists sought to hold the government accountable for its actions in Southeast Asia and the expenditure of life and treasury for what they considered to be ill-defined purposes. Challenges to the authority of the government and the insistence on change permeated the times and penetrated the dynamics of local politics and community relations with existing city, state and academic institutions.

The New Haven community was in a state of crisis as many feared that violence would erupt. The tensions were exacerbated by the rhetoric of national and local politicians as well as the protesters themselves. Leaders within the new CMHC became involved in efforts with local community leaders to defuse the tensions. Many of these meetings were held in the Center. The process revealed a number of issues including what level of participation and control would the community have in this emerging center which had been mandated to serve the community's needs. This included discussion about the level of diversity within the Center, in terms of both the population it served and the people it hired. Some community leaders were dubious about the contemplated mission of the CMHC because of the operational alliance between the State of Connecticut and Yale University. In some quarters Yale University was perceived as a self interested, elitist institution with little concern for the surrounding community. This perception was, perhaps unintentionally, fostered by the organizational structure of the Center in which its leaders were Yale faculty and appointees and the line staff were mostly state employees.

When the CMHC acquired a grant to create the Hill-West Haven Division, a new era of catchmented services began. The Hill-West Haven Division was a gerrymandered strip of geography that encompassed a mostly African-American population in the Hill section of New Haven, Connecticut and a mostly low-income white portion of West Haven, Connecticut. In keeping with the original intent of the CMHCC Act of 1963, the Hill-West Haven Division was conceived to provide care to the socially, culturally and economically disadvantaged. The Hill-West Haven Division provided both substance abuse care and routine inpatient and outpatient care for those within its mandated catchment area. As its service delivery evolved, the Hill-West Haven Division embraced a philosophy of providing comprehensive care to its population on the local level.

An important aspect of the initiative creating the Hill-West Haven Division was the concerted effort to recruit and train members of the local community as mental health workers, thereby creating a more culturally diverse workforce. Another important aspect was the establishment of a Board of Directors with local community members on it that had oversight for the Division and had a say in some personnel decisions. The Hill portion of the Hill-West Haven Division no longer exists except for the prevention component that has morphed into the Consultation Center. A clinic in West Haven, affiliated with the CMHC, continues to operate and to serve the socially disadvantaged citizens of that town.

Cultural competency

Cultural competency has emerged as a powerful buzz phrase within organizations seeking to develop more effective strategies to deal with prominent health disparities between whites and various ethnic groups. In its executive summary and final report, the President's New Freedom Commission (2003) cited cultural competency as one of the mechanisms for eliminating health care disparities. There is tremendous theoretical potential in this model for improving health care outcomes for ethnic minorities, but it has not yet been tested empirically. Cultural competency is defined as "a set of congruent practices, skills, attitudes, policies, and structures which come together in a system, agency, or among professionals and enable that system, or those professionals to work effectively in cross cultural situations" (Cross et al., 1989). In their final report the President's New Freedom Commission called for improving access to care that is culturally competent while acknowledging the lack of research and evidence on its effectiveness. It appears almost intuitive that cultural competency, as an organizing principle for service delivery, can make a difference in closing the health care and outcome gaps between whites and other ethnic minorities, but only rigorous empirical evaluations will confirm this (Brach and Fraserirector, 2000).

In 2001, the Commissioner of the Connecticut Department of Mental Health and Addiction Services (DMHAS) issued "The Multicultural Clinical/Rehabilitation Best Practices." This document represents the culmination of several years of efforts to define and put forth guidelines for implementing culturally competent care throughout the DMHAS system. DMHAS noted their intention to make these guidelines contractual standards with required measures and outcomes with a principal focus on access, engagement and retention of patients in treatment. The aim of these efforts is closure of the gaps between ethnic minorities and whites within Connecticut's behavioral health care system. The Office of Multicultural Affairs (OMA), created within DMHAS in 1997, has the primary task of monitoring these multi-cultural practice outcomes for services to people from diverse backgrounds and from traditionally underserved groups. OMA's strategic plan for 2007–2010 has five goals (Connecticut Department of Mental Health and Addiction Services, 2001). The strategic goals of OMA include: (1) developing policies, structures, environments and values that are inclusive of cultural competency; (2) establishing an overall strategy for multi-cultural workplace development; (3) revising cultural competence standards; (4) enhancing clinical assessments throughout the system of care; (5) initiating training for the prevention and elimination of institutional racism throughout the care system.

Cultural competency as a concept has a number of dimensions involving the individual provider and organizational and systems aspects. Cultural competency involves much more than periodic seminars and workshops on cultural sensitivity or awareness. It is a model dedicated to system-wide, scrupulous monitoring of an organization's effectiveness in cross-cultural situations and the development of programs to address deficiencies. OMA's strategic plan and goals address the critical domains of cultural competence, which is needed for a state and nation that are becoming increasingly diverse.

Another important aspect of cultural competency lies in the education of professionals to be respectful of and sensitive to cultural patterns that influence care. Accreditation bodies now require that persons in training demonstrate an ability to deliver culturally competent care. The Hispanic Clinic, for example, has a track for psychology trainees designed to provide mentorship, practicum placements with monolingual patient populations and coursework on cultural competency. Within the Department of Psychiatry, coursework on the significance of ethnicity and the meaning of ethnic identity has been a mainstay of the training curriculum. Ezra Griffith and Sergio Mejia developed and taught a seminar on Special Populations and Diversity that was an important aspect of psychiatric residency training throughout the 1970s and 1980s. This seminar provided a penetrating look into a variety of populations and went beyond traditional examinations of race and culture to include issues related to such topics as sexuality and physical disability. In recent years the lead author of this chapter (HCB) has given lectures to the PGY-2 class of psychiatry residents and has taught a year-long seminar in the Division of Mental Hygiene for post-doctoral fellows in psychiatry and psychology and post-graduate fellows in social work on "The Meaning of Different-ness" which examines identity development and its impact on the therapeutic process. Blue and Gonzalez (1992) have written in more detail about the latter issue. Griffith, Gonzalez and Blue have also contributed chapters on the Principles of Cultural Psychiatry for the 3rd and 4th editions of the *American Psychiatric Press Textbook of Psychiatry* (1999, 2003). Former Department of Psychiatry and CMHC staff members, Lillian Comas-Diaz and Frederick Jacobsen, developed ethno-cultural psychotherapy that examines how race and ethnicity come to manifest themselves in the dynamics of interpersonal relationships and psychotherapy. Comas-Diaz and Griffith co-edited an important book, *Clinical Guidelines in Cross-Cultural Mental Health* (1988). As more and more demands are placed on the departmental training curriculum, less time has been devoted to these topics. This may be an impediment to the aim of developing culturally competent professionals.

Future challenges

The central challenge for academic programs is to test empirically the tremendous potential of cultural competence to improve access of ethnic and cultural minorities to services and the outcomes of those services. The fundamental question is whether cultural competence improves outcome of treatment and can reduce the disparities in outcomes of care now widely observed in the mental health system. Assuming this evaluation proves the power of cultural competence to make a difference, another challenge is to educate the mental health workforce in the theory and practice of cultural competence. Finally, academic programs, in partnership with the state, can help develop categorical services targeted at conspicuously underserved groups, as has been done in the past for Latinos and disadvantaged individuals.

Conclusion

The CMHCC Act of 1963 generated hope that people with mental health concerns would receive comprehensive and high-quality care regardless of race, ethnicity, national origin or ability to pay. Over the past forty years, that hope has eroded somewhat in the face of changing priorities and financial constraints. As more local mental health agencies have shifted their focus on providing care primarily for the seriously mentally ill, those with less serious mental health issues have faced less available services. This has led to increasing levels of unmet needs with ethnic minorities faring worse than their white counterparts. The persistent disparities in access, utilization, and health outcomes between whites and non-whites must be addressed aggressively. As the population of this nation changes and the number of minorities increases, the general health care and mental health care system must develop more effective strategies to close these gaps. Patient education, outreach and enhancement of the cultural competency of providers will be crucial to this enterprise.

References

Abad V, Ramos J, Boyce E: A model for delivery of mental health services to Spanish speaking minorities. Am J Orthopsychiatry 44:584–95, 1974

Alarcon RD: Culture and psychiatric diagnosis: impact on DSM-IV and ICD-10. Psychiatr Clin North Am 18:449–65, 1995

Andersen R, Newman JF: Societal and individual determinants of medical care utilization in the United States. Milbank Q Health and Society 51:95–124, 1973

Atdjian S, Vega WA: Disparities in mental health treatment in U.S. racial and minority groups: implications for psychiatrists. Psychiatr Serv 56:1600–2, 2005

Atkinson DR, Poston CW, Furlong MJ: Afro-American preferences for counselor characteristics. J Counseling Psychology 33:326–30, 1986

Atkinson DR, Poston CW, Furlong MJ, et al.: Ethnic group preferences for counselor characteristics. J Counseling Psychology 36:68–72, 1989

Bernal G, Scharron-del-Rio MR: Are empirically supported treatments valid for ethnic minorities? Toward an alternative approach for treatment research. Cultur Divers Ethnic Minor Psychol 7:328–42, 2001

Blue HC, Gonzalez CA: The meaning of ethnocultural difference: its impact on and use in the psychotherapeutic process. New Dir Ment Health Serv 55:73–84, 1992

Brach C, Fraserirector I: Can cultural competency reduce racial and ethnic disparities? A review and conceptual model. Med Care 57(suppl.1):181–217, 2000

Brown ER, Ojeda VD, Win R, et al.: Racial and ethnic disparities in access to health insurance and health care. Los Angeles: UCLA Center for Health Policy Research and the Henry J. Kaiser Family Foundation, 2000

Cheung FK, Snowden LR: Community mental health and ethnic minority populations. Community Ment Health J 26:277–91, 1990

Comas-Diaz L, Griffith EEH (eds.): Clinical Guidelines in Cross-Cultural Mental Health. New York: John Wiley & Sons Ltd, 1988

Connecticut Department of Mental Health and Addiction Services (DMHAS), 2001. Multicultural Clinical/Rehabilitation Best Practices, 2001. Available at: http://www.ct.gov/dmhas/lib/dmhas/omabestpractices.pdf. Accessed October 29 2007

Connecticut Department of Mental Health and Addiction Services, 2007. Office of Multicultural Affairs Strategic Plan 2007–2010. Available at: http://www.ct.gov/dmhas/lib/dmhas/omastrategicplan.pdf. Accessed October 29, 2007

Cooper-Patrick L, Powe NR, Jenckes MW, et al.: Identification of patient attitudes and preferences regarding treatment for depression. J Gen Intern Med 12:431–8, 1997

Cross T, Bazron B, Dennis K, et al.: Toward a culturally competent system of care: a monograph on effective services for minority children who are severely emotionally disturbed. Washington, DC: Georgetown University Child Development Center, 1989

Cutler DL, Bevilacqua J, Bentson HM: Four decades of community mental health: a symphony in four movements. Community Ment Health J 39:381–98, 2003

Diala C, Muntaner C, Walrath C, et al.: Racial differences in attitudes toward professional mental health care and in the use of services. Am J Orthopsychiatry 70:455–64, 2000

Geiger JH: Race and health care—an American dilemma? New Engl J Med 335:815–6, 1996

Griffith EEH, Gonzalez CA, Blue HC: The basics of cultural psychiatry, in The American Psychiatric Press Textbook of Psychiatry, 3rd Edition. Edited by Hales RE, Yudofsky SC, Talbott JA. Washington, DC: American Psychiatric Press, 1999, pp 1463–92

Griffith EEH, Gonzalez CA, Blue HC: Introduction to cultural psychiatry, in The American Psychiatric Press Textbook of Psychiatry, 4th Edition. Edited by Hales RE, Yudofsky SC, Talbott JA. Washington, DC: American Psychiatric Press, 2003, pp 1551–83

Holzer CE, Goldsmith HF, Ciarlo JA: Effects of rural-urban county type on the availability of health and mental health care providers, in Mental Health, United States. Edited by Manderscheid RW, Henderson MJ. Rockville, MD: Center for Mental Illness, 1998

Hu TW, Snowden LR, Jerrell JM, et al.: Ethnic populations in public mental health: service choice and level of use. Am J Public Health 8:1429–34, 1991

Isaac RJ, Armat VC: Madness in the Streets: How Psychiatry and the Law Abandoned the Mentally Ill. New York: Free Press, 1990

Karger HJ, Stoesz D: American Social Welfare Policy: A Pluralist Approach. New York: Longman, 1994

Kessler RC, Berglund P, Bruce ML, et al.: The prevalence and correlates of untreated serious mental illness. Health Serv Res 36:987–1003, 2001

Leaf PJ, Bruce ML, Tischler GL, et al.: The relationship between demographic factors and attitudes toward mental health services. J Community Psychol 15:25–38, 1987

Lillie-Blanton M, Brodie M, Rowland D, et al.: Race, ethnicity, and the health care system: public perceptions and experiences. Med Care Res Rev 57:218–35, 2000

Lindsey KP, Paul GL: Involuntary commitments to public mental institutions: issues involving the overrepresentation of blacks and assessment of relevant functioning. Psychol Bull 106:171–83, 1989

Mayberry RM, Milli F, Ofili E: Racial and ethnic differences in access to medical care. Med Care Res Rev 57(suppl.1):108–45, 2000

National Center for Health Care Statistics, 1996

Padgett D, Struening EL, Andrews H, et al.: Predictors of emergency room use by homeless adults in New York City: the predisposing, enabling, and need factors. Soc Sci Med 41:547–56, 1995

PBS, Frontline: The New Asylums, Interview with Reginald Wilkerson. Airdate May 10, 2005. Written, produced, and directed by Navasky M, O'Connor K. Available at: http://www.pbs.org/wgbh/pages/frontline/shows/asylums/interviews/wilkinson.html. Accessed August 12, 2006

Pingitore D, Snowden LR, Sansone R, et al.: Persons with depression and the treatments they receive: a comparison of primary care physicians and psychiatrists. Int J Psychiatry Med 31:41–60, 2001

President's New Freedom Commission on Mental Health: Achieving the promise: Transforming mental health care in America. DHHS Pub. No.SMA-03–3832. Rockville, MD, 2003

Robins LN, Regier DA: Psychiatric Disorders in America: The Epidemiologic Catchment Area Study. New York: The Free Press, 1991

Rochefort DA: Origins of the "third psychiatric revolution": the Community Mental Health Act of 1963. J Health Polit Policy Law 9:1–30, 1984

Rogler LH: Research on mental health services for Hispanics: targets of convergence. Cultur Divers Ethnic Minor Psychol 2:145–56, 1996

Rogler LH, Malgady RG, Costantino G, et al.: What do culturally sensitive mental health services mean? The case of Hispanics. Am Psychol 42:565–70, 1987

Ruiz P: Issues in the psychiatric care of Hispanics. Psychiatr Serv 48:539–40, 1997

Salazar TA, Valdez JN: The need for specialized clinical training in mental health service delivery to Latinos. Academic Exchange Quarterly 4:92–8, 2000

Snowden LR, Holschuh J: Ethnic differences in emergency psychiatric care and hospitalization in a program for the severely mentally ill. Community Ment Health J 28:281–91, 1992

Snowden LR, Hu TW, Jerrell JM: Emergency care avoidance: ethnic matching and participation in minority serving programs. Community Ment Health J 31:463–73, 1995

Sue DW, Sue S: Barriers to effective cross-cultural counseling. J Counseling Psychology 24:420–9, 1977

Sue S: Psychotherapeutic services for ethnic minorities: two decades of research findings. Am Psychol 43:301–8, 1988

Sue S, Fujino D, Hu LT, et al.: Community mental health services for ethnic minority groups: a test of the cultural responsiveness hypothesis. J Consult Clin Psychol 59:533–40, 1991

Sussman LK, Robins LN, Earls R: Treatment-seeking for depression by black and white Americans. Soc Sci Med 24:187–96, 1987

Takeuchi DT, Cheung MK: Coercive and voluntary referrals: how ethnic minority adults get into mental health treatment. Ethn Health 3:149–58, 1998

Talbott JA: Deinstitutionalization: avoiding the disasters of the past. Hosp Community Psychiatry 30:621–30, 1979

Torrey EF: Nowhere to Go: The Tragic Odyssey of the Homeless Mentally Ill. New York: Harper Row, 1988

U.S. Census Bureau. Connecticut's population projections: 1995 to 2025. Available at: http://www.census.gov/population/projections/state/ 9525rank/ctprsrel.txt. Accessed November 27, 2005

U.S. Census Bureau, 2004. U.S. Interim Projections by Age, Sex, Race, and Hispanic Origin. Available at: http://www.census.gov/ipc/www/usinterimproj. Accessed September 28, 2007

U.S. Census Bureau. 2004 American community survey. Available at: http://factfinder.census.gov. Accessed September 14, 2005

U.S. Census Bureau: Annual Estimates of the Population by Sex, Race, and Hispanic or Latino Origin for Connecticut: April 1, 2000 to July 1, 2004. SC-EST2004-03-09, 2005

U.S. Department of Health and Human Services. Mental health: culture, race, and ethnicity—a supplement to mental health: report of the surgeon general. Rockville, MD: U.S. Department of Health and Human Services, Public Health Service, Office of the Surgeon General, 2001

United States Public Health Service. Office of the Surgeon General. SAMHSA. Center for Mental Health Services. Mental Health: A Report of the Surgeon General 1999. Rockville Pike: National Institute of Mental Health

Wang PS, Demler O, Kessler RC: Adequacy of treatment for serious mental illness in the United States. Am J Public Health 92:92–8, 2002

Weinick RM, Zuvekas SH, Cohen JW: Racial and ethnic differences in access to and use of health care services, 1977 to 1996. Med Care Res Rev 57:36–54, 2000

Williams DR: African American health: the role of social environment. Journal of Urban Health: Bulletin of the New York Academy of Sciences 75:300–21, 1998

Zylstra RG Steitz JA: Public knowledge of late-life depression and aging. J Appl Gerontol 18:63–76, 1999

7

A public–academic partnership at the Connecticut Mental Health Center

Wayne F. Dailey, Thomas A. Kirk, Jr., Robert A. Cole and Paul J. Di Leo

Yale University and Connecticut state government each has a rich history and tradition. This chapter examines how the traditions, missions, and values of Yale and the state have influenced and defined the public–academic partnership at the Connecticut Mental Health Center. This micro-history examines the evolution of behavioral health services and public sector psychiatry in Connecticut and elsewhere. It explores how multiple factors, which include people in key positions, fiscal resources, political realities and institutional culture have sculpted the partnership. Finally, the authors speculate about how present-day forces are aligning in the nation's behavioral health care system and the role public–academic partnerships can play in shaping this future.

The Connecticut Mental Health Center (CMHC) and its associated community behavioral health programs are the progeny of a relationship that evolved between an old and venerable academic institution and an equally well-rooted state government. Yale University, established in 1701, and Connecticut, first colonized in 1633 and admitted as the fifth state to the union in 1788, both have commanding histories and traditions. These traditions, missions, and values have influenced the relationship between Yale and the state, and have shaped the operation of the Center and the evolution of behavioral health services and public sector psychiatry in Connecticut and elsewhere. Other factors have shaped the public–academic partnership, including people in key positions, fiscal resources, political realities and institutional culture. These views reflect the perspective of the authors, all of whom have extensive experience working in state government. In addition, one author (RAC) also has considerable experience as a Center administrator employed by the university.

Mental health care in Connecticut

Connecticut's government has been involved in supporting people with mental illness since colonial times. This role has its origins in the English Common Law concept of

40 Years of Academic Public Psychiatry. Edited by Selby C. Jacobs and Ezra E. H. Griffith
© 2007 John Wiley & Sons, Ltd.

parens patriae, under which the state accepted responsibility for persons with mental disabilities who could not fend for themselves. Early government efforts were modest, and by today's standards seem harsh and misguided. They may be better understood, however, when seen in light of yesteryear's culture, when people with mental illness were thought to be possessed by the devil, idleness for any reason was scorned, and individual productivity was seen as linked to community survival.

In order to provide support for "the insane," in 1699 the General Court of Connecticut passed An Act for the Relieving of Idiots and Distracted Persons making the towns financially responsible for indigent people who were judged *non compos mentis* (Hoadley, 1868). Just over a decade later, the support role of families of people with mental illness was defined, and penalties were added for relatives who failed to assist if they had the means to do so (Public Document No. 72, 1922). In 1727, Connecticut's government ordered that a workhouse be constructed for "rogues, vagabonds, common beggars, and other lewd, idle, dissolute and disorderly persons, and for setting them to work." Although the law does not specifically mention persons with mental illness, its intent was to encompass the mentally ill along with homeless persons and dangerous individuals. This law also specified that people committed to workhouses could be whipped ". . . not to exceed ten stripes at once . . . ," and that food could be withheld ". . . until they are reduced to better order." Shackling of uncooperative workhouse residents also was permitted (Hoadley, 1868). During a four-year period beginning in 1793, Connecticut law permitted the jailing of persons with mental illness who were judged dangerous to the community. Conditions of confinement were deplorable, and included holding people in cages and pens, or shackling to restrict movement. In 1797, statutory language that permitted jailing was repealed (Hoadley, 1868).

In 1814, and again in 1821, the State Medical Society initiated studies to determine the prevalence of mental illness in Connecticut. With the help of local clergy who provided information from towns and villages, the Society concluded that there were at least 1000 people with serious mental illness in the state. This was at a time when the state's total population was little more than 275,000. Recognizing that care and support for those with mental illness left much to be desired, in 1822 the General Assembly appropriated $5000 to sponsor development of The Connecticut Retreat for the Insane. Additional funds were raised through private contributions. This facility later became known as The Hartford Retreat, and today is Connecticut's esteemed Institute of Living. While the new facility offered humane, palliative care, its 50 beds were insufficient to address demands of the state's growing population (Public Document No. 72, 1922). Nevertheless, decades would pass before another such institution was built. During the 1850s, despite mounting pressures on Connecticut's legislature from the State Medical Society and the directors of the Hartford Retreat, the legislature failed to act until these groups joined forces with an articulate and well-known social reformer from Massachusetts—Dorothea Lynde Dix. Working with local advocates as she had done in several other states (her advocacy work led to the founding of 32 mental hospitals in 18 states), Dorothea Dix convinced Connecticut's General Assembly in 1866 to build a hospital for poor people with serious mental illnesses. The new 450-bed facility located in Middletown opened its doors in April 1868. It was called General Hospital for the Insane. Later its name would be changed to Connecticut Valley Hospital (CVH) (Carini et al., 1974).

At its peak in 1936, the CVH had expanded to accommodate more than 3000 patients. Two other large state-operated inpatient psychiatric facilities had also been built: Norwich State Hospital in 1904, and Fairfield Hills Hospital in 1933. By the early 1950s, the combined capacity of the three facilities had grown to over 9000 patients at a time when the state's total population was little more than half of its present 3.5 million residents. For the next few decades, these institutions formed the mainstay of mental illness treatment in Connecticut, offering services similar to those provided in state hospitals throughout the nation—mostly custodial care, work-based therapies in which patients were paid token wages to assist with operation of the hospital's farm, and for the most seriously ill, interventions that in hindsight were tragically misguided (e.g., hydrotherapy, insulin coma therapy, involuntary sterilization and surgical lobotomies) (Carini et al., 1972). Despite many shortcomings, the hospitals were not devoid of compassion. Indeed, attendants, nurses and doctors offered many individual kindnesses to patients, and worked hard to relieve their pain. Even the architectural features of hospital buildings were meant to convey dignity and respect. In Page Hall at the CVH during the 1920s, white tablecloths covered dinner tables, and an orchestra played softly from a balcony while patients ate their evening meal. Yet long-term psychiatric hospital care fell far short of providing effective treatment for its patients. Thousands languished in these bucolic settings, some for their entire adult lives, in stultifying monotony. Although the hospitals would begin to operate satellite outpatient clinics in several Connecticut communities, the needs of people with mental illness living outside the hospital walls remained largely unmet.

In the 1950s the tide began to turn, ushering in a new era in the treatment of serious mental illness. In 1952 it was discovered that chlorpromazine relieved positive symptoms of schizophrenia. The FDA approved its use in 1954. It was also shown that a common mineral, lithium carbonate, could relieve the manic and depressive symptoms of bipolar disorder. Some of the early research on lithium was conducted at Connecticut's Ribicoff Research Facilities now located at the CMHC. Discovery and initial use of the first psychotropic medications came at approximately the same time as several other important developments. First, journalistic exposés about the treatment of patients in state hospitals raised public awareness and concern (Deutsch, 1948; Ward, 1946). Second, the psychiatric rehabilitation of people with serious mental illness was becoming better understood (Lamb, 1994). Third, coverage under the federal Medicaid program was extended to nursing home care, and private insurance companies began paying for inpatient psychiatric treatment in general hospitals. Fourth, several landmark federal district court rulings were issued during the 1960s and 1970s regarding the rights of people with mental illness. In *Wyatt v. Stickney* (1972), *Rouse v. Cameron* (1966) and *Donaldson v. O'Connor* (1974), though subsequently weakened by the U.S. Supreme Corrt, which skirted the right to treatmen tissue (*O'Connor v. Donaldson*, 1975), the courts found that psychiatric patients had a constitutional right to treatment. *Lake v. Cameron* (1966) further affirmed that treatment should be provided in the least restrictive setting. This combination of factors led to the deinstitutionalization of hundreds of thousands of psychiatric patients throughout the United States. Many of these patients were transferred to nursing homes as states shifted the financial burden of their care to Medicaid.

Mental health care in Connecticut was also beginning to change. In 1954 at a time when the population of state hospitals in Connecticut and elsewhere in the nation was near its peak, the State of Connecticut established the Department of Mental Health (DMH). This new agency was created to exercise greater control over Connecticut's state hospitals, which were operating as independent fiefdoms, and to begin developing a service delivery system. Eventually, the DMH would include a Division of Community Services, an Alcohol and Drug Dependence Division, and a Division of Children's Services. The latter two were eventually divested from the DMH, until the return of substance abuse prevention and treatment services led to the creation of the Department of Mental Health and Addiction (DMHAS) in 1995. While support for inpatient care remained the priority at the DMH, some DMH officials and a growing number of mental health advocates saw a need to develop community-based services for people with mental illness. Their concerns stemmed from the simple fact that, with the exception of small, hospital-based psychiatric outpatient programs, community mental health care for people with serious disorders in Connecticut was virtually non-existent.

Fredrick "Fritz" Redlich, chairman of the Department of Psychiatry at Yale at the time (later appointed dean of the School of Medicine) shared this concern with a group representing the Connecticut Mental Health Association. They met with newly elected Governor Ribicoff, in 1955, in the offices of DMH. According to Ribicoff, Redlich asked: "Governor, what do you plan to do about mental health?" Not wishing to be put on the spot, the governor responded by asking: "Well Fritz, what is Yale going to do about mental health?" This famous exchange was the beginning of many conversations between representatives of the state and Yale, which ultimately led to a decision in 1959 that the two entities would collaborate in the establishment and operation of a mental health facility in New Haven. Later in this chapter, we will discuss some of the conflicts and tensions that arose between the parties at certain points during the history of the CMHC. To a large degree, these tensions are inherent in the organizational structure, given its joint governance, multiple missions and unique staffing arrangement. It is noteworthy that concerns about ownership, financing, lines of authority, and balance between the service and academic missions were discussed between and among the parties at great length, long before the first brick was laid for the building. Such discussions date back to as early as 1956 when Commissioner Blasko and his state hospital superintendents expressed grave concern that Yale would dominate any joint venture and that research and training would take priority over patient care in such an arrangement. In 1963 when construction funding became available through passage of the federal *Community Mental Health Centers Act* (PL 88-164), Yale and the DMH took immediate steps to secure these funds. In 1963 the General Assembly passed Public Act 579, S.1. authorizing creation of the Connecticut Mental Health Center. (Present operation of the Center is governed by §17a-460a through §17a-460f of Connecticut General Statutes.) Construction of the CMHC facility at 34 Park Street, New Haven began in 1964 and the Center opened its doors in September 1966. Resources for the project came from a combination of federal, state, and Yale University funds. (The opening of the CMHC was followed by construction of the Greater Bridgeport Community Mental Health Center in 1970.)

Roles and responsibilities of Yale and the state as they pertained to the operation of the CMHC were codified in a memorandum of agreement that was executed between the parties. This document served as the foundation for the relationship. Each year, a staffing contract was negotiated between Yale and the state, under which the state would provide financial support for Yale faculty and staff who were responsible for managing most aspects of the Center's operations, including a wide range of direct-care, training and research programs. In addition, the state provided a significant number of employees who functioned in direct-care and support capacities, including a limited number of managerial positions. Under the terms of the memorandum of agreement, all such faculty and staff, whether employed by Yale or the state, were accountable to the Center's director. Annual budget allocations from the state have also covered the majority of non-personnel costs of the Center.

Establishment of the CMHC had a beneficial effect in the greater New Haven area, and created awareness about the value of community mental health services that would eventually spread across the entire state. However, supporters of inpatient care, including the state psychiatric hospital superintendents and the DMH commissioner, were concerned that community-based services would divert resources and attention from the hospitals. They were reluctant to make a commitment to community mental health, and resisted implementation of Public Act 75-563 Connecticut statute (PA 75-563) that created a regional administrative structure designed to integrate inpatient and community-based services. A report to the Connecticut General Assembly in 1979 found that state hospital inpatient programs continued to dominate Connecticut's mental health landscape and utilized most of its financial and staffing resources. Community mental health services were in short supply in most areas, and inpatient and community programs were generally not well coordinated (Connecticut General Assembly, Legislative Program Review and Investigations Committee, 1979). Despite the venture into community mental health at the CMHC in New Haven and in a few other parts of the state, the DMH leadership was still predominately focused on psychiatric inpatient care. Whereas many states made extensive use of federal construction and operations grants, community mental health center development in Connecticut proceeded rather slowly. In the early 1980s when the federal government finally halted the application process for new centers, several Connecticut catchment areas still had no access to community mental health center services.

Personnel, fiscal resources and political realities

The hard work of community mental health advocates was about to pay off. In 1981 the DMH commissioner, Eric Plaut, resigned and was succeeded by a charismatic psychiatrist named Audrey Worrell. Prior to becoming commissioner, Worrell had been a faculty member at the University of Connecticut's Department of Psychiatry. She also had served as the interim director of Hartford's Capitol Region Mental Health Center. She understood the value of community mental health services and had let it be known that she intended to push for their development. Worrell was committed to encouraging the work of community mental health advocates. Her mandate to realign service delivery in Connecticut came from the State Board of Mental Health, the body that had recommended her for appointment by the governor. She was about to initiate the most sweeping reform in Connecticut's mental health system since the days of Dorothea Dix. Although she believed Connecticut still had too many state-run psychiatric beds, she promised not to neglect the quality of public sector inpatient services as she worked to reduce the inpatient census.

Changing Connecticut's mental health system would not be easy; many of the key players still clung to the status quo, and community services had not been sufficiently developed to demonstrate their full potential. State hospital staff, and their associated labor unions, viewed the move toward community mental health with considerable suspicion, believing that union jobs were threatened. These staff asserted that state hospital census reductions during the 1960s and 1970s had already resulted in the discharge of all patients capable of leaving. Those who remained were too severely disabled for community living, and no amount of outside support would change that fact. Meanwhile, some senior managers at the DMH worried that during tight fiscal times, it would be easier to defend the budgets of highly visible "brick-and-mortar" state facilities than a diffuse array of small programs run by dozens of private non-profit agencies.

The medical and administrative leadership of Connecticut's general hospitals also were concerned, if not outright antagonistic toward the DMH (Tamayo et al., 1990). Emergency department chiefs complained they were experiencing significant delays in obtaining access to state inpatient beds. Adults in psychiatric crises often spent days in emergency rooms, sometimes strapped to gurneys in hallways, waiting for state beds to become available. General hospital chiefs of psychiatry were equally distressed. They were under pressure from hospital administrators to transfer financially burdensome, long-stay psychiatric patients to state beds. Their worries intensified when Commissioner Worrell capped the census of the state hospitals because of her concerns about patient and staff safety in these facilities. The commissioner argued that improving access to community mental health care would enable people to avoid hospitalization. General hospital leaders rejoined that more state inpatient beds were needed, and that Commissioner Worrell's policies were making matters worse. The Connecticut Hospital Association (CHA) sued the DMH over the emergency department logjam (*Connecticut Hospital Association Inc. v. Audrey Worrell, MD*).

Worrell's term as commissioner (1982–1986) stirred significant controversy. She had clashed with the chairman of the University of Connecticut's Department of Psychiatry, and thus could not rely on his support in her role as commissioner. Despite her credentials as a psychiatrist, she lacked support from many key individuals in Connecticut's psychiatric community. In order to survive and achieve her vision, she needed to strengthen her support and establish a well-articulated strategic plan. She responded by recruiting new professionals to the DMH, and by relying on senior faculty at the Yale Department of Psychiatry for advice. Several faculty, including the CMHC's director, Boris Astrachan, functioned as a de facto think-tank and privy counsel, offering suggestions to help her address complex conceptual, ideological and political questions. Astrachan was well suited to the task. He was widely recognized as a senior statesman in public psychiatry, and nationally known for his work in depression, schizophrenia, group process, systems theory and psychiatric administration. His visible support for Worrell, coupled with the backing of other senior medical school faculty at Yale, increased her clout and steadied her political footing. As a result of the strong relationship between the two, Worrell gave Astrachan a free hand to set the research and training agenda at the CMHC.

Worrell's vibrant personality attracted the attention of Connecticut's General Assembly. In legislative committee hearings, she gripped their interest with dramatic clinical vignettes, some humorous, some touching or tragic, describing community life for people with serious mental illness. As part of a strategic process, she convinced the state's governor to establish a Blue Ribbon Task Force on Mental Health in 1982. The task force report supported her assertion that more community programs were needed. As a result of these efforts, and buoyed by strong support from the governor and the general economic prosperity in the state, the mid-1980s became a major growth period for community mental health services in Connecticut. During this time, case management programs, vocational services and psychosocial rehabilitation programs based on the popular Fountain House model (Beard et al., 1982) were created in many parts of the state. Additionally, funds were obtained to establish pilot crisis intervention programs in each of the state's five regions. These initiatives were designed to stabilize people in psychiatric emergencies and divert them from general hospital emergency rooms and inpatient care. The success of those programs helped to facilitate a settlement of the *CHA v. Worrell* lawsuit. Worrell also determined that mental health service providers should help clients find safe and affordable housing. Although this idea seems rather unremarkable today, at the time many service providers believed that helping clients solve housing problems was beyond the scope of their work.

Worrell made other important contributions to community mental health in Connecticut. For example, she implemented a system of care that unified control over state hospitals and community support programs using regional directors. This structural change was essential in moving the system toward a focus on community-based care, and toward improved continuity and integration of service delivery (Wolf, 1990). Perhaps her most important legacy was that she clarified and narrowed the DMH mission. In doing so, she acknowledged that while DMH had a broad legislative mandate encompassing all Connecticut adults with mental illness, it was constrained by finite resources. Therefore, Connecticut needed to focus its attention and assets on providing effective services to poor people with the most serious psychiatric disorders, and on those at risk of hospitalization.

After five and one-half tumultuous years of change marked by significant accomplishments, Worrell resigned in 1986 and was succeeded by Deputy Commissioner Michael Hogan.

As commissioner, Hogan maintained the policy direction and consolidated the gains of his predecessor. He also added many new programs, including assertive community treatment (ACT) teams, some with staff reallocated from the ever-shrinking state hospitals (Essock and Kontos, 1995), and residential programs—supervised apartments, supported apartments and group homes. He devoted considerable attention to communicating the DMH mission and philosophy, and to strengthening the training of private non-profit providers through a Human Resources Development Initiative. Additionally, using staff from DMH regional offices throughout the state, he began developing "managed service systems" designed to improve continuity of care and collaboration among community providers, and between inpatient and community services. During this period the CMHC was designated the "lead agency" for the managed service system serving New Haven and the towns of Hamden, Bethany and Woodbridge. As we discuss later, this designation ultimately led to the formation of a highly collaborative inter-agency care system for the state's priority service population, led by the CMHC. Hogan also increased the emphasis on program monitoring and performance measurement by adding quality assurance directors to each DMH regional office, and he fostered development of consumer organizations, such as the Connecticut Alliance for the Mentally Ill, now NAMI-CT.

Crisis in leadership at the CMHC (1987–1989)

Although Commissioner Hogan appreciated the significant contributions of the CMHC and Yale to community mental health in Connecticut, problems emerged that caused a setback in the partnership between Yale and the state. Early in his tenure, an unfavorable audit report regarding the state contract with Yale made it politically necessary for Hogan to adopt a more distant posture in his relationship to the university. Soon afterward Astrachan left the CMHC to become chairman of psychiatry at the University of Illinois in Chicago. In the search for a new Center director, tensions between DMH and Yale grew as each attempted to assert its perceived authority over the selection process. The partnership was experiencing an uncharacteristic period of uneasiness. The selection standoff was resolved when the dean of the Yale School of Medicine nominated and Hogan appointed Ezra Griffith as the CMHC's new director. Griffith is a nationally recognized expert in forensic psychiatry. In addition, his African-Caribbean-American background contributed to his strong interest in cultural psychiatry, and in exploring the role of African-American churches and clergy in the delivery of urban health and mental health services. As the CMHC director, Griffith's thoughtful leadership helped to sustain the relationship between the DMH and Yale while the two organizations struggled over audit and contract details as well as program priorities.

The positive relationship between Yale and the DMH that had characterized the Worrell years was not restored during Commissioner Hogan's tenure. When the state's economy slowed and the budget tightened in 1989, the DMH and the CMHC leaders began disagreeing about operational priorities for the Center, particularly regarding the amount and percentage of funds that should be devoted to research, training and direct-care services, as well as how any such decisions would be made. A significant outgrowth of this period of tension and budget struggles was the development of strong, independent relationships between the leadership of the CMHC and key members of the New Haven legislative delegation. Over the years, the existence of these relationships has made it possible, at times, to influence legislative budget decisions directly regarding the funding of the annual staffing contract, as well as other policy matters important to the operation of the Center's programs. In more recent years, as tensions between the parties abated and a collegial partnership reemerged, the CMHC's interactions with the legislative delegation have been more closely coordinated with the strategic direction and legislative communications of the commissioner and his staff.

In 1990 Lowell P. Weicker, Jr., a Yale alumnus, was elected governor of Connecticut. Soon afterward, Commissioner Hogan resigned to become commissioner of Mental Health in Ohio. Later, he would serve as chairman of the President's New Freedom Commission on Mental Health under President George W. Bush. During the Worrell and Hogan years, Connecticut's mental health system had undergone substantial change; for example, state expenditures for community support services had grown from less than $5 million in state fiscal year 1983, to nearly $48 million in fiscal year

1991, an increase of 90%. Additionally, although total DMH expenditures had more than doubled during that time period (from $127.3 million to $265.4 million), inpatient care had decreased from 72% to 50% of total expenditures, and spending on community support programs, largely in private non-profit agencies, had grown from 13% to 30% of expenditures (Mental Health Expenditures SFY 1983–SFY 1991).

With the departure of Hogan, Governor Weicker appointed Yale's renowned child psychiatrist, Albert J. Solnit, to serve as Connecticut's new DMH commissioner. In this capacity, Solnit emphasized clinical excellence, professional accountability and patient rights. Although he held the highest post in the state mental health system, he was always accessible to consumers and their families. He personally conducted dozens of clinical case conferences throughout the state, in which the most complicated and intractable client care, organizational, and systems problems were tackled head-on. Under his leadership, these conferences served as an extraordinary teaching tool, and they conveyed his personal expectation that everyone in the system would work diligently to solve difficult problems.

During his tenure, Solnit presided over several major changes in the state's mental health system. These included development of a statewide system of local mental health authorities (LMHAs), which built on the foundation laid by Commissioner Hogan's managed service system initiatives; closure of two large state hospitals; transfer of many inpatient staff to community positions; and reintegration of mental health and addiction services within a single state agency.

Connecticut's system of LMHAs was based on a conceptual model proposed by the Robert Wood Johnson Foundation (RWJF) (Shore and Cohen, 1990). Recognizing that service coordination and continuity of care were important to achieving successful treatment outcomes for people with serious mental illness, the RWJF recommended creation of locally based mental health authorities throughout the nation that would have clinical and administrative responsibility for all people with serious mental illness living within defined geographical regions. As DMH began to develop this system in Connecticut, the CMHC was the obvious choice to become the LMHA for the greater New Haven community. In this capacity, the CMHC would serve as the hub of clinical care and would lead collaborative efforts among all DMH-funded community-based programs in the area. These other agencies would function as affiliates of the Center. Additionally, the CMHC crystallized formal relationships that coordinated inpatient care provided at the Center and at the CVH with outpatient and community support services that were needed to sustain community tenure for people with serious mental illness leaving inpatient settings.

By 1995 the combined census of Connecticut's three large state hospitals had declined to the point where it no longer made economic sense to operate these massive facilities. Prior to the closure of Norwich and Fairfield Hills hospitals, the three large state hospitals had a combined census of about 750 patients. Meanwhile, community-based mental health care had become more comprehensive and better accessible. This, coupled with stagnation in the state's economy during the first half of the 1990s and pressure to reduce state spending, led to a decision to close two state hospitals. Fairfield Hills Hospital closed in December 1995, followed by Norwich Hospital in October 1996. Some patients from these facilities were discharged to community programs while others were transferred to CVH. Although some staff layoffs occurred, most employees were offered and accepted transfers to state-operated community-based programs. While this was a difficult transition period, Solnit remained an unwavering advocate for quality care and fought pressure within state government to curtail spending on community-based services.

In 1995 after nearly a decade of operating as separate agencies, mental health and substance abuse services were combined within a single state authority called the Department of Mental Health and Addiction Services (DMHAS). This was followed in 1996 by the recommendations from a Governor's Blue Ribbon Task Force on Substance Abuse, which led to the creation of the Alcohol and Drug Policy Council (ADPC) and set the stage for changes that would strengthen the role of addiction services in Connecticut. Yale faculty at the CMHC's Substance Abuse Treatment Unit (SATU) would play an important role in helping to realize these gains. In contrast to most parts of the state, where collaboration in addressing the complex needs of people with co-occurring psychiatric and substance use disorders was slow to catch on, the CMHC led the way. The Center had a long-standing tradition of integrated mental health and substance abuse treatment. Additionally, it is noteworthy here that during Solnit's tenure, the CMHC was selected to lead a local service system for substance-abusing persons receiving state general assistance benefits.

As a follow-up to the landmark 1999 U.S. surgeon general's report on mental health, and in response to concerns about gaps in the state's service system, Connecticut Governor John Rowland appointed a Blue Ribbon Commission on Mental Health in 2000. The commission report revealed that although significant progress had been made in developing community mental health services in Connecticut, much remained to be done, particularly in the area of improved access to children's mental health care, and in use of federal Medicaid support for adult services under the Rehabilitation Option. David Kessler, honorary chairperson of the commission and dean of the Yale School of Medicine, was believed by many to have inspired the report's extraordinary candor. The commission's report led to creation of the Mental Health Policy Council, with an adult issues subcommittee co-chaired by Griffith.

After nine years as commissioner (a longer tenure than all but one of his predecessors), in 2000 Solnit returned to the Yale Child Study Center and to his cherished clinical practice as one of America's great child psychiatrists. Deputy Commissioner Thomas Kirk, Jr. succeeded him. While the contributions of the current administration will be better understood with the passage of time, some observations can be made at present.

Early in his administration, and based on growing evidence that such an approach was needed, Kirk, assisted by former DMHAS Deputy Commissioner Arthur Evans, Jr. began developing a statewide recovery-oriented system of behavioral health care for adults with serious psychiatric and substance use disorders. In order to facilitate this work, Kirk strengthened the connection between the DMHAS and the Yale Department of Psychiatry and engaged Yale's formidable brain trust in conceptualizing ways in which recovery principles could be translated into everyday practice. The creative talents of Larry Davidson, founding director of Yale's Program on Recovery and Community Health (PRCH) were central to this effort. The DMHAS provided funding for PRCH to develop a training academy that became known as the Recovery Institute. Later, the DMHAS Division of Education and Training assumed many of these educational activities. As of this writing, hundreds of staff throughout the state have been trained in recovery-oriented concepts and practices. As part of the Recovery Initiative,

Yale played a leadership role in developing a Recovery Self-Assessment instrument. Service providers throughout Connecticut are using this tool (now in its second revised edition) to evaluate how far they have come toward achieving a recovery orientation. Supported by the public–academic partnership, Yale faculty worked collaboratively with consumers and providers in an effort that led to the development and dissemination of DMHAS Recovery Practice Standards.

Connecticut's work on the Recovery Initiative attracted national attention. In September 2005 Connecticut became one of only seven states to receive a competitive Mental Health Transformation State Incentive Grant from the federal Substance Abuse and Mental Health Services Administration (SAMHSA). This five-year, $13.7 million grant award resulted from an application developed by the DMHAS, and is meant to assist the state in achieving the goals set forth by the President's New Freedom Commission on Mental Health (2003). Each of the seven recipient states is focusing on different aspects of the transformation process. Connecticut's contribution will be to demonstrate how a recovery-oriented system can improve the lives of people with mental illness. This approach recognizes that recovery is about hope, choice, active participation in community life, jobs, education, healthful relationships, safe and affordable housing, and access to high-quality, culturally competent treatment and supports. Work on the Recovery Initiative led the National Alliance on Mental Illness (NAMI) to rate Connecticut with a "B+" for "recovery supports" (NAMI, 2006) and for having started developing its recovery vision prior to the President's New Freedom Commission recommendations in this area.

The impact of organizational missions and cultures

In evaluating the four-decade partnership between Yale and the state at the CMHC, we might ask, "What have we learned from this alliance, and how might these lessons help forecast our future or be of use to others involved in public–academic partnerships?" As described above, people, economic conditions, and political realities were instrumental in shaping the relationship. Other forces also were key. In each instance, the molding influence of people, resources, and politics took place through interplay with the distinct organizational missions and cultures of the university and of the state agency. Sometimes these forces drew the partners closer together, and sometimes they pushed them apart. These dynamics perhaps can be better understood by examining the core missions and cultures of the university and of the state behavioral health authority.

The Yale University School of Medicine has a tripartite mission encompassing teaching, research and service. While public service is unquestionably of significance, as with most academic centers, teaching and research remain important foci. They are the dual engines for expanding and refining the body of scientific knowledge, and for educating and training professionals in theories, research methods and evidence-based practices.

By comparison, throughout the history of the DMHAS (and its predecessor the DMH), the primary mission has been to function as a safety net for medically indigent persons with behavioral health disorders. In the state agency, public service is paramount.

The DMHAS/Yale partnership at the CMHC has enabled the state and the university to assist each other in attaining important organizational goals. The CMHC has served as a nexus at which the university has increased its profile of community involvement by serving economically disadvantaged and disabled people living in diverse racial-cultural neighborhoods. Concurrently, the state has enhanced the quality of behavioral health care in a major urban area and has obtained access to nationally recognized scientists and researchers for training, consultation, and assistance with identifying and disseminating evidence-based practices. These activities continue to improve quality at all levels within a complex statewide service system. Meanwhile, the combined political clout of the university and the state has been instrumental in helping to accomplish fundamental reform in community mental health in Connecticut.

Experiences similar to those seen in the State of Connecticut–Yale University relationship have been noted elsewhere. For example, in 1986, the American Psychiatric Press published a book, edited by John Talbott and Carolyn Robinowitz, entitled *Working Together: State-University Collaboration in Mental Health* (1986). The penultimate chapter of that text discusses lessons learned from a number of such collaborations across the country. The authors express the view that: "Probably the most important single ingredient to the success of state-university collaborations is strong and committed leadership on both sides." Further, they observe: "Not only must numerous frank and open meetings take place between involved parties, but there must be recognition that staff support will have to be assiduously cultivated in both systems, and that progress will be reviewed at regular intervals as well as on an as-needed basis, to resolve problems as they arise." The authors also point to what they describe as the "principle of jointness" or, in other words, the degree to which the partnership is truly mutual and collaborative, characterized by "a similar set of values, goals, and views of the solutions to the attendant problems." On a related note, there is reference to the important role of "bridging persons" between the two entities, including "at least one or more individuals who have worked in the state system and know its realities. Further, those who have proven themselves in both cultures—university and state system—will quickly gain the confidence of both sides." While these observations and conclusions were written twenty years ago, with no specific reference to the CMHC, the lessons learned are nonetheless applicable to the Yale–state experience in Connecticut. In addition, other authors have described lessons learned from public–academic partnerships (Talbott, 1991), including why some fail (Barter and Langsley, 1986), pitfalls of joint ventures (Gaylin and Loutsch, 1986), what works and doesn't work (Talbott and Greenblatt, 1986), and how general systems theory can be used to understand complex organizational dynamics (Yank et al., 1992).

In the present discussion, we offer a simple model, displayed in Figure 7.1, to illustrate the relative importance of teaching, research and service delivery as subcomponents of the mission of an academic institution such as Yale University, compared with a typical state behavioral health agency such as DMHAS.

As can be seen, the service mission is dominant in the state agency. Training is used to enhance workforce skills for existing employees, create career development opportunities, and to assist with the recruitment and retention of qualified personnel, particularly those from diverse racial and cultural groups.

Although the research and training functions have a strong foundation at the DMHAS (in April 2006 the Yale Department of Psychiatry presented the Mental

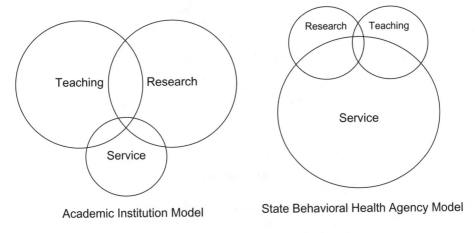

Academic Institution Model   State Behavioral Health Agency Model

Figure 7.1 *Comparative focus on mission subcomponents*

Health Research Advocacy Award to Commissioner Kirk for supporting innovations in neurobiological and treatment research in the areas of mental illness and substance abuse, and in recognition of the contributions this research makes to his emphasis on recovery), this has not always been so. In the past, and to a lesser extent at present, some stakeholders in public sector behavioral health have seen research as a luxury that drains resources away from the primary service mission. During periods of economic prosperity, support for research activities generally continues unchallenged. However, when the economy slows, and state revenues decline, it forces a state agency to protect its core service mission. At these times critics of research spending may gain the upper hand, causing research to be targeted for budget reduction. Training also may be jeopardized because it is commonly perceived as less critical than direct service, and because the provider agency may not be able to afford the cost of replacement personnel needed to "backfill" posts of employees participating in training events. Private non-profit service providers must make difficult decisions knowing that if an employee post is not backfilled it might adversely affect safety or the ability to generate revenue needed to support ongoing program operations. During economic hard times, the trade-off between quality care supported by training on the one hand, and reducing personnel costs on the other, becomes a "Sophie's choice" for behavioral health agency leaders.

Figure 7.2 shows how the CMHC has adjusted its mission to create greater balance among the subcomponents. In truth, this figure overstates the equality of the three parts. By any objective measure, such as budget or staff time allocation, the service mission subcomponent at the CMHC is always larger than that of training or research. It also should be noted that this configuration is dynamic, not static, and, at any single point in time, it is not uniform across all operational units of the Center. Thus, for example, the relative emphasis on various aspects of the Center's mission may shift from time to time to accommodate the planning and implementation stages of a new research grant, or the arrival of new residents or trainees.

This model may explain some of the dynamic tension at the CMHC, which has a mission configuration that differs from the state and the university. When the state

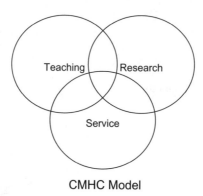

CMHC Model

Figure 7.2   *Balancing the mission at the CMHC*

enters a period of fiscal restraint, strong support for research and training are required from both the state behavioral health authority and the university in order to counterbalance forces that see these functions as expendable.

In addition to differences in the missions of the state agency and the university, many important differences in organizational culture also influence relationships at a community mental health center where the state and university work in partnership.

First, let us consider the university setting. The most senior personnel in the university are its administrators, deans and tenured professors. Tenure rewards faculty members for their achievements, granting them a predictable and stable future, and enabling them to plan and execute ambitious intellectual projects and large-scale or long-term lines of scientific inquiry. As faculty integrate the art and science of clinical education, a great deal of emphasis is placed on the use of reliable and valid data. Conclusions derived from analysis of high-quality data can be safely shared with other members of the scientific community or used in applied settings, and incorporated into clinical education.

In contrast, the most senior leaders in mental health (or behavioral health—here we will use the term mental health to connote both) within state government are its commissioners and deputy commissioners. These individuals are appointed by, and "serve at the pleasure" of the governor. Unlike some state agency commissioners who are selected because of well-established political connections, mental health commissioners in Connecticut tend to be picked because of their specialized subject-matter expertise. Their political connections may be somewhat tenuous. Possibly as a consequence, the tenure of commissioners of mental health is typically brief. Nationwide data reveal that their median term of office is a mere 20.4 months (Lutterman, 2006), leading some to quip that they are among "the highest paid migrant workers in the United States." While the last five mental health commissioners in Connecticut have enjoyed longevity far exceeding the national median, each new arrival recognizes from the outset that accomplishing anything meaningful and lasting means doing it quickly.

The press to move quickly influences the change process and how day-to-day decisions are reached. Although considerable effort is made in the state agency to use high-quality data to guide decision-making, as a practical matter decisions must be reached without enough data, or by using data of questionable reliability and validity. Thus, while data quality and use of data in decision-making are important in both the state agency and in the university, data quality and the kinds of statements or decisions that are made from data differ widely across the two settings. Generally accepted standards of scientific inquiry require researchers in academic settings to be very cautious about the conclusions they reach based on data, whereas in the state agency, this constraint (or luxury) simply is not possible.

These differences in organizational culture and priorities can cause tension and require negotiation and compromise regarding operations and decision-making at the community mental health center setting. Thus, for example, in a mental health center operated under a public–academic partnership, for scientific reasons faculty-clinicians might wish to form a treatment group that includes clients who meet the specific requirements of a research protocol. Meanwhile, state agency clinicians, with whom the faculty interact, might argue that other high-need or high-risk clients should be treated first.

There are very real and visible differences between the hiring practices, productivity standards, compensation and benefit plans, and reward systems of the university and the state civil service. When university faculty and state employees work side-by-side in the same organization, these differences are readily apparent and, at times, become a source of internal tension. Care must be taken lest this characteristic of institutional culture becomes misinterpreted as indicating that some employees are more important and trusted or more highly valued than others.

Some thoughts on the future

Several contextual items set the stage for the consideration of future challenges. First, in his 1999 report, U.S. Surgeon General David Satcher concluded that a range of effective treatments exists for most mental disorders (Report of the Surgeon General, 1999). Second, in 2001 the Institute of Medicine found that it takes an astounding average of 17 years for new knowledge generated through randomized controlled experimental trials to be incorporated into clinical practice, and even then these "evidence-based practices" are not consistently applied in field settings (Crossing the Quality Chasm, 2001). Third, the President's New Freedom Commission called for "transformation" of the mental health system based on its assessment that problems in the current system were too extensive to be solved through incremental change or simple reform (President's New Freedom Commission on Mental Health, 2006). Fourth, despite over 40 years of community mental health development in the U.S., in its 2006 report card on public mental health systems, NAMI gave the country an overall performance rating of "D" (NAMI, 2006). Connecticut and Ohio shared the highest ratings of public mental health systems in the nation—both states scored "B." And finally, programmatic shifts contained in the 2006 Deficit Reduction Act (DRA), P.L. 109–171, that are designed to generate cost savings in the Medicaid, Medicare and Temporary Assistance for Needy Families programs, have prompted concern regarding the potential adverse impact on people with serious mental illness who are heavily reliant upon these programs (Bazelon, Center for Mental Health Law, 2006).

In summary, we can see at the national level that while significant progress has been made in developing effective treatment technologies and supports for people with serious mental illness, this process has been slow, and successful practices have been unevenly applied. While Connecticut has fared better than most states, over the past several decades incremental advancement of community mental health care in the United States has not produced satisfactory results, and now a looming funding crisis threatens to damage an already fragile system. This in turn could exacerbate the current trend toward criminalization of mental illness and may raise new obstacles for people who already face many challenges in their efforts to achieve recovery from psychiatric disabilities.

Yet, even with these problems, there is cause for guarded optimism about the future. The recommendations contained in the report of the President's New Freedom Commission (2006) and in Transforming Mental Health Care in America (2006), and transformation activities under way in many states, show movement in a positive direction. In order to continue this progress, several fundamental issues must be addressed. These include:

- Ensuring the delivery of high-quality, culturally competent, behavioral health care, that is directed toward the identification and elimination of health disparities;

- Ensuring the adequacy and stability of funding for services and supports;

- Supporting excellence in the preparation of the behavioral workforce;

- Promoting person-centered, consumer-driven care that supports consumer efforts to attain a better education, paid employment or participation in volunteer activities, and safe and stable housing;

- Supporting psychoeducation for families of people with serious mental illness; and

- Improving safety for consumers and for the communities in which they live.

Strong public/academic partnerships, such as the one that has evolved at the CMHC between Yale University and the State of Connecticut are helping to address many of these problems. Significant participation of scientists, teachers and clinical experts, including some who have extensive credentials in all three areas, is common in the CMHC partnership setting. The public/academic partnership is also adept at leveraging resources through research, service enhancement, demonstration projects, and other grants involving federal and private sources. For example, in Connecticut fiscal year 2006, state general fund expenditures at the CMHC of approximately $3.5 million for research leveraged $21.0 million (direct cost only) in additional federal and other grants. A long-standing Yale–state indirect cost recovery agreement resulted in reimbursements of nearly $1 million to the state as a direct result of these research activities at the CMHC.

As we look to the future, we encourage state mental health authorities and universities throughout the nation to develop new alliances and strengthen existing ones. In addition to their proven ability to promote excellence and innovation in mental health care, these partnerships can serve as platforms to spread awareness of mental health as perhaps the nation's most significant public health issue. Finally, as partners, states and universities can use their combined political clout to ensure the adequacy of financial support for research, training and services.

Conclusion

The forty-year joint venture between Yale University and the State of Connecticut at the CMHC is itself a statement about the viability of such arrangements. With its mix of teaching, research and service, the Center has created a uniquely stimulating environment. Each day professional staff are challenged by the combination of a service—population comprising of people with some of the most complex psychiatric, medical, social, economic and legal problems seen in any public behavioral health setting—by the requirements of ongoing research and training, and a large complement of inquisitive and creative trainees and psychiatric residents. An expectation of quality care and the rigorous pursuit of excellence permeate the Center's atmosphere. At every level, the Center's activities communicate its commitment to the future of public sector behavioral health professions. Despite multiple challenges, the relationship has stood the test of time, proving over and over that the benefits it yields for the partners, for the community, and for public psychiatry are well worth the effort.

References

Barter JT, Langsley DG: University-state collaborations: why some fail? in Working Together: State University Collaborations in Mental Health. Edited by Talbott JA, Robinowitz CB. Washington, DC: American Psychiatric Press, pp 135–50, 1986

Beard JH, Propst R, Malamud TJ: The Fountain House model of psychiatric rehabilitation. Psychiatr Rehabil J 5:47–55, 1982

Carini E, Douglas D, Heck L, et al: The mentally ill in Connecticut: changing patterns of care and the evolution of psychiatric nursing 1636–1972. State of Connecticut, Department of Mental Health. Hartford, Connecticut, 1974

Connecticut General Assembly, Legislative Program Review and Investigations Committee. Mental health in Connecticut: services in transition. Hartford, Connecticut, 1979

Connecticut Hospital Association, Inc. v. Audrey Worrell, M.D., Commissioner, Department of Mental Health. Docket No. CV 84-0290158 S, Superior Court, Judicial District of Hartford/New Britain at Hartford.

Crossing the Quality Chasm: A New Health System for the 21st Century. Washington, DC: Institute of Medicine of the National Academies, 2001

Deutsch A. The Shame of the States. New York: Harcourt, 1948.

Donaldson v. O'Connor, 493 F 2d 507 (5th Cir. 1974)

Essock S, Kontos N: Implementing assertive community treatment teams. Psychiatr Serv 46:679–83, 1995

Gaylin S, Loutsch E: Pitfalls of joint ventures between state and academic institutions: the New York experience, in Working Together: State University Collaborations in Mental Health. Edited by Talbott JA, Robinowitz CB. Washington, DC, American Psychiatric Press, pp 151–64, 1986

Hoadley CJ: The Public Records of the Colony of Connecticut, August 1689–May 1706. Press of Case. Lockwood and Brainard, Hartford, Connecticut. pp 285–6, 1868

Judge David L Bazelon: Center for Mental Health Law: What deficit reduction means for people with mental disabilities. Bazelon Center Mental Health Policy Reporter V(2):1–13, March 21, 2006

Lake v. Cameron, 267 F. Supp. 155 (1967)

Lamb RH: A century and a half of psychiatric rehabilitation in the United States. Hosp Community Psychiatry 45:1015–20, 1994

Lutterman T: NASMHPD Research Institute, Personal communication, January 2006

Mental Health Expenditures SFY 1983–SFY 1991. Department of Mental Health, Hartford Connecticut

NAMI: Grading the States 2006: A report on America's health care system for serious mental illness. National Alliance on Mental Illness. Washington, DC. Available at: http://www.nami. org/gtstemplate.cfm?section=grading_the_states&lstid=701. Accessed May 16, 2006.

O'Connor v. Donaldson 422 U.S. 563, 1975

President's New Freedom Commission on Mental Health. 2003. Washington, DC. Available at: http://www.mentalhealthcommission.gov/. Accessed May 16, 2006

Public Document No. 72. Report of the State Psychopathic Hospital Commission to His Excellency the Governor of Connecticut, State of Connecticut. 1922 Appendix A, pp 25–6

Report of the Surgeon General. Office of the Surgeon General, Department of Health and Human Services. Washington, DC, 1999. Available at: http://www.surgeongeneral.gov/ library/mentalhealth/home.html. Accessed May 16, 2006

Rouse v. Cameron, 125 U.S. App. D.C. 366, 373 F. 2d 451 (1966)

Shore MF, Cohen MD: The Robert Wood Johnson Foundation program on chronic mental illness: an overview. Hosp Community Psychiatry 41:1212–6, 1990

Talbott JA: The Pew project: national effort to improve state-university collaborations. Hosp Community Psychiatry 42:70, 1991

Talbott JA, Greenblatt M: Lessons learned: what works and doesn't work, and how to overcome resistances, in Working Together: State University Collaborations in Mental Health. Edited by Talbott JA, Robinowitz CB. Washington, DC: American Psychiatric Press, pp 195–208, 1986

Talbott JA, Robinowitz CB (eds): Working Together: State-University Collaboration in Mental Health. Washington, DC: American Psychiatric Press, 1986

Tamayo L, January J, Peet M, et al: The system impact of an urban mobile crisis team, in Psychiatry Takes to the Streets. Edited by Cohen N. New York: Guilford Publications, pp 121–33, 1990

Transforming Mental Health Care in America: The Federal Action Agenda: First Steps. Substance Abuse and Mental Health Services Administration, Washington, DC. Available at: http://www.samhsa.gov/Federalactionagenda/NFC_execsum.aspx. Accessed June 2, 2006

Ward M: The Snake Pit. New York: Random House, 1946

Wolf J: Chronicle of change: a case study of the Connecticut mental health system. Adm Policy Ment Health 17:151–64, 1990

Wyatt v. Stickney, 344 F. Supp. 387 (M.D. Ala. 1972)

Yank GR, Spradlin WW, Porterfield PB: General systems approaches in mental health administration. Acad Psychiatry 16:59–71, 1992

8

Public psychiatry training and education at the Connecticut Mental Health Center

Jeanne Steiner, Nancy Anderson, Richard Belitsky, Michael Hoge, Martha L. Mitchell, William H. Sledge and Sophie Tworkowski

The history of the Connecticut Mental Health Center (CMHC) can be partly understood by studying the origin and progression of its training programs over the past four decades. The basic values of understanding patients within the context of their communities, collaborating with other professionals and translating the most current knowledge of the field into the care of the patients have been core elements throughout the history of the Center. Each of the major professions—psychiatry, nursing, social work and psychology—has participated in the development of training programs that have prepared and inspired young professionals to work with the special populations served in the public sector and to appreciate the nature of effective interdisciplinary collaboration. Each professional group has its own story to tell. However, the broad theme is the special dedication and expertise that have been evident over the past 40 years and the commitment to carry forth this vision for the future.

Since its inception, the Connecticut Mental Health Center (CMHC) has been committed to the training of mental health professionals—particularly psychiatric residents, clinical psychologists, social workers, psychiatric nurses and medical students. This was in recognition of the academic mission of the institution, as well as the expectation that many of the trainees would remain in Connecticut, providing clinical service and contributing to the workforce of mental health programs in the state (CMHC Programs and Plans, 1966). The tradition has been upheld over the past 40 years, with no wavering of resolve from the state or the university in their support of the key mission of education. The CMHC is both a local and a national resource for future clinicians, researchers, and educators well versed in their areas of practice and expertise.

Each of the disciplines has concentrated its attention on the understanding and treatment of individuals who suffer from serious mental illness and/or addictive disorders. Many of the core services and programs of the Center have been built on community-based treatment for the primary "target population" of the Department of Mental Health and Addiction Services (DMHAS), defined as individuals who are

40 Years of Academic Public Psychiatry. Edited by Selby C. Jacobs and Ezra E. H. Griffith
© 2007 John Wiley & Sons, Ltd.

indigent and who experience "severe and persistent" illness. However, over the years, the CMHC's mission has shifted to include other special populations, such as young adults, individuals who have been exposed to trauma, and patients who have had involvement with the criminal justice system.

From the beginning, a central tenet of the CMHC's treatment and training programs has been the appreciation of each individual patient within the context of his or her social environment. Although historically the field of social work has emphasized this aspect of assessment and care most consistently in its programs, the staff and trainees from all disciplines at the CMHC have been taught the critical role of institutional, community, cultural and family context as they consider an individual who is seeking care. The trend to treat individuals who are severely ill in community-based settings and to mobilize and enhance their natural supports has been a fundamental aspect of the CMHC's clinical services and training programs. Public sector practitioners must become adept not only in assessment and treatment modalities for those with serious disabilities, but also must be able to facilitate the integration of evidenced-based treatment and rehabilitation and to advocate for service system development that will meet patients' needs and provide opportunities for them to achieve success in the community.

Another critical component of the training programs within the CMHC has been the interaction of faculty and trainees from the various mental health disciplines. This immersion in an interdisciplinary educational experience fosters the development of interprofessional respect and collaboration, which is particularly relevant for practice within the public sector. Although each of the disciplines represented at the CMHC has promoted and mentored trainees in their development of a professional identity and provided discipline-specific expertise in their teaching and supervision, the value of learning together and from individuals of other professional groups has long been a consistent institutional value. Social workers have taught family therapy theory and practice to residents in psychiatry, and advanced practice nurses have enhanced their knowledge of the prescription of medication by participating in seminars taught by psychiatrists. Service system development and the management of systems of care have been taught by many notable CMHC administrative leaders and psychiatry faculty; in the past 10 years, this has become an area of expertise for many faculty psychologists. This latter group has also filled key leadership positions in the CMHC's activity as a lead mental health agency (LMHA) in the greater New Haven area. As the medical needs of the patient population have become a more prominent concern and focus of attention, the nursing faculty have been in a position to teach trainees from many disciplines the key components of physical health screening, counseling and facilitation of care. Faculty psychiatrists have provided lectures and case conferences for the trainees in their seminars and clinical sites covering a wide range of diagnostic and treatment topics based on the best available evidence in the field and have been role models for leadership, scholarship and clinical care. The trainees at the CMHC, therefore, have had an extraordinary exposure to an interdisciplinary approach to the care of individuals who experience serious illness in the context of multiple social burdens. In addition to the valuable teaching that is imparted by role models from different fields, the trainees at the CMHC are educated in an environment where novel research is performed and results translated into the care of patients. It is important to note that the patients themselves have had much to teach the CMHC's trainees.

It is also worth emphasizing that the CMHC faculty and other senior staff have been providing continuing education to professionals who hold staff positions in the Center. This is an important contribution to workforce development. Seminars and intensive workshops that reflect such efforts in the field of public psychiatry and the changing needs of the patient population have included, for example, brief therapies, cultural competence, integrated treatment for substance abuse and mental health disorders, and recovery-oriented systems of care. These initiatives have enriched the clinical environment, enhanced job satisfaction for staff and added to the vibrancy of the academic milieu.

Residency training

At the CMHC, the structure and direction of training for psychiatric residents have paralleled the evolving missions and core values of the institution. Consequently, residency training has included general education and training as well as specialty education for advanced residents along certain thematic lines. Residency training has always been interdisciplinary and continues to be so today. It emphasizes the teamwork and multidisciplinary skills and knowledge necessary to provide effective community and public sector services. During the almost two decades of Boris Astrachan's leadership of the CMHC, he highlighted the capacity to operate in complex social systems as an essential element of the general training and education for professional students in the core mental health disciplines of psychiatry, psychology, social work and nursing. This vision of education included learning the role of consultant as well as primary psychiatric provider so that residents could function well in either activity after graduation.

This approach fit well with the Yale Department of Psychiatry's innovative core and track system implemented in 1971 in which the three years of psychiatric residency training were divided into an 18-month core and an 18-month specialty track experience. The core included three six-month rotations, which were unique in their management of the initial experiences of psychiatry residents. In the PG 2 year, there were six-month inpatient and outpatient experiences, both of which emphasized the phenomenology of psychiatric syndromes, diagnosis and therapeutics. In PGY 3 the core experience was six months working as a consultant in emergency psychiatry, consultation liaison in a general medical setting and community consultation. Half of PGY 3 and all of PGY 4 were spent in a specialty track experience. Initially there were two tracks located at the CMHC: the social and community psychiatry track and the neurobiological research training track. A follow-up study demonstrated that early experience in these tracks had correlated substantially with subsequent career activity in terms of academic productivity as well as clinical work settings and modalities (Sledge et al., 1990).

For the Yale general psychiatry residency, this meant that the teaching content during core clinical rotations at the CMHC included not only traditional topics such as etiology, diagnosis and treatment modalities of psychiatric conditions, but also addressed the social context in which illness occurred and treatment was being provided. There was substantial emphasis on experiences in group relations, spearheaded by Daniel Levinson, Peter Newton, Edward Klein and others in the early years, and

Marshal Edelson and others later. For instance, all residents participated in group relations training, and residents at the CMHC had the opportunity to participate in and observe (through one-way mirrors) group therapy with patients and to examine these experiences through supervision. This was complemented by a rich offering of high-quality didactic sessions, which included discussion of theories and experiences of group dynamics (Bion, 1961; Yalom, 1970). In addition, there was attention to the impact of the ward milieu and the relationships between and among unit staff through specific teaching activities, such as a seminar in which residents presented to senior faculty the CMHC leadership dilemmas and difficulties related to the work environment. In one version such a seminar included study of representative literature related to group and organizational dynamics (Newton and Levinson, 1973).

In the last 20 years, as the mission of DMHAS increasingly focused on the provision of clinical services to a "target" population (those who are poor and severely mentally ill) and less on the work of community mental health, the CMHC shifted its clinical and service focus as well to the provision of high-quality, innovative services to the target population in the New Haven area. Consequently, the CMHC-based training and education shifted attention away from the role of the psychiatrist as consultant and expert in social systems and more toward direct service to patients with severe and persistent mental illness. This reflected the emphasis of DMHAS and the leadership of the new director, Ezra Griffith, as he took the reins of the institution in 1987. This focus also paralleled another shift in educational paradigm for residents in the Department of Psychiatry: to emphasize more clinical core and less specialty track experiences, resulting in a revised core of 24 months (a year of inpatient and a year of outpatient) with a 12-month concentration rather than an 18-month specialty track. This emphasis on clinical service included shorter inpatient stays with a focus on symptom reduction and discharge planning and large outpatient caseloads with an emphasis on pharmacologic treatment, case management and novel ways of engaging patients [assertive community treatment (ACT) and outreach to the homeless]. Training on clinical rotations for psychiatric residents at the CMHC has evolved accordingly. Now in 2006 three three-month inpatient rotations, together with a three-month research/academic selective constitute PGY 2, and a year-long outpatient placement in PGY-3 highlights the diagnosis and treatment of individuals with serious (and often co-morbid) mental illness and limited resources. Advanced training now focuses on clinical and administrative skills through chief residency positions in PGY 4 that prepare psychiatrists for leadership in both academic and public sector settings.

Advanced training opportunities in forensic, neurobiological research, and addiction psychiatry have paralleled the development of exceptional basic and clinical research facilities and specialized clinical services at the CMHC. For example, the Ribicoff Clinical Neuroscience Unit and related clinics and laboratories have been the site of residency training for both general psychiatry residents and advanced research fellows. In addition, a federally funded Biological Scientist Training Program (BSTP) grant has supported the Neuroscience Research Training Program for more than 20 years. This specialized track of the general residency (which includes rotations on an inpatient research unit, in outpatient research clinics and laboratories) has fostered the research careers of several generations of psychiatrists. The Law and Psychiatry Division, which provides court-ordered forensic evaluations for the State of Connecticut and consultation to attorneys in the public and private sectors, provides training experiences in the general residency and has a nationally acclaimed ACGME-accredited residency program in forensic psychiatry. Similarly, The Substance Abuse Treatment Unit, which is the site of the CMHC's clinical care and research in addiction psychiatry, provides training in the general residency and participates in the Yale ACGME-accredited residency program in addiction psychiatry.

Psychology

As a discipline and a training program, clinical psychology had a major presence at Yale when the CMHC opened in 1966 as a collaborative endeavor of the State of Connecticut, Department of Mental Health and the Department of Psychiatry, Yale University. Thus, it was natural for psychology to be a strong partner among the professions that were assembled to provide leadership and to develop teaching and research programs at the Center. A chief of psychology was appointed, faculty members were hired and a training program was implemented, drawing on the training tradition that had been established at the Yale Psychiatric Institute.

Training levels

The doctoral preparation of clinical psychologists typically involves five years of graduate study. After the first year, it is common for students to engage in part-time clinical rotations or practica, while simultaneously completing coursework and research. A full year of pre-doctoral clinical internship must be completed prior to the conferring of the doctoral degree, and typically occurs in the fourth or fifth year of graduate study. Supervised, post-doctoral experience is required for subsequent licensure and can be gained through post-doctoral training fellowships or through supervised employment.

Since its opening, the majority of psychology training at the Center has involved the one-year, full-time, pre-doctoral clinical internships. These have been part of an accredited internship program that is managed by the Psychology Section of the Yale Department of Psychiatry, which, in addition to the CMHC, places students at the Yale-New Haven Psychiatric Hospital and, historically, at the Yale Psychiatric Institute and Waterbury Hospital.

Data on the number of psychology students trained at the CMHC are readily available only for pre-doctoral interns and only for the past 15 years. From July of 1992 through June of 2006, a total of 165 students were trained in the pre-doctoral internship program. The annual class size has varied due to funding fluctuations, ranging from 9 to 15 students and averaging 11 per year. Extrapolating from these figures, a reasonable estimate is that more than 350 pre-doctoral fellows have completed their training at the CMHC since its opening.

Post-doctoral psychology training also began at the Center when it opened, although it has remained more loosely organized, much smaller until recently in terms of number of students, and more research-oriented in focus, particularly because early funding for post-doctoral clinical training from the National Institute for Mental Health ceased to be available. Accreditation did not exist for post-doctoral programs until recently and still remains optional. As a result, the post-doctoral experiences have been individually negotiated and tailored, based on the common interests of an applicant and the faculty member who supports the fellow through research grants or clinical revenues.

In the past several years, the NIH-funded post-doctoral training programs in research have significantly augmented the more individually tailored post-doctoral positions. Post-doctoral experiences have been a common and effective stepping stone to a junior faculty position within the Department of Psychiatry and the CMHC for many of the most promising psychologists.

Practicum students were not trained at the CMHC early in the Center's history. Such trainees only devoted part-time to clinical rotations, tended to have minimal skills and required intensive supervision, thus making their integration into the Center too labor-intensive. However, there has been a trend over the past half-dozen years to accommodate such students, particularly those keenly interested in the population served at the CMHC. Their training experience has focused on basic skill-building and increasing the confidence and comfort of these budding psychologists in clinical, interdisciplinary settings.

Theoretical roots

While the psychoanalytic and psychodynamic perspectives had been prevalent in psychology at Yale, the birth of the Center occurred in part because of growing social consciousness and commitment among the faculty. Thus, while the psychodynamic traditions provided a firm foundation for early training and still have a detectable influence, there quickly emerged an emphasis on community and social psychology, group processes, and organizational dynamics that shaped faculty activities and permeated their teaching. This continued to evolve into the strong emphasis on community psychology training that took firm root in the Center and is exemplified today by The Consultation Center, which annually trains a large group of pre- and post-doctoral psychologists in prevention, early intervention and health promotion.

Population focus

A fundamental change occurred in community mental health in the 1970s and 1980s with the federal, state and local emphasis on providing improved, community-based care for individuals with severe and persistent mental illness. As the Center went through a wrenching shift in terms of its population and service focus, so too did the training programs begin to transform their focus. Students increasingly learned about severe illness, case management, and short-term inpatient and day hospital care. As the faculty began to embrace this work, the training became a more creative dynamic in relation to this population focus, through innovations involving outreach, rehabilitation, community reintegration, recovery, the development of systems of care, and program evaluation.

In a parallel fashion, faculty became interested and committed to treating persons with addictive disorders and built a variety of service and research programs focused on this population. A dedicated treatment unit for addiction disorders was opened within the CMHC and has been a long-standing training site for pre- and post-doctoral psychology fellows. Almost all fellows now receive training and clinical experience in addictions, given the prevalence of individuals with co-occurring disorders in all of the Center's programs.

Psychologists receive training in the care of other major populations, including the following: children and their families, through the West Haven Mental Health Clinic; the elderly, through programs at The Consultation Center; and monolingual Latinos, through the Center's Hispanic Clinic. Throughout all of these theoretical and population-based shifts, training in psychological assessment has been a routine part of the educational experience. However, it has changed substantially in focus as well, starting with an emphasis on dynamic assessment as a tool for understanding and teaching about psychopathology, to the current emphasis on neuropsychological assessment as a tool for evaluating cognitive functioning and as a guide to cognitive remediation.

Roles and contributions

Psychology fellows at the CMHC have obtained their training in a rich interprofessional environment that involves placement on interdisciplinary teams, supervision from faculty in other disciplines and participation in multidisciplinary seminars. These experiences have been complemented by a core set of department-wide seminars offered annually that are exclusively for psychologists, designed to help them build their discipline-specific skills and identity. The Center has provided a supportive context in which fellows have shaped their individual identity as psychologists, choosing to emphasize or combine roles in assessment, treatment, prevention, consultation, program development and management, policy development, program evaluation, and research.

Examined from the perspective of public sector behavioral health, the Center has played a substantive role in educating a large number of psychologists who are now in the workforce. Specifically, it has fostered the education and training of psychologists in treatment, prevention, and research related to the care of persons with severe mental and addiction disorders. It has helped to provide a highly skilled professional workforce in Connecticut's system of services and in those systems beyond the state's borders. Further, it has helped to train a cadre of leaders who now shape behavioral health policy, service provision and research across the nation.

Nursing

The history of nurses' training at the CMHC is a complex story in several ways. First, the history of nursing education arises from the CMHC's tripartite mission and joint linkage to the state and university, which since 1966 were grounded on the academic side in both the Yale School of Medicine and the Yale School of Nursing. Second, by a selective focus on training, the vision of its interrelations with the changing practice of psychiatric nurses within the CMHC organization and beyond may be obscured. Third, from the CMHC's inception, its nurses have included Yale-CMHC joint appointees as well as state nursing employees. This dual composition is a distinctive fact for this discipline at the CMHC and enlarges the scope and complexity of the discussion of nursing training.

Background and formative years

The Yale University School of Nursing (YSN) was founded in 1923 with funding and an endowment by the Rockefeller Foundation. Since its creation in 1949, the YSN master's degree program in psychiatric nursing has been a fulcrum for leadership in the specialty and the discipline at large. Professor Ida Jean Orlando (1954 to 1961) is acknowledged as one of three psychiatric nurses in the U.S. whose theory base for practice has had the greatest developmental influence on psychiatric nursing (Burgess, 1985). In the formative years of the CMHC, from about 1965 to 1971, the YSN faculty roster included psychiatric nurses Rhetaugh Dumas, Rachel Robinson, Donna Diers, Judith Krauss and M. Angela McBride, all with exceptional national achievements during their careers. Education for advanced practice has long been the central curriculum goal at the masters' level at the YSN. Indeed, the mission of the YSN is one of commitment to the integrated endeavors of practice and scholarship, with appreciation for the centrality of practice in generating theory and knowledge in the discipline (Bulletin of Yale University School of Nursing, 2005–2006).

From 1959 to 1966, the school was led by Dean Florence Schorske Wald, a psychiatric nurse whose acumen about effecting change through collaboration has been one of her great enduring gifts. In 1965, she played a key role as one of the Yale and the state leaders who developed the Position Paper on Staffing for the CMHC, in which nursing joint appointments were a pivotal feature. In the 1965 and 1966 staffing documents, all of the Center's senior nursing personnel, including the director of nursing, assistant directors and clinical specialists, held YSN–CMHC joint appointments (Position Paper on Staffing, 1965; Programs and Plans, 1966). At the YSN, these nurses held faculty term appointments, and thus were subject to periodic reviews of their service, teaching and research activities. The CMHC staffing plans also called for nurses in state civil service positions to be assigned to all units, in generous supply by staffing standards then, let alone today. In those early CMHC years, the climate of excitement was palpable among nurses—faculty, students, Yale and state alike—and the learning curve through the give-and-take among all disciplines sloped sharply upward. From a national historical perspective, the opportunity was unprecedented for the CMHC nurses to fulfill such non-traditional roles and responsibilities within the context of the organization's integrated structures for nursing practice and education.

The readiness of nursing for the new CMHC enterprise was exemplified by the first and second directors of nursing. Rachel Robinson, the first director, inspired a legend about her exquisite competence and professional presence for all nursing personnel during the years of preparation and start-up. Thereafter, Rhetaugh Dumas held dual positions as the director of nursing at the CMHC and the YSN psychiatric nursing chairperson. An eminently gifted leader, she left Yale in 1972 and became the director of the NIMH Psychiatric Nursing Training Branch and thereafter deputy director of the NIMH.

The 1970s and 1980s

A sign of the transition from the early formative years to a second phase in nursing's teaching–learning endeavors at the CMHC rests in the waning motivation to revise the annual memorandum of agreement between the YSN and the CMHC. The first such memorandum was approved in 1967 by Dean Wald for the YSN and Gerald Klerman, director of the CMHC. It was an extension of the original 1964 memorandum entered into by the State and Yale, made specific to nursing's experiences and disciplinary responsibilities in this joint endeavor. Revised between 1968 and 1975, the content in the memoranda between the YSN and the CMHC primarily addressed the collaboration expected for the joint appointee positions and students at the CMHC. By 1975 the novelty of collaborating in these matters was supplanted by more reliable, patterned interactions by the CMHC administration and the YSN leadership. The memoranda said little about responsibilities of senior nursing personnel—i.e., the joint appointees—for nursing in-service and staff development, in contrast to the emphasis in the 1965 and 1966 CMHC staffing documents on this issue.

By the early seventies, the trend was under way for the boundaries of the CMHC service units to become less permeable and their service ambitions more consistently intramural in nature. The West Haven satellite clinic with its child, family and consultation components was a notable exception. The YSN–CMHC clinical specialists worked in their advanced practice roles on these units where they supervised students—typically one to three graduate psychiatric nursing trainees—each academic year from September to May. Learning to carry out psychiatric clinical assessments with skillful application of the nursing process and theories about human behavior was a mainstay in these placements; as was learning psychotherapy, crisis intervention and case management techniques. In addition, many students received instruction from faculty of other disciplines on an impromptu basis and participated in interprofessional supervision and seminars. Likewise, the units' clinical specialists and state head nurses often taught psychiatric residents or other trainees about concepts such as the skillful management of behavioral crises.

During their two-year master's program, many nursing students had some stipend and tuition support from the NIMH nursing training grants. Training support for nurses phased out completely during the 1980s, except for a subset of students electing to concentrate on care of persons with chronic psychiatric disorders, under an NIMH training initiative for this population. In addition, from the mid-1970s, the YSN also had briefer placements at the CMHC.

Outcomes and Outlook

Over time the YSN–CMHC relationship in this joint academic–public sector institution has deeply influenced the organizational culture. Interprofessionally, the comprehensiveness of care, quality of client outcomes and ethos of collaboration have profited. In time, more cooperative teaching–learning endeavors developed between the joint appointees and state nurses—with mutual benefits. In the 1980s, a more integrated nursing department structure furthered this goal. A reciprocal benefit has been the upgrading of professional credentials and career development. The YSN's presence influenced many state nurses at the CMHC (and elsewhere in Connecticut) to obtain graduate degrees in their field through full- or part-time study, often at the YSN. In turn, many YSN masters' program graduates sought state positions. Within the past two years alone, five YSN graduates and faculty have held top management and senior clinical positions at the CMHC, positions not specifically pertaining to nursing. Statewide, all the DMHAS facilities and community programs have employed YSN graduates in their administrative, clinical, educational and research endeavors.

In the policy realm, the YSN–CMHC joint appointees and graduates who trained at the CMHC have influenced policies in wide-ranging endeavors, within Connecticut, the region and nationally. It can easily be said that the CMHC has had a conscious policy-influencing orientation, and the multi-professional climate has fostered the attitudes of partnership and mutual respect that are essential to sound policy making. The CMHC's own internal policies reflect these same attitudes for credentialing in the CMHC's medical and professional staff.

The interorganizational arrangements between the CMHC and the YSN began in the 1960s and became familiar in the 1970s and 1980s. Recently, however, they have undergone substantive change. The annual number of nursing trainees at the CMHC has dropped significantly. Whereas previously an average of 15 to 20 students specializing in the care of adults and children with serious mental illness came to the CMHC, now there are only four to seven master's level nursing students. This may be related in part to the changes in advanced practice nursing, with the expansion of psychiatric nurse practitioner roles and the obtaining of prescriptive authority.

As a hybrid organization (not just state, not just Yale, but both), the CMHC has a long tradition of flourishing with a busy mix of individuals and groups, having varied career interests, incentive systems and professional competencies. The mutual benefit to the CMHC and the YSN of the commitment to collaborating for nursing training is an intrinsic part of that tradition.

Social work

In planning for the CMHC, professionals charged with conceptualizing the mission identified training as one of the Center's primary goals. The unique partnership with Yale University brought access to faculty and students from its medical school and school of nursing, and there was a structure in place that facilitated this training task. In social work, however, the protocols and academic relationships had to be developed because Yale University did not have a school of social work. The proposed staffing plan called for several of the CMHC social work positions to be filled as Yale positions, including the director of social work. Martin Schwartz initiated the social work training program as the first director of social work from 1966 to 1970.

There were key social, political and fiscal forces that influenced our service system over the past 40 years, necessitating new programs to serve persons with mental illness in their communities. The five forces that most influenced social work training were: (1) the licensing of clinical social workers in 1986; (2) the closing of Connecticut state psychiatric hospitals; (3) the reduction in the length of inpatient and outpatient stays; (4) the increase in the number of patients with long-term disabilities and co-occurring disorders; and (5) changes in the socioeconomic and geographic catchment area criteria for service eligibility. This important shift to community- based treatment models had a major impact on staff and intern training.

Staff development

At the CMHC, the social work staff were assigned to various service units. Most clinical services utilized a treatment team approach based on the medical model. Initially, social work interventions were primarily method specific: casework, group work, or community organization. Charles Robinson directed the department from 1970 to 1992 as social work roles evolved from this method-specific perspective. In the late 1960s and 1970s, social work practice included competencies in individual, group and family therapy, psychosocial assessments, aftercare planning, community liaison and support, and community program development. Within this context, social work practice focused on the person in his/her environment.

With deinstitutionalization and the downsizing of Connecticut state psychiatric hospitals in the 1980s, new training challenges emerged that incorporated community-based models. Over the next decade, social work services expanded to include case management, assertive community treatment (ACT) teams, and outreach and engagement programs targeting homeless persons with major mental illness and addiction disorders. Licensed clinical social workers on ACT teams were now authorized and trained to initiate emergency hospitalization certificates for clients in crisis situations.

Given the evolving skills required of public sector social workers, ongoing staff training was a necessity, not only for acquiring new clinical competencies but also to articulate and support the social worker's changing role and expectations. Staff development was conducted on two tracks: social work department-specific and interdisciplinary Center-based. As a teaching facility, the CMHC had the faculty and professional staff resources, both Yale and state, to address these training needs. Social workers took the lead in the case management training and supervision of 10 bachelor-level case managers. Ninety percent of these case managers completed their MSW degree while employed at the CMHC.

In-service training was a critical component in supporting our staff to gain new competencies as programmatic changes were implemented. This was especially true as our mandate emphasized serving the behavioral health needs of the urban poor. Training modules focused on crisis intervention, collaborative and clinical case management, group treatment, psychosocial rehabilitation, support group development, brief treatment, treatment of co-occurring disorders, motivational enhancement therapy, post-traumatic stress disorders, dialectic behavioral therapy, cultural competence, family psychoeducation, collaborative treatment planning, consumer and family education, forensic issues, and recovery models.

During the past decade, there was an effort to prioritize and consolidate the spectrum of training initiatives due to time constraints. Managed care, staff productivity, treatment authorization and documentation, and the reduction in staff and fiscal resources became a reality at the CMHC. Edna Aklin is the current director at a time when role flexibility and managerial responsibility are increasing and influencing social work practice at the Center. Presently social workers hold major roles as clinical managers including team directors in ambulatory services, the director of services for inpatient and sub-acute services, and the Center's director of clinical operations.

Social work intern training

Social work intern training always has been part of the Center's training mission. Initially, graduate social work students were selected from the Smith College School of Social Work due to its clinical focus and block placement schedule. The reputation of the CMHC as a unique community mental health facility began to attract students from other social work graduate schools. Students were interested in a setting that valued training, provided quality learning and supervision, and presented opportunities for professional experience with a clinically and culturally diverse caseload.

In addition to the University of Connecticut and Southern Connecticut State University, the CMHC met the needs of students who were Connecticut residents attending graduate schools in New York City or Massachusetts, but looking to do a field practicum in Connecticut. There was significant growth in the intern pool with students from Columbia University, New York University, Fordham University, Hunter College and Springfield College. For a brief period in the early 1980s, we collaborated with Atlanta University so as to attract more African-American interns to the training program and subsequent staff positions.

Sophie Tworkowski was director of social work from 1992 until 2003. In 1992 she initiated an integrative seminar entitled "Social Work Practice in the Public Sector" for the CMHC social work interns. The seminar was deemed necessary to ensure that all interns would learn key models of service delivery and develop the skill competencies for effective social work practice in public sector community mental health. The seminar enabled the interns to integrate their experience in a supportive environment and to be trained by senior social work clinical faculty and staff in addition to their site supervisor.

The training experience focused on core and individualized skills depending on the service unit hosting the intern. Depending on their academic practice area concentrations, interns were able to select from various placements which over time included inpatient/outpatient units, substance abuse treatment, community outreach programs, day hospital, law and psychiatry, or administrative and program development experiences within the Care Management Unit and The Consultation Center. The design and content of the social work interns training evolved due to the same factors as discussed in the Staff Development section. New service programs were initiated, and others were consolidated, depending on the changing client needs and gaps in community service.

In summary, the Social Work Department has successfully addressed the training goal stated in a 1966 CMHC position paper: "To develop mental health personnel who will be prepared to staff mental health centers throughout the state and the country." The Center has trained over 125 Yale and state professional social workers and more than 700 social work interns since 1966. A significant number of the interns transitioned into social work positions at the CMHC. Other staff and interns assumed clinical and administrative positions in Connecticut and other state community mental health and residential programs.

Future directions

As training at the CMHC has changed during the past 40 years, the commitment to developing the careers of future mental health professionals has not wavered. As we take stock of the current trends and future directions in public psychiatry, it is clear that the Center continues to provide an extraordinary site for education and training in the context of a rich clinical and research environment. Leaders in the field of public-sector education and practice have identified critical components for the effective delivery of public sector care, and among the top tasks are the ability to work within and across the boundaries of complex systems and to develop appropriate roles on multidisciplinary teams (Yedida et al., 2006). These tasks are inherently part of the daily work at the CMHC, and an explicit part of the training mission.

The trainees are taught by individuals who are deeply involved in developing greater insight into the causes and effective treatments for individuals who suffer from serious mental illness and addiction disorders, and whose lives are complicated by social and environmental stresses that render them among the most vulnerable of populations. Although the emphasis on certain populations and special needs of patients has shifted over the decades, the trainees and staff at the CMHC have learned in an environment where community-based care, cultural competence, and hope for an individual's future have been embedded continuously in the values and practice of the institution. They have experienced the richness of working within a multidisciplinary team where interprofessional respect and collaboration are valued and promoted; they have seen that the complex needs of the patients served at the CMHC can be best understood and addressed when different perspectives are considered.

Recently implemented initiatives that trainees will carry with them into their careers include the constructs of best practices, and evidence-based practice. These examples of workforce development and effectiveness involve models of care that incorporate the skills and values of lifelong learning in order to assimilate and translate the key discoveries of what works best for patients into direct practice. The emphasis on understanding individuals in the context of their culture and community, the importance of integrating treatment and rehabilitation, and the critical role of mental health providers in facilitating appropriate medical care for psychiatric patients are fundamental principles that CMHC trainees have learned to appreciate. As the field of public psychiatry has been invigorated by the recovery movement, which emphasizes a more hopeful and consumer-driven or patient-centered system of care, the CMHC is poised to inculcate that perspective in the next generation of professionals.

Workforce development activities are likely to receive increasing attention nationally, in Connecticut, and in the Greater New Haven area over the foreseeable future. There is growing recognition of a workforce crisis in behavioral health that is marked by the following: difficulties recruiting individuals for selected disciplines, geographic areas and positions; problems retaining employees, as turnover rates may exceed 50% annually in some organizations and jobs; and concerns about the relevance and effectiveness of pre-service and continuing education (Hoge and Morris, 2002). The President's New Freedom Commission on Mental Health (2003) concluded that a more concerted focus on workforce development is essential if transformation of mental health care in America is to be achieved. The Substance Abuse and Mental Health Services Administration has commissioned a national strategic plan on workforce development, with Yale faculty playing a major role in its formulation. The CMHC, through its faculty and staff, are positioned to intensify efforts to translate science to services through increased educational efforts with behavioral health professionals and with the many paraprofessionals that comprise from 40% to 60% of the staff in most public sector systems of care.

In 2006 the CMHC launched two new fellowship programs that embody the continued commitment to career development for young professionals. One is a two-year, federally funded fellowship in research education on chronic mental illness, which will train individuals in research methodology and teach them about the major problems in caring for the CMHC's target population. The second program is a state- and community-funded fellowship that offer advanced training to early career psychiatrists who are interested in the clinical, organizational and policy aspects of public psychiatry; this fellowship should facilitate their development as future leaders in the field. It is clear that the field of public psychiatry encompasses many areas of competency and knowledge that are broader than that which is found in many general residency programs (Yedida et al., 2006), such as a clear understanding of the interlocking residential and vocational systems of care, the treatment of co-occurring mental health and addictions disorders, and the assessment of function and disability. Fellowships in public psychiatry offer additional experience and mentorship in these areas and the opportunity to develop the critical skills of effective participation in and leadership of interdisciplinary teams and agencies. One might argue that those individuals who complete such fellowships should be eligible for added qualifications in public psychiatry.

In summary, the training programs at the CMHC have evolved over the past 40 years and continue to flourish in their depth, breadth, and ability to remain both relevant and future-oriented. The interdisciplinary collaborations that form the backbone of the care that is provided and the excellence of the scholarly endeavors conducted at the CMHC have promoted a uniquely exciting environment in which to share knowledge with trainees.

We expect that new initiatives and training programs will develop in the coming decades and that these will reflect the strong tradition of educating nurses, psychologists, social workers and physicians in how best to improve the lives of people with severe mental illness and addictive disorders. The faculty and staff of the CMHC have fostered the professional growth of countless individuals who have become practitioners, researchers, educators, leaders, and policy-makers throughout the State of Connecticut and the nation. This is an extraordinary tradition of dedication to improving the lives of those in need of help and sharing that commitment with others.

Acknowledgments

The authors thank the following individuals for reviewing material for this chapter: nurses Donna Diers and Florence Wald; social workers Edna Aklin, Peggy Bailey, Karen Conaway, Annette Ladner, Charles Robinson and Jane Sturges; and psychologists Sidney Blatt and David Snow.

References

Bion WR: Experience in Groups. London: Tavistock, 1961

Bulletin of Yale University School of Nursing, 2005–2006

Burgess AW: Psychiatric Nursing in the Hospital and Community. Englewood Cliffs, NJ: Prentice Hall, p 118, 1985

Connecticut Mental Health Center Programs and Plans, March 1966

Hoge MA, Morris JA: Behavioral health workforce education and training. Adm Policy Ment Health 29(4/5):297–303, 2002

Newton PM, Levinson DJ: The work group within the organization: a sociopsychological approach. Psychiatry 36:115–42, 1973

Position Paper on Staffing for the Connecticut Mental Health Center. Presented to officials of the State of Connecticut and Yale University, November 1965

President's New Freedom Commission on Mental Health: Achieving the promise: transforming mental health care in America. Final report (DHHS Pub. No. SMA-03–3832), Rockville, MD, 2003

Programs and Plans for the Connecticut Mental Health Center, pp 2–3, 32–3, 1966

Sledge WH, Leaf PJ, Fenton WS, et al: Training and career activity: the experience of the Yale advanced track program. Arch Gen Psychiatry 47:82–8, 1990

Yalom ID: The Theory and Practice of Group Psychotherapy. New York: Basic Books, 1970

Yedida MJ, Gillespie CC, Bernstein CA: A survey of psychiatric residency directors on current priorities and preparation for public-sector care. Psychiatr Serv 57:238–43, 2006

9

The future of academic public psychiatry

Selby C. Jacobs and Ezra E. H. Griffith

The editors offer an overview of the forces that have shaped public psychiatry since the community mental health center movement began in 1963. Summarizing main points from the
chapters, they highlight the contributions made by academic programs at the Connecticut
Mental Health Center to progress in public psychiatry. Reciprocally, they review the essential
contributions made by public psychiatry to the Yale Department of Psychiatry and, by extension, to academic psychiatry in general. They discuss the management of the relationship
between Yale University and the State of Connecticut as a foundation for the success of the
partnership. After reviewing the current context of public psychiatry, they offer a view of future
challenges. They conclude that public psychiatry has an essential role and promising future.
Further, they emphasize that academic programs, through advance of knowledge and dispas-
sionate evaluation of new ideas, will make vital contributions to the future of the field.

At the dedication of the Connecticut Mental Health Center on September 30, 1966,
Frederick Redlich said, "these three endeavors—service, training, and research—
could form an ambitious program for the . . . new institution." This was the first official statement of the multiple missions of the Center. He went on to identify three
"specific academic tasks" through which the CMHC could make important and badly
needed contributions. They were epidemiological study, evaluation of the effects of
mental health efforts, and educational innovation.

Over the past 40 years, much, but certainly not all, of the academic effort at the
CMHC stems from this vision. Chapter 5 describes the stimulus that Redlich's view
provided to psychiatric epidemiology, services research and public health scholarship
at the CMHC. Beyond those, virtually all of the academic programs at the CMHC,
some of which Redlich did not foresee, such as addictions and forensic psychiatry,
utilize a population (epidemiologic) perspective to place their work in context. Indeed,
the community mental health center movement of the 1960s, of which Redlich was a
part, stimulated momentous changes in psychiatric services and practice. It also provided a crucible for the development of the academic programs at the Center.

Academic pursuits at the CMHC do not occur in a vacuum. The evolution of academic programs depends on both the intrinsic development of each intellectual discipline and the real-world challenges confronting policy makers, program managers

40 Years of Academic Public Psychiatry. Edited by Selby C. Jacobs and Ezra E. H. Griffith
© 2007 John Wiley & Sons, Ltd.

and practitioners. In other words, a dialogue about the future cannot be merely an academic exercise that draws solely on expert, professional or investigator opinion. It must address the political pressures, the economic realities, and the competing demands of other elements of health and human services. Public discussion occurs within the arena of psychiatric services, in the general health care field, and in conversations with individuals and their families about the services they need.

We believe that the academic programs of the CMHC have catalyzed progress in public psychiatry over the past 40 years. Reciprocally, participation in public psychiatry has sustained essential commitments of the CMHC academic programs. Here we review the preceding chapters of this book to help understand future directions of public psychiatry and academia's role in it.

Forces that shaped contemporary public psychiatry

The 1960s opened with two major, largely parallel movements set in motion. One, stemming from optimism about community-based approaches to care, was the community mental health movement. This movement contributed to the development of the CMHC itself. The other movement, the deinstitutionalization of chronically ill patients from state asylums into the community, was a reaction to deplorable conditions in many institutions and the appearance of new treatments and mechanisms of financing. The relationship between these two professional and social movements dominated public psychiatry over the next 40 years. In the 1980s the agendas and needs of the community mental health movement, which failed to focus adequately on seriously ill individuals in the community, and deinstitutionalization, which was placing many seriously ill individuals on the streets of the community, collided. The result was emergence of a political and professional focus on chronically ill individuals in the community. This led to development of new programs, interventions and community systems for serving individuals in the community. The Community Support Program of NIMH and the projects it funded stimulated rapid progress in care of chronically ill patients. New treatments, outreach programs, community supports, the recovery philosophy and empowerment of consumers were products of this development.

The emphasis on secondary and tertiary care of the seriously ill individual eclipsed the theoretical approaches to preventive programs introduced during the 1960s and 1970s. Slowly, during the 1990s, mental health specialists defined a foundation for scientific, psychiatric prevention designed to place preventive interventions on the same evidence-based footing as clinical interventions. With the publication of the New Freedom Commission Report, which noted the large national investment in tertiary care for psychiatric disorders, prevention and early intervention were placed back on the agenda.

Analogously, as efforts to serve ethnic minorities and the poor flagged during the 1980s, attention to cultural competence rose in order to serve diverse groups better in the systems of care designed for seriously ill persons. Still largely untested, cultural competence became a major strategy among others such as increasing access and developing categorical services, to reduce disparities in psychiatric care outcomes among minority groups.

Patient rights emerged in the 1960s in the circumstances of the war on poverty and the civil rights movement. Not only have patient rights been expanded and refined over the years, it is reasonable to see them as a prelude to the "consumer" empowerment movement of the 1990s. Also, the patient rights movement, including the American Disabilities Act in 1990, set the stage for the recovery movement that rose subsequently.

A gigantic expansion of mental health professionals, each discipline with its special educational systems, set the stage for interdisciplinary practice. This workforce expansion, which began in the 1960s, included psychiatrists, psychologists, nurses and social workers, as well as efforts to improve the preparation of paraprofessional workers. The large expansion in the number of clinicians increased access to services. Access has improved particularly in ambulatory settings and general hospitals. A challenge remains to cover service shortage areas, both in rural and urban poor areas. This workforce expansion concomitantly led to more intense inter-professional rivalries over scope of practice and a need to define professional roles more clearly.

The community mental health movement represented a major investment of the federal government in the care of mentally ill patients in the 1960s. In addition, the federal government enacted Medicaid for disadvantaged people and Medicare health care insurance for the elderly and disabled. Medicaid and Medicare completed this period of remarkable, federal policy initiative. Cost-shifting strategies about who paid for care between state and federal governments played out throughout the remainder of the 40-year period. For example, in 1982, block grants to states for mental health ended categorical, federal funding for community mental health. Block grants signaled a major shift of cost over time from the federal government to the states. In response, during the 1980s, states began to "Medicaid" their services in order to gain federal reimbursement for covered services and alleviate the fiscal burden on their general funds. By 2001, states faced fiscal crises during an economic downturn, when Medicaid as a part of state budgets was growing and had become second only to education costs. States began to advocate for Medicaid reform. The federal government was glad to respond in the framework of a strategy to cap federal Medicaid reimbursement and shift costs back to the states. Medicaid reform is now an active process and will continue to shape public services over the next few years. The most recent expression of this is the 2006 Deficit Reduction Act, which essentially offers more flexibility to states in defining eligibility, benefits and co-pays in order to control state costs in exchange for more predictability in federal costs.

In the 1970s, biologic psychiatry surged as a powerful model for understanding psychiatric disorders. This occurred partly in reaction to the dissipating hegemony of psychoanalysis. Clinical research developed new treatments for schizophrenia, depression, obsessive-compulsive and other disorders. The development of the Diagnostic and Statistical Manual picked up steam. The manual arguably has been one of the most fundamental forces over the past 40 years. It has shaped how psychiatric professionals understand disorders and how they practice psychiatry. Historic and environmental phenomena have given rise to the modern definition of post-traumatic stress disorder and a range of appetitive or addictive disorders (including problem gambling). Perhaps more fundamental, a biologic orientation, predicated on basic science and clinical research, has established a knowledge base for psychiatry. As with other medical specialties, evidence-based practice is now a realistic goal.

The subspecialty of addiction psychiatry flowered in the 1970s. In the early stages, in reaction to viewing substance abuse as a moral weakness, there was progress in understanding addictions as brain disorders. While this progress continued into the 1980s, nevertheless, as part of the fight against a cocaine epidemic and as a function of a politically conservative tide that emphasized punishment instead of treatment, the criminalization of addictions mounted. Also, unfortunately, as individuals with chronic mental illness adjusted to life outside of institutions, substance abuse was a high risk. Co-morbidity of mental illness and addiction became commonplace and currently is the modal clinical presentation in many community settings.

The criminalization of addictions, in turn, paved the way to a whole new domain of psychiatric practice connected directly or indirectly to the criminal justice system. Deinstitutionalization and other forces also impinged on this development. Courts required expertise in evaluation, disposition, and services for mentally ill and addicted people entering the judicial system. The new forensic psychiatry services included evaluations of competence, court diversion programs, alternatives to incarceration, and reentry programs from prison, which currently demand resources. In addition this new field tackled the problem of risk assessment and management in the community.

Homelessness appeared and grew as a major social problem in the 1980s as a result of several forces including inadequate affordable housing, poverty and other factors. The occurrence of homelessness aggravated the mental illnesses and addictions of individuals living in the community. It demanded recognition as a problem that should be addressed in plans of care. Residential services and homeless shelters were developed to respond to this need. Considerable effort focused on garnering these resources, while also addressing the serious illnesses of homeless individuals. Consequently, clinical and housing services had to be coordinated.

In the 1990s, in response to concern about the rising costs of psychiatric care, policy makers turned to privatization of the financing of services. Managed care strategies used in the private sector, it was assumed, would control costs in the public sector. Underlying privatization was market place theory with its attention to value, cost, effectiveness, supply, demand and incentives. These variables slowly replaced consideration of systems and system coordination as the policy focus. In part, this movement was driven by the motivation of some state governments to give up providing services and develop their role as a payer. Attention shifted from financing of public services to parity of health insurance coverage for psychiatric disorders as a means of financing care. Currently, personal responsibility and ownership policies, predicated on market-place theory, are concepts that advance a shift from governments to individuals for health care.

After September 11, 2001, yet another important and novel agenda was added to those described above. Appropriately, in the aftermath of the terrorist attack, states turned to their health and mental health departments to develop disaster readiness plans. Hurricane Katrina in 2005 revealed a lack of preparation to cope with a natural disaster of such magnitude and the consequences of providing mental health and substance use services. More recently, mental health plans have been developed for coping with an epidemic from new strains of influenza.

Though the historical picture we portray above is oversimplified, we believe it is essentially accurate. We contend that these major forces and agendas over the past 40 years in public psychiatry, whether old, new, cyclical or dialectical, whether professional, social or political, are still active. If this assumption is true, it emphasizes the complexity of the present mission of public psychiatric institutions. No matter how challenging the task of public psychiatry was in the 1960s, the mission seems more complex at present. No matter how challenging the effort to serve deinstitutionalized, chronically ill persons in the community may have seemed in the 1980s, continuing commitment to that goal, among other demands, seems more complex at present. For many years in the 1980s and 1990s, individuals with serious mental illness were an exclusive target population. Though admittedly a heterogeneous group, this target population was reasonably well defined. Presently the target population is not only the seriously ill, but also individuals with substance use disorders and co-morbid disorders, individuals deeply embroiled in the criminal justice system or exiting incarceration, and individuals who are homeless. On top of an expanded target population, a broad agenda exists including prevention, disaster readiness, acute clinical care, tertiary care, forensic services, categorical services for monolingual Latinos, and community supports.

The contribution of academic programs to change in public psychiatry

Over the years, as documented in the preceding chapters of this volume, academic programs of the CMHC have played a major role in formulating strategic responses to the challenges facing the Center and the field of public psychiatry. When the community mental health movement brought a community and social perspective to hospital and outpatient-based treatments, psychiatric epidemiology, services research and prevention science were the tools for evaluating central tenets of the new point of view. New goals included increased access, early intervention and prevention, equity in outreach to individuals from minority populations, and community-based treatment. As public psychiatry evolved in the 1980s, academic substance use programs and law and psychiatry programs forged new knowledge bases of diagnosis, treatment and risk management. Cross-cultural research kept alive an original commitment of the community mental health movement to serve ethnic minorities and the disadvantaged. As the mission of public psychiatry progressively focused on serious mental illness in the 1980s, an academic program on chronic mental illness emerged and sustained this core mission. This focus has been essential in more recent years by providing a platform for advocacy for tertiary care tasks, in order to balance acute care and other competing demands. Law and psychiatry programs developed the expertise and services for collaborating with the criminal justice system in serving seriously ill individuals in courts and prisons.

All of the CMHC's academic programs also have educational ramifications, which have been instrumental in development of specialized psychiatrists and other mental health professionals, who are prepared to meet the challenges of contemporary practice and, in particular, the challenges of practice in public psychiatry. There are several unique aspects of the educational programs at the Center: the interdisciplinary approach of education, the consideration of personal and environment experience in relation to mental illness, and the focus on challenges in public practice over the years, including most recently, the need for dual competency of clinical staff to treat both mental health and substance use disorders. These educational programs have contributed substantially to the preparation of new cadres of psychiatrists and other mental health professionals suited to contemporary public psychiatry. Progress on development of high-quality mental health and substance use services has depended on effective workforce education built into academic programs.

The future of public psychiatry

Public psychiatry must survive as it is so intrinsically linked to the future for some of our society's most vulnerable members. For the past 150 years, states have been the unit of social organization in American society most consistently concerned with the seriously mentally ill. State budgets for mental health services, with the exception of the community mental health era, have been a foundation for public psychiatry. States must not abandon this historic role. At present, Medicaid is emerging as a dominant mechanism for financing public services. Medicaid, a federal and state partnership, changes and simultaneously reinforces the state role, through the development of state plans, which are reviewed by the federal Center for Medicaid and Medicare Services.

Given the size of the public domain in psychiatry, it is hard to imagine its being supplanted by alternate systems. Cost data from 2001, including Medicaid and costs by state governments, indicate that 52% of all mental health and substance abuse expenditures fall in the public arena. Medicaid reimbursement rates historically are low and unfavorable to covering costs in solo private practice. For this reason, we do not foresee any migration of private practitioners into the public arena.

Until effective treatments for serious mental illnesses are discovered, individuals with chronic mental illness and disabilities are going to require special care. We know the consequences of ignoring or criminalizing the behavior of the vulnerable individuals with mental health or addiction disorders. The result is high numbers of individuals with serious mental illness and addictions in prisons or among the homeless people living on our streets.

In our view, the core mission of public psychiatry must be one of providing mental health and substance abuse services in the community to a target population of low-income (disadvantaged) individuals, which includes the seriously and chronically mentally ill. In many cases, the responsibility extends to medical care, given the shortened life expectancy of those with chronic mental illnesses. For individuals with chronic illnesses and disabilities, psychiatrists often are the principal caregivers, either providing general medical care themselves or actively coordinating it.

In addition to treating the seriously and chronically mentally ill, public psychiatry now has a larger and differentiated population to serve: those with addictions, those in the criminal justice system with mental illness and substance use, those individuals with illness transitioning out of prison, the homeless insofar as they suffer from mental illness and addictions, young adults at risk, and the general population through a public health agenda that includes disaster preparedness, early interventions, prevention and community development.

The partnership between the federal government and states to finance the care of a vulnerable mentally ill population may prove to be a strong approach. Sharing the cost of care for the core population of individuals with chronic mental illness and other high risk, needy groups eases the burden of both levels of government. The partnership places the financing in part on a broad risk pool and locates the planning of services close to the communities in which these people live. A more effective federal–state partnership may stabilize the oscillating cost-shifting and policy initiatives between federal and state levels of government.

In the introductory chapter, we offered a definition of public psychiatry. As we noted, it is hard to tell where public and private sectors begin and end as a result of the varying patterns of services reimbursed by payers in the public sector. Among "public" payers, Medicaid and state general funds are the most prominent. Between these two, Medicaid is progressively the most dominant payment mechanism. Roughly, these two payers currently circumscribe the services offered in the public sector. Medicaid progressively is the vehicle for reimbursing acute care. State funds progressively are targeted at long-term, community-based rehabilitative and support services. They also are used to target special, high-risk populations, such as persons who are chronically ill, homeless, or transitioning out of prison. We believe that current processes of Medicaid reform, both through policy developed by the Medicaid Commission and budget strategies such as the 2006 Deficit Reduction Act will progressively define the relationship between these two payers.

Although we believe in the logic of public psychiatry, present and future, we emphasize that the field will have to earn its future. We do not believe it will or should survive by default. Virtually all the political and health care reform scenarios that we envision will challenge public psychiatry to demonstrate its value. The large private non-profit component of the system will perennially challenge the government-owned parts to offer high value, that is, to be efficient, productive and of high quality. In turn, the public-owned system will challenge the private, non-profit sector to share responsibility for the most difficult patients. This reciprocal relationship between private and public sectors was played out recently in the privatization movement of the late 1990s, when the question arose of whether state-funded services might completely fold into a private model.

There is a future for public psychiatry, but it must meet several contemporary challenges. Among these are: transformation and recovery, quality and patient safety, integration with general health care (insofar as public psychiatry is a carve-out), and the implications for Medicaid eligibility, benefits and co-payment of expanding this federal form of health insurance to the uninsured.

Public psychiatry and its current context

Change in American society poses challenges to the whole of medicine and psychiatry, and in particular, public psychiatry. Recently, momentous shifts in the organization, delivery and financing of health care promise to transform the delivery of mental health care. In the past seven years, the Surgeon General (SG) has issued three reports. The first report in 1999 noted substantial progress in establishing the efficacy of psychiatric treatments. It concluded that services were provided in a de facto non-system, which had grown as new mental health initiatives sprouted over the years. Further, in order to deliver effective treatments to the public, the report recommended a major goal of implementing evidence-based practice throughout the system. Two years later in 2001, the SG issued a call to reduce suicides, thereby providing the first national public health message on a major source of mortality from psychiatric disorders. In another report, the same year, he directed attention to disparities in health care outcomes for members of minority populations. He then reinforced a call for culturally competent care originally mentioned in his first report.

Also recently, the Institute of Medicine published its landmark report, Crossing the Quality Chasm, which laid out an agenda through evidence-based practice for improving patient safety and quality of care. The Joint Commission on Accreditation of Healthcare Organizations carried this agenda forward by establishing quality improvement and patient safety as core elements of their review criteria. Information technology now, more than ever before, can provide the tools for monitoring quality and also makes quality information available to the public via the Internet. Pay-for-performance strategies, already being piloted by Medicare, may provide further incentive for delivering optimal care.

The President's New Freedom Commission on Mental Health (2003), the first presidential commission on mental health in a quarter century, concluded that the mental health system was a "patchwork relic" and was "in shambles." These words echoed the United States Surgeon General from a few years before and all national commission reports since the Kennedy era. The Commission, recommended a transformation of the system of care built upon a foundation that emphasized six fundamental goals. They are (1) public education to reduce stigma and highlight the centrality of mental health to overall health; (2) consumer- and family-driven care; with consumers and family fully involved in treatment planning and system development; (3) the elimination of disparities in services through improving cultural competence and access to care; (4) establishing early screening, assessment and referral as common practice, across the lifespan and in primary care and school settings; (5) assuring the delivery of excellent health care, particularly into underserved areas, through dissemination of evidence-based practices and accelerating research into recovery, trauma, acute care and disparities; and (6) the use of technology to enhance access to care as well as health information through the development of integrated electronic psychiatric records and personal health information systems. In 2005, the Substance Abuse and Mental Health Services Administration (SAMHSA) issued a transforming federal action plan and awarded demonstration grants to seven states including Connecticut. As part of the "new federalism," states have considerable latitude in developing local solutions within the framework defined by the Commission.

The "ownership" policies of the Bush administration hold potential for becoming an overriding theme that drives system change for the time being. These policies, ultimately a strategy for controlling government costs, are partly a reaction to the fact that managed care has exhausted its cost-cutting potential and partly a function of using marketplace mechanisms (supply, demand, cost, incentives) to shape and manage health services. They are designed to transfer responsibility, choices, and costs for health care to individual consumers through ownership and control of personal health insurance. Ownership and personal responsibility are advocated by disparate constituencies. Recovery advocates see these themes as premises for empowering recipients of care. Payers see them as a strategy to shift costs to individuals. Managed care executives see them as a tool for controlling payer/contractor costs.

A movement toward universal health insurance provides another opportunity to fulfill a mental health policy goal for 15 years of insurance parity for mental health and substance use disorders. This goal has depended on establishing the scientific basis and effectiveness of psychiatric treatments, while demonstrating the ability to control costs through managing care. The emphasis of the Surgeon General reports and the New Freedom Commission on evidence supports the goal of parity. In addition, repeated analyses have established the feasibility and low cost of achieving parity in a managed system. As part of the discussion of universal health insurance which is shaping up, the stage now appears set, in contrast to the last national debate in 1993, for ultimate success on this goal.

Emphasis on health insurance for acute care might reinforce narrowly defined models of medical practice that give short shrift to long-term care for chronic disease, which are essential foci for effective public, psychiatric practice. A focus on acute care can also lead to diminished attention to prevention. Under such circumstances, chronic disease management and chronic care models provide important antidotes to the diminished focus upon rehabilitative services and long-term care. Attention to public health interventions emphasizes prevention, screening and early interventions as essential parts of service systems.

For public psychiatry, Medicaid has now emerged as a leading financer of health services. With Medicaid as the leading budget line item in many states, questions are now being raised about limiting eligibility, benefits and utilization. Medicaid reform has been set in motion for the purpose of the federal government's capping its costs and states controlling theirs. Reform looms as an important current development to watch for its implications for financing mental health and addiction services in public psychiatry. The Deficit Reduction Act (DRA) of 2006 introduced new flexibility for states to change the traditional nature of Medicaid. The tools given to states to pursue reform include "limited benefit" and "fixed contribution" plans. Already, concern has emerged that limited benefits and fixed contributions may be inimical to development of high-quality, safe systems of care. Also, the optional benefits (under the DRA) for chronically ill, disabled psychiatric patients might be compromised by making access to these special services very difficult.

On the state level in Connecticut, current policy is reflected in the strategic vision for the State of Connecticut's Department of Mental Health and Addiction Services (DMHAS), articulated by the commissioner and his leadership team. This policy envisions a value-driven, recovery-oriented system of evidence-based and culturally competent care. In addition, DMHAS, while striving for organizational and management effectiveness, is developing a quality of care management system and new resources (non-state) to support these goals. A centerpiece of this policy agenda is the commissioner's intent to have Connecticut, in collaboration with SAMHSA, lead the nation, with emphasis on recovery, in transforming the psychiatric service system, as called for in the New Freedom Commission Report.

Academic challenges in public psychiatry

Research on severe and persistent mental illness demands the convergence of qualitative and quantitative techniques if progress is to be achieved. For example, it will be a challenge to integrate the perspectives of basic research on rehabilitation with the tenets of the recovery movement. As long as the seriously ill individual remains the core target of public services, academic programs should support the state agency in the pursuit of a transformation agenda with recovery as a central theme. Academic programs can help facilitate integration of clinical services, rehabilitation and recovery. This can be done not only intellectually but practically (e.g., through observations from studies of patient-centered care).

Academic addictions programs should remain involved in the development and implementation of interventions for co-occurring disorders, which are now the modal clinical presentation in many community clinics. Coincident with this, there is educational pressure to prepare mental health professionals to treat both mental illnesses and addictions. Effective pharmacological treatments need to be developed for cocaine and methamphetamine dependence. Also, there are opportunities to bring special drug interventions to mentally ill populations, such as smoking cessation for chronically ill patients. New models of care, introduced into primary care in order to extend the reach of addiction services, need to be evaluated. The search for better interventions for substance use must continue. Discoveries necessitate prompt translation into practice, a process for which the CMHC program already has an outstanding record. New interest in improving access to addiction services is another domain that requires evaluation by systematic study.

The development and evaluation of new services for the waves of individuals with mental health and substance use disorders who are leaving prisons and jails are important. There are crucial questions that need to be evaluated about the best approaches to sexual offenders now crowding into psychiatric hospitals. The strategic management of risk relating to the suicidal and potentially violent patient is another area where forensic psychiatry can contribute to community care.

The translation of new discoveries into practice is a unique challenge for neurobiologists. The CMHC research program focuses on disorders of central importance to the public sector, such as schizophrenic illness, depression (especially because of its contribution to remedial burden of disease) and substance abuse. Fundamental discoveries about the etiology or mechanisms of psychiatric disorders probably have the largest potential for efficiently and effectively reducing burden of disease as well as costs of treating mental health and substance use disorders.

Risk factor research that integrates social and biological variables holds promise for development of early interventions, if not prevention. The descriptive epidemiology of mental illness in prisons is important for understanding the magnitude and nature of the problem. Studies of the course of illness, in contrast to acute illness, will help to better understand how to reduce the burden of disease. Services research has a critical agenda ahead to refine and develop both institutional and individual measures of outcome and quality for monitoring performance and public consumption. As a counterbalance to acute disease models of care, the strategies of disease management and chronic disease models of care need evaluation. Perhaps of greatest importance is the challenge of evaluating the consequences of the reform of Medicaid and Medicare that are rippling throughout the system of health care. A busy agenda is also ahead for prevention research in expanding the scientific basis of preventive interventions, including risk/protective factor studies, testing of interventions and evaluating the diffusion of interventions into the general population.

A key challenge for cross-cultural scholars is to maintain attention to disparities in outcome. The contributions of cultural competence, categorical service development and other interventions to reducing those disparities need evaluation in relation to each other. There is a need to evaluate systematically assumptions about cultural competence, as an independent strategic solution to the problem of disparities in outcome.

The educational activities of public academic units are under pressure to teach the principles and practice of evidence-based medicine. This helps clinicians develop a foundation for lifelong learning, as well as a strategy for rapidly translating new discoveries about diagnosis and treatment into practice. Given the multiple agendas competing for attention in the public arena, new education programs on serious mental illness and non-acute phases of illness hold the promise of keeping attention focused firmly on a core target population for public psychiatry. Central among educational challenges is the question of whether the field of public psychiatry should come together, perhaps led by university centers with academic public psychiatry programs, to discuss and move toward the certification of added qualifications in public psychiatry, as a subspecialty of general psychiatry.

As the service system begins to respond to federal and state transformation initiatives, two main educational goals seem inevitable. The first is education of psychiatrists for a transformed system. Public psychiatry requires special knowledge about managing chronic illness and disability; about coordination of the system in which care occurs; and cooperation among multiple systems such as mental health, criminal justice and housing. Interdisciplinary education creates an early predisposition and knowledge for team practice in the public sector.

The other goal is manpower development to prepare the existing public workforce for practicing in a transformed, mental health system. For example, the principles of recovery, evidence-based medicine, knowledge of forensic issues in clinical practice, inclusion of prevention and early intervention, skills in integrating community treatment and rehabilitation, and the capacity to intervene effectively in co-occurring mental and substance use disorders need wide dissemination. Finally, as new educational strategies and packages emerge, an academic institution can catalyze the translation of novel, more effective educational techniques into broad practice for the state.

Fundamental to all these academic activities is our belief that academic discovery and knowledge must be translated expeditiously into the public arena of practice. We pursue this objective via internal and external paths. Internally, we carry out annual scans of new knowledge for the purpose of putting new best practices into effect. Externally, we actively participate in public policy discussions as a key to introducing academic knowledge and expertise into development of future public sector practice. A broad array of public policy expertise anchored in academic programs exists at the CMHC. In our interactions, whether they are with mental health consumers, advocates and activists or federal, state and local government officials, we recognize that we are but one voice among many that are seeking to influence public policy.

In the broadest sense, academic programs can and ought to contribute to public psychiatry by a fundamental commitment to the creation and support of quality in practice. Quality is enhanced by new knowledge of diagnosis, more effective and efficient treatments, best-practice packages, efficient translation and evidence-based medical practice. We hope the CMHC will be in a position 40 years from now where it will point back proudly to developments in emerging areas, as we now look back on past developments in substance abuse treatments and law and psychiatry. Indeed, new knowledge and improved quality may lead, along with parity and value-driven services, to a new era in psychiatric services, not only for the public sector but for all of psychiatry.

Even if scientific progress in developing quality and the achievement of parity of insurance benefits and federal entitlements lead to a new era of psychiatric services, the reform in bringing enhanced mental health and substance use insurance benefits to the mentally ill might not provide well for the chronically ill, disabled person, whose needs are related to long-term rather than acute care. In our view, biologic, service system and financing agendas of the past 20 years have diffused service to the chronically ill population. It is precisely for this purpose that state–academic partnerships of the type embodied in the CMHC, reflecting a joint Connecticut–Yale commitment, may be most important. Their mission is to understand, serve and protect the interests of these vulnerable individuals in society. Despite advances in insurance benefits for treating acute mental illnesses, there may well remain a need for categorical programs and funding to serve chronically ill, disabled individuals. This role has been the time honored mission of state departments of mental health since the mid-19th century. Academia, as a partner of states over the past 40 years, enhances the mission of reaching this most vulnerable and perennially underserved population of psychiatric patients.

Public psychiatry and academia

Although the main task of this volume has been to consider the contributions to public psychiatry of academic programs at the CMHC, it is useful to consider the contributions of the academic programs at the CMHC to the Yale Department of Psychiatry. We point out that the CMHC has made contributions to the Yale Department of Psychiatry, equal in importance to those it has made to DMHAS.

The State of Connecticut's support of the CMHC both through the general fund budget and a faculty/staff contract provides vital underwriting of a large number of faculty positions, research programs and education. The existence of this support of academic departmental programs has influenced significantly the economic viability and stability of the department over several decades. The faculty contract has shrunk over the years and has been attacked periodically by competing interests in the state. Nevertheless, it has provided a more stable source of support than sole reliance on revenue-generating clinical services in the private sector, which have experienced enormous pressure under managed care.

Additionally, the clinical mission of the CMHC, in particular its core mission to serve chronically ill and disabled patients, serves as a reference point for the academic programs at the CMHC and by extension the Department of Psychiatry. In 1966, when the CMHC opened in the context of a largely psychoanalytically oriented department, many faculty members recognized the CMHC as a threat to what they valued most. Faculty members of the Yale Department of Psychiatry at the CMHC, while pursuing the intrinsic intellectual developments in their respective fields, have had to demonstrate over the years the relevance of their endeavors to the clinical mission of the CMHC. This need fosters a balanced research portfolio and education program. Balance might not be achieved in the absence of such a facility as the CMHC in the department. Indeed, we have cited the rise of substance use programs and law and psychiatry programs as examples of initiatives that arose in response to challenges in public psychiatric practice. These might not have developed as robustly in the Department of Psychiatry, absent the CMHC. Ultimately the clinical mission of the Center, while meeting academic standards, has become one of the major departmental, medical school and university commitments to serving the community in which they reside, a fact of considerable advantage to the university in its community relations.

Management of the state–academic partnership

As Chapter 7 on the state–academic partnership emphasizes, both partners in this productive collaboration of the Connecticut and Yale bring unique histories, cultures, motives and methods to bear on the facility called the CMHC. The CMHC by extension integrates both state government and university cultures under the roof of one facility. In order to accomplish the goals of both the State of Connecticut and Yale University, it is essential that this complex partnership be wisely managed, something that we concede has not always occurred during the last four decades.

The CMHC is a partnership between the state and Yale, codified in a memorandum of agreement and state law. The state owns the CMHC. It contracts with Yale to manage and to provide medical and professional services. Leadership of the CMHC is accountable to two authorities. One is the state for clinical services through the Commissioner of Mental Health and Addiction Services. The other is Yale University for teaching and research through the Dean of the School of Medicine and the Chairman of the Department of Psychiatry. The Dean of Yale's School of Medicine nominates and the Commissioner appoints the Director of the Center. These individuals are central figures in making the partnership work, and they depend on many talented individuals to accomplish their goals.

The CMHC is a unique organization that functions as an academic community mental health center. Its four missions are clinical services, education, scholarship and community development, the latter as part of being a good, responsible institution in the city. There is an obvious need to manage the missions: to integrate them cohesively as much as possible, to resolve conflict and to balance them. This forges a unique culture for the institution. Yale not only provides management for the Center but also makes essential contributions, which include important resources derived from the acquisition of federal and foundation grants. As a result, both Yale and the state make substantive fiscal contributions to the work done at the CMHC.

These mutual contributions and advantages are often misunderstood by outsiders and sometimes the partners themselves. Chapter 7 highlights the tension that is palpable when an organization is constructed and managed through a partnership. For example, following the leadership of one director, both partners seemed to lose sight of their joint interests and the obvious advantages to be gleaned from the partnership. The new CMHC director, to little avail, went through fruitless exercises to assure each partner that its demand for unilateral allegiance (either to the state or to Yale) made little practical sense. The new director then focused on pursuit of the four CMHC missions of service, education, research and community development that were mutually beneficial to both partners. He concentrated on pointing out repeatedly how CMHC activities benefited patients, both locally and nationally. He argued insistently that the cardinal reason for the CMHC resided in its being a powerful intellectual vehicle that could contribute to the solving of problems encountered by local and distant communities. He implemented this idea, in part, by a renewed involvement with New Haven's police, the school system and the clergy. With time, community observers, legislators and political advocates began to take renewed notice of the CMHC as a state–academic entity and sought its help in different ways. In this light, the Yale–state disputes eventually subsided. A vibrant institution was reborn, and that is what we have today.

The basic tenet of the CMHC is that all the missions are larger and better together than alone. For example, the integration of the academic and clinical services missions is important because it makes translation easier. It also contributes to the quality of staff and practice outcomes. Often, academic programs lead in the arena of program development in the public sector, as in the cases of law and psychiatry and substance abuse, which have become core programs. CMHC management advocates for and protects the missions when a particular mission, usually the academic mission, is targeted for budget cuts. The fact of multiple missions requires that managers communicate continually with policy makers, stakeholders, faculty and staff about the total picture.

Given the essential contributions of effective management to sustaining the future of the CMHC as a model of academic public psychiatry, echoing to a large extent Chapter 7, we would emphasize several desiderata. Success of the partnership will be optimal if the institution and its parent authorities consistently pay attention to providing effective leadership, developing and maintaining shared purpose, and employing faculty and staff who are experienced, competent, and respected in both the cultures of the university and the state. Both the CMHC, though its mission is broader as an academic institution, and the DMHAS as a state agency face the same basic challenges, outlined in Chapter 7, including evidence-based practice, recovery-oriented care, cultural competence to reduce disparities in health care outcomes, and the need to maintain and develop human and funding resources. In addition, while the state and the university may differ in cultures and primacy of particular missions, they share common interest in meeting the challenges facing the whole field of behavioral health. These include promotion of excellence, public education, workforce education, advocacy for the field of mental health and substance abuse, and the development of new technology to support quality monitoring and patient safety. At the CMHC, this sentience is embodied recently in a joint state–Yale commitment to develop new space in a building addition to house program components reflecting the multiple missions of the Center, now housed in inadequate or off-site, leased space.

Conclusion

Given the changing circumstances of health and mental health care, the future academic agenda is both long and challenging. We believe that the field of public psychiatry faces new challenges that merit the scholarly and scientific study that academic programs can bring to a subject. The daunting public psychiatry agenda discussed throughout this book argues for the importance of research and development as part of a comprehensive public strategy (and budget) for promoting knowledge-based change through demonstration projects, evaluative studies, clinical research, preclinical inquiry and public health investigation. Indeed, public psychiatry can usefully turn to academic disciplines to provide a scientific knowledge base for its practice and system development. A scientific foundation is consistent with professionalism and tempers philosophical and political debates that inevitably shape policy. Small investments in research and development will create the foundation for sustainable progress.

At the official opening of the Connecticut Mental Health Center on September 30, 1966, Redlich articulated for the first time a tripartite mission of the CMHC. He said "these three endeavors—service, training, and research—could form an ambitious program for the . . . new institution." He then continued, "I believe, however, that more is expected of the Connecticut Mental Health Center." Indeed, demanding as a tripartite mission may be, the challenge of those words, "more is expected" endures today as we face the future. We believe that academic programs have made and will continue to make vital contributions to public discussion, evaluation and the direction of public psychiatry. We and our co-authors have argued throughout this volume that the agenda is complex and challenging. We are optimistic that progress will continue and academic programs will make vital contributions to that progress.

Epilogue: Academic–public partnership from a British perspective

Ajoy Thachil and Dinesh Bhugra

The overarching role of the National Health Service (NHS) in delivering health care and that of public funds in supporting higher education means that, in essence, almost all academic psychiatry in the U.K. is academic public psychiatry. Substantial variations exist between geographical areas in the extent of academic activity and the type and range of services available. Most of these discrepancies can be explained by historical anomalies of funding. Some of the differences can also be explained by when the academic units were set up. In historical terms, the Maudsley Hospital has played a significant role in training future academics not only in the U.K. but also in places as far away as Australia, Malaysia and the Indian subcontinent. However, the historic and continuing association of Academic Departments of Psychiatry, University Medical Schools, NHS teaching hospitals, District General Hospitals, Mental Health Units and other local mental health services serve to reinforce the centrality of the core model.

This model represents a symbiotic collaboration between services and academic interests with the mental health needs of the public and health care delivery as its prime focus. From its inception, there has been a clear recognition that advancing psychiatric knowledge and training students of the mental health professions are key to ensuring the model's sustainability. The development of this service model has been characterized not by a single-stage adoption of policy and structures, but by a process of gradual reform and development over more than fifty years. Further, this process has had a significant impact on psychiatric service models because of the very nature of its organizational identity, as a publicly funded enterprise serving public interests.

In this, the parallels between the Connecticut Mental Health Center (CMHC) and U.K. models are striking. Whereas the CMHC model represents a hybrid that is in many ways unique in the United States, the pre-eminence of its counterpart in British psychiatry attests to the relevance and applicability of the American model in diverse socio-cultural contexts.

40 Years of Academic Public Psychiatry. Edited by Selby C. Jacobs and Ezra E. H. Griffith
© 2007 John Wiley & Sons, Ltd.

Historical context

The genesis of academic public psychiatry in the U.K. can be traced back to Dr. (later Sir) Frederick Walter Mott's (1853–1926) visit to Kraepelin's clinic in Munich in the first decade of the 20th century, although the Royal Medico-Psychological association existed and had academic meetings on a regular basis. Ideas about the treatment of the mentally ill were changing, and there was considerable support for the separation of early curable cases and their treatment in small units. Receiving houses, for observation and short-term treatment, were advocated on the lines of such units that had been introduced successfully in Australia and the Charité Hospital in Berlin. The London County Council (LCC), established in 1889, had taken over the asylums previously established by Surrey and Middlesex County Councils and the City, along with those created for mental handicap by the Metropolitan Asylums Board. In the new Claybury (Essex) asylum, which opened in 1893, it took the initiative of equipping research laboratories (opened in 1895). It was against this backdrop that the Council appointed Frederick Mott, a noted medical scientist with a research interest in Neuro-syphilis, as the first director of the mental hospital pathology laboratory in 1895.

Mott returned from his visit gripped with the idea of a university psychiatric clinic devoted to early treatment, research and post-graduate education. He used the preface of his research report, published in a 1907 issue of the Archives of Neurology, to put forward this idea and linked it to the scheme for a Receiving House, which the London County Council had just abandoned after an unsuccessful seven years trying to promote an enabling Bill. With his knowledge of the working of the LCC, Mott was able to induce Henry Maudsley, his erstwhile teacher and mentor at University College, London, to offer £30,000 to the LCC to build such a hospital provided it was associated with the University of London. His offer was accepted in 1908 but, for reasons that are discussed below, the Maudsley Hospital did not open until 1923. It was confirmed as a university medical school in 1924.

The Maudsley became the only post-graduate psychiatric hospital and for several years had the distinction of being a special health authority offering tertiary clinical services for the rest of the country. The latter day incarnations of those institutions are the Institute of Psychiatry (IoP) at King's College, London and the South London and Maudsley NHS Foundation Trust (SLaM). They represent the pre-eminent example of the academic public psychiatry model in the U.K. For this reason, the rest of this chapter will use the IoP/SLaM experience as a template to explore the evolution of this concept and its parallels to the CMHC experience.

From St. Mary of Bethlehem to south London and Maudsley: 1377–2007

In 1247, Simon Fitzmary, an Alderman and Sheriff of London, founded the Priory of St. Mary of Bethlehem outside Bishopsgate, in the East End of London. By 1329, it was being used as a hospice and had received a license to collect alms for the poor and needy of the area and the Mother Church in Palestine. This was probably a significant source of funding.

In 1375, the Priory was taken over by the Crown and became a Royal Hospital. In 1377, it began the care of mentally ill patients. "Care" included such patients being chained to the wall and, when violent, being whipped or ducked in water. Patient numbers steadily increased, and records show that it was being called "Bedlam" by 1450. (Both Bedlam and Bethlem are medieval variants of Bethlehem and these two names have since passed into popular parlance with reference to the Hospital.)

The Priory was dissolved in 1547, and Henry VIII granted Bethlem a charter as a hospital for the insane. The government (and revenues) of the hospital was granted to the City of London, thus making it a City Institution as well as a Royal Hospital. The management was granted to the City in 1557, which promptly transferred it to the Governors of Bridewell Hospital. Bridewell had originally been a palace, but its position next to the Fleet River meant that it was soon deserted. It then became a hospital, but was primarily used as a prison.

The Governors left the management of Bethlem to "keepers," who made what they could from those funding the upkeep of individual patients. Payments came from the patient's parish, livery companies, or relatives. The charges depended on what the keeper thought the market would bear. At this time, Bethlem was the only fee-paying, specialized hospital in London and one of the first of its kind anywhere in the world. The Governors gave most of their attention to Bridewell, and the patients of Bedlam suffered terrible neglect. By the early 17th century, Bethlem, the only hospital for the insane in the country, was overcrowded, squalid and dilapidated.

Not surprisingly, the buildings had become so decrepit by the middle of the 17th century that it was decided to move the hospital to new, modern premises. An appropriate site in the East End was identified at Moorfields, for the first purpose-built hospital for the insane in Britain. The hospital moved to its new premises in 1675. The practice of charging an entrance fee started around this time, and a constant stream of visitors came to watch the patients. This persisted until 1770, when better sense seems to have prevailed.

However, by the end of the 17th century, the new hospital had become as dilapidated and unsafe as the old. It was not until 1815 when it was moved, this time to a new building south of the river, at St. George's Fields in Southwark (now the site of the Imperial War Museum).

In 1838, extra wings for the criminally insane were added, and punishment rather than treatment remained the norm. However, by this time, other institutions for the mentally ill had been established, with private asylums being much in demand to avoid the public provision at Bethlem. Despite this, the treatment policy remained unchanged until the mid-19th century, when the hospital came under regular government inspection. After two inquiries that were severely critical of the system, punishment began to be replaced by treatment. Patients were given jobs to occupy them, and medical treatment with drugs such as Chloral Hydrate and Digitalis was instituted. Wards were furnished with more consideration for patient comfort and keepers were replaced by nurses. With these positive changes came the penniless middle-class lunatics; the common poor being increasingly cared for at local (usually publicly funded) asylums in their home counties. These changes coincided with the efforts of Dorothea Dix in the United States, to bring to public attention the benefits of "moral psychiatry," which had in turn, led the opening of large private hospitals such as the Institute of Living in Connecticut. In 1864 the criminal patients at Bethlem were moved to the new

Broadmoor Hospital in Berkshire, which was built to replace the cramped and prison-like criminal wings at Bethlem.

Meanwhile, the seeds of a new kind of Psychiatric Hospital were being sown else-where in London. As noted above, Frederick Mott put forward the idea of a university psychiatric clinic linked to a Receiving House and he managed to persuade Henry Maudsley, who offered £30,000 to the London County Council (LCC), to build such a hospital. The LCC accepted the offer, but did nothing about it for several years until Maudsley threatened to revoke his gift, when the LCC found a site on Denmark Hill south of the river near Camberwell, opposite King's College Hospital. Though the buildings were completed in 1916 and Mott moved his laboratories there, the outbreak of World War I saw Army casualties and the Ministry of Pensions moving into the new premises.

The Maudsley Hospital for nervous and mental diseases opened in 1923, drawing largely from LCC clinicians previously associated with Long Grove Asylum (an LCC hospital that had opened in 1907). Edward Mapother from Long Grove was the first Medical Superintendent. It is germane to the subject of this chapter that at its formal opening as a public institution by the Ministry of Health in 1923, Mapother told the press that "it is the first institution of its kind to be founded in Great Britain on the lines of the neurological and psychiatric clinics of the Continent and America, designed for the combined treatment and investigation of organic nerve diseases, neuroses and incipient psychoses."

Neuroses and incipient psychoses were suitable for outpatient treatment, and a clinic had been opened at St. Thomas' Hospital in nearby Waterloo as early as 1889. The Mental Treatment Act of 1930 empowered local authorities to set up (publicly funded) outpatient psychiatric clinics, and the medical staffs of their mental hospitals started outreach work in the community, reaching patients with non-psychotic illness, a model that had become well established by 1936.

Meanwhile, right from its inception, the Maudsley Hospital had begun to accept groups of LCC asylum medical officers for three months clinical teaching each. Later, it began to run six-month lecture courses in preparation for the Conjoint Diploma in Psychological Medicine (DPM) which was open to any doctor who could pay the fees. It was confirmed as a university school in 1924, and Mapother became Professor in 1926. In 1929, Dr. A. J. Lewis arrived from Australia, after a Rockefeller Fellowship had taken him to the United States and Germany. He was followed by Dr. Eliot Slater in 1931. From 1933 onwards, several psychiatrists fleeing Nazi persecution arrived, including Mayer-Gross, Guttmann and Alfred Meyer. Dr. Aubrey Lewis became Clinical Director of the hospital in 1936, and Professor of Psychiatry at London University at the Maudsley in 1946 and was knighted for his services to psychiatry.

In 1930, The Bethlem Royal, still a Charitable Hospital, and situated barely three miles away from the Maudsley, moved again. London was becoming unhealthy to live in, and Southwark was not considered socially acceptable for the educated ladies and gentlemen who were receiving treatment there. Its destination was another purpose-built site based on the independent "garden villa system," on an old country estate set amongst acres of woodland, in Monks Orchard, at Beckenham in Kent. In 1948, the Bethlem severed administrative ties with Bridewell, and merged with the Maudsley Hospital, now about eight miles away. Their joint administration was taken over by the new, publicly funded National Health Service (NHS). In the same year, the Maudsley Hospital Medical School joined the British Post-Graduate Medical Federation, as the Institute of Psychiatry (IoP) at London University.

The years between 1932 and 1967 saw a tremendous expansion of both clinical and academic infrastructure; with the addition of a garden villa for acutely disturbed (1932), an outpatient block (1936), a children's wing (1939), a neurosurgical unit jointly with Guy's Hospital (1952), and the introduction of opportunities for students to attend the Brixton Child Guidance Clinic, Remand Homes and six-month secondments to the National Hospital for Neurology and Neurosurgery at Queen Square. Further developments included the introduction of wards for disturbed adolescents, old age psychiatry and metabolic studies, an outpatient psychotherapy department with Freudian, Jungian and eclectic therapists, an EEG Department, and biochemistry, physiology and pharmacology laboratories. The discipline of psychology became important and grew to be a large department in its own right, collaborating in everyday clinical diagnosis and pursuing research in human and animal psychology, while retaining a focus on training clinical psychologists.

The latter half of this period coincides with the genesis of the CMHC project in Connecticut following discussions between Fritz Redlich, then Chairman of the Yale Department of Psychiatry, and Abraham Ribicoff, the Governor of Connecticut. Their idea of creating an academic, state institute for clinical demonstration projects and research was inspired by the New York State Psychiatric Institute model. This was similar to the Maudsley model, itself inspired by earlier European and American models. The codifying of the relationship between the State of Connecticut and Yale University in a memorandum of agreement at the CMHC's opening, which served to define its missions and the responsibilities of the two partners, was similar to the contract between the publicly funded NHS and the Institute of Psychiatry at London University, which came into effect in 1948.

In 1997, the Institute of Psychiatry (IoP) at the Maudsley became a school of King's College, London. In 1999, the Bethlem and Maudsley NHS Trust (providing public services to the London Borough of Croydon and South Southwark) merged with the Lewisham and Guy's Mental Health Trust (serving the London Borough of Lewisham and North Southwark) and the Lambeth Healthcare NHS Trust (serving the London Borough of Lambeth) to form a new trust called the South London and Maudsley NHS Trust (SLaM), which is the largest mental health trust in the United Kingdom. It serves a huge, multicultural swathe of South London a catchment population of over 1.2 million and its major hospitals are the Bethlem Royal, the Maudsley, Lambeth (the erstwhile Southwestern Hospital at Landor Road), the York Clinic of Guy's Hospital, the Adamson Centre of St. Thomas's Hospital and the Ladywell Unit of Lewisham University Hospital. In 2006, SLaM became an NHS Foundation Trust, named the South London and Maudsley NHS Foundation Trust. National Health Service Foundation Trusts are the face of the U.K. Government's new policy of decentralization of public services and the creation of a "patient-led" NHS. NHS Foundation Trusts are a new type of NHS Trust in England and have been created to devolve decision-making from central government control to local organizations and communities so they are more responsive to the needs and wishes of their local people. Such Trusts have more financial independence, while retaining access to public funding.

Academic work and clinical care: an integrated model

The Institute of Psychiatry (IoP) and the South London and Maudsley NHS Foundation Trust (SLaM) have a Statement of Common Purposes that reads:

"The Institute of Psychiatry and the South London and Maudsley NHS Trust work together to establish the best possible care for people who experience mental health problems. A key joint aim is promoting excellence in research, development and teaching in the sciences and disciplines key to the understanding and treatment of mental disorders and related disorders of the brain. This knowledge and the skills thus gained will be applied to prevention of these disorders, finding the most effective treatments and developing the best service models for the community."

It is evident that the relationship of the CMHC to the Connecticut Department of Mental Health and Addiction Services and the Yale Department of Psychiatry continues to define the Center. It is this State–University collaboration that guides and defines the multiple missions of the CMHC, as the relationship between SLaM and the IoP shapes the goals of that institution. The major missions of the CMHC are the provision of clinical services, education, research and community development. The last mission is a function of the Center's location in an urban setting with social problems that influence both illness and pathways to care. The multiple missions give the Center its particular character as an academic community mental health facility. All of the above facts have direct parallels with the IoP/SLaM experience.

Most of the IoP's teaching programs have a research component; with research accounting for 70% of the Institute's income (it has an annual turnover of approximately £63 million). In the last United Kingdom Research Assessment Exercise (RAE 2001), the IoP achieved the highest possible rating of five stars. The main purpose of the Research Assessment Exercise (RAE), conducted jointly by the Higher Education Funding bodies in England, Wales, Scotland and Northern Ireland is to enable the funding bodies to distribute public funds for research selectively on the basis of quality. Institutions conducting the best research receive a larger proportion of the available grant so that the infrastructure for the top level of research in the U.K. is protected and developed. The RAE assesses the quality of research in universities and colleges in the U.K. Ratings range from one to five stars, according to how much of the work is judged to reach national or international levels of excellence. Higher education institutions that take part receive grants from one of the four Higher Education Funding bodies in England, Scotland, Wales and Northern Ireland.

The staffing contract between the State of Connecticut and Yale University provides for the leadership and a multidisciplinary staff complement at the CMHC to be hired by Yale University. All of these professionals are also faculty in Yale's Department of Psychiatry or the School of Nursing. By virtue of this, the CMHC serves as the principal location of faculty in the Department of Psychiatry who concern themselves with academic public psychiatry. However, most nurses and other operational personnel are state employees.

Clinical activities linked to the NHS Trust (SLaM) account for approximately 20% of the Institute's income. In its educational endeavors, the IoP's relationship with SLaM is a key factor. This is attributable to the Trust's staff possessing a wide range of expertise (clinical, training and research) and because the Trust has historically held a pivotal role in addressing the U.K. government's mental health priorities. A substantial proportion of IoP teaching staff are involved in the everyday clinical care of patients and the Institute consults patient representatives about the planning and design of research.

Taught programs account for the remaining 10% of the Institute's income. These are primarily in-depth post-graduate programs in specialist areas related to psychiatry, psychology, and basic and clinical neurosciences. Teaching by staff with research and clinical expertise allows students to gain specialist knowledge and thus to develop their careers as clinicians, therapists, researchers and trainers. This is facilitated by appropriate generic and specialist clinical placements with SLaM. Service user involvement in research and training represent a further area of synergy between the academic institution and the clinical service.

SLaM, as mentioned in the previous section, provides mental health and substance misuse services to people from the London Administrative Boroughs of Croydon, Lambeth, Southwark and Lewisham, and substance misuse services in Bexley, Greenwich and Bromley. This includes generic Community Mental Health (Case-management) Teams, Crisis Resolution Teams, Assertive Outreach Teams, Community Rehabilitation Teams, Early Intervention in Psychosis Teams, Child and Adolescent Mental Health Services, Psychiatric Liaison Services, Inpatient Services, Mental Health Teams for the Homeless, Addiction Services, Psychotherapy and Clinical Psychology Services in each Borough. The Trust also provides National Specialist services to people from across the U.K. National Specialist Services include Adult Attention Deficit Hyperkinetic Disorders (Adult ADHD), Affective Disorders, Anxiety Disorders, Autism, Behavioral Disorders, Behavioral Genetics, Trauma, Chronic Fatigue, CBT, Couple and Sexual Therapy, Eating Disorders, HIV, Brain injury, Psychotherapy, Memory Disorders, Mental Impairment, Peri-natal Psychiatry, Neuropsychiatry and various areas of Psychosis. As with the CMHC and Yale, not all SLaM employees hold academic contracts at the IoP and vice versa.

Just as the passage of the Community Mental Health Centers Act in 1963 created incentives for Connecticut and Yale University to seek federal support for a "catch-mented" center (serving a specific geographic area), the creation of the NHS in 1948 led to a demarcation of mental health "catchment areas" throughout the U.K. And, as the federally funded center known as the Hill-West Haven Division and federal policies under the 1963 Act dominated the evolution of clinical services at the CMHC, public funding via local Primary Care Trusts in each Borough dictated the evolution of services within that part of SLaM. These clinical services, at both the Center and at IoP/SLaM, have also influenced the agenda for education and research. A case in point is the development of a medical anthropologist-led Cultural Competency and Conflict Resolution Service in the highly multicultural London Borough of Lambeth.

Just as block grants in 1982 and the reemergence of the Connecticut Department of Mental Health led to the CMHC's realigning its clinical programs and academic missions with the goals of the state agency, SLaM, its precursors and the IoP have had periodically to realign their strategic objectives with those of the U.K. Department of Health, which oversees the NHS.

Within the historical framework outlined in earlier chapters, the CMHC is a state-owned community mental health center located in a medium-sized urban setting. The Center delivers a variety of clinical programs. The majority of the patients in treatment have disabilities, co-occurring substance abuse problems and legal problems. The clinical programs include acute inpatient services; sub-acute, transitional services to housing; research beds; a walk-in, evaluation service; an outreach service to homeless persons and to individuals in crisis; a classical, assertive community treatment team; and ambulatory treatment and case management, organized into diagnostic teams. In addition, through satellites, the Center has a clinic treating substance abuse and a culturally competent clinic dispensing care to monolingual Latinos. The satellites include three community-based clinics in local communities. In one satellite, the Center provides services to children and families. Further, the Center is a lead mental health agency for 16 community-based agencies that provide vocational and psycho-social rehabilitation, residential services, case management, and family education and support services. In this and much else, its model of service delivery closely parallels that of the IoP/SLaM alliance, albeit on a smaller scale.

Conclusion

Similar models have emerged around the country where medical schools have students, attached to various departments, who learn on the job in hospital settings. The post-graduate training is overseen by a new organization called Post-Graduate Medical Education and Training Board with serious input from the Royal College of Psychiatrists. In universities across the land, various courses are run for training, and the clinical input by and large comes from publicly funded clinical services. The relationship between universities and clinical services is very close, to the degree that for consultant appointment panels representatives of the university are a must. There is no doubt that such close relationships create problems at times, although at others these can make clinical training much easier.

Index

Note: page numbers in *italics* refer to figures

40 Years of Academic Public Psychiatry. Edited by Selby C. Jacobs and Ezra E. H. Griffith
© 2007 John Wiley & Sons, Ltd.